Clinical Application
of Acupuncture
and Moxibustion Technique
（Chinese-English Edition）

实用临床
针灸技法
（双语版）

主 审　孙国杰　王 华
主 编　杜艳军
编 委　（按姓氏笔画排序）
王 丽　王述菊　王静芝　刘 青　刘欣媛
杜艳军　宋 杰　张晓明　周 华　徐派的
程井军　游 敏　瞿 涛

Chief Referees Sun Guojie　Wang Hua
Chief Editor Du Yanjun
Editorial Board Members （Listed in the Order of the Number of Strokes in the Surnames）
Wang Li　Wang Shuju　Wang Jingzhi
Liu Qing　Liu Xinyuan　Du Yanjun　Song Jie
Zhang Xiaoming　Zhou Hua　Xu Paidi
Cheng Jingjun　You Min　Qu Tao

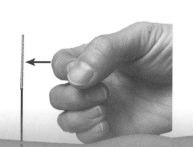
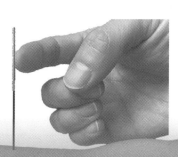

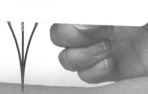

华中科技大学出版社
http://www.hustp.com
中国·武汉

内 容 简 介

本书除绪论外共二十九章，分为基础篇和应用篇。基础篇主要介绍针灸技术的基础知识、操作步骤及要领、适应范围和注意事项，并配有操作技术的图解；应用篇主要介绍部分针灸技术的特色应用，以进一步体现针灸技术的实用性、灵活性、可操作性与安全性。

本书适用于各级针灸医务工作者、科研人员、医学院校学生及国内外针灸爱好者。

图书在版编目（CIP）数据

实用临床针灸技法：双语版：汉英对照/杜艳军主编.—武汉：华中科技大学出版社，2022.1
ISBN 978-7-5680-7629-6

Ⅰ．①实…　Ⅱ．①杜…　Ⅲ．①针灸疗法-汉、英　Ⅳ．①R24

中国版本图书馆 CIP 数据核字（2022）第 020214 号

实用临床针灸技法（双语版）
Shiyong Linchuang Zhenjiu Jifa（Shuangyu Ban）

杜艳军　主编

策划编辑：汪飒婷
责任编辑：汪飒婷　张　曼
封面设计：廖亚萍
责任校对：张会军
责任监印：周治超
出版发行：华中科技大学出版社（中国·武汉）　　电话：（027）81321913
　　　　　武汉市东湖新技术开发区华工科技园　　邮编：430223
录　　排：华中科技大学惠友文印中心
印　　刷：武汉科源印刷设计有限公司
开　　本：880mm×1230mm　1/16
印　　张：14.25
字　　数：531 千字
版　　次：2022 年 1 月第 1 版第 1 次印刷
定　　价：59.80 元

前　　言

　　针灸技法是我国古人在与疾病长期斗争中创造发明的一种外治医疗方法,几千年来在我国医疗保健事业中发挥了重大作用,是祖国医学宝库中的一颗璀璨明珠。2010 年中医针灸纳入联合国教科文组织《人类非物质文化遗产代表作名录》,中医针灸的普及率日益提高,逐步走向世界,已成为"世界针灸"。

　　针灸治病的有效性,除了取决于辨经、辨证取穴外,最重要的是其技术操作,它直接关系到针灸治病疗效的优劣。规范化的针灸操作技术是针灸疗法发展与创新的基础,也是针灸国际化交流的重要内容之一。

　　面对"一带一路"助力中医针灸走出去步伐的加快,面对包括针灸在内的中医药对外教育的不断发展,面对国际化中医针灸人才的不断需求,我们在撰写此书时结合长期针灸临床实践和多年的针灸及其双语教学经验,重在围绕经典又实用的临床针灸技法,期望通过中英双语形式更好地促进中医针灸技法在全球的普及与传播。

　　本书分为基础篇和应用篇。基础篇主要介绍十几种针灸技术的基础知识、操作步骤及要领、适应范围和注意事项,并配有操作技术的图解;应用篇主要介绍部分针灸技术的特色应用,以进一步体现针灸技术的实用性、灵活性、可操作性与安全性。参加本书编写的人员均来自高校和医疗单位,不仅有世界针联教育工作委员会成员,还有世界针灸学会联合会中医针灸传承基地(中国武汉)的成员。本书虽然受篇幅所限,但仍注意理论的完整性,尽量保持刺法灸法学的自身体系。

　　本书适用于各级针灸医务工作者、科研人员、医学院校学生及国内外针灸爱好者。由于编写时间仓促,编者编写经验不足,英语水平有限,书中难免有不足与疏漏之处,敬请广大读者提出宝贵的批评与指导意见,以助本书今后的修订和完善。

　　本书中《黄帝内经》的英译文主要参考了文树德(Paul Ulrich Unschuld)先生的译著,在此特别致谢。

编　者

Preface

Acupuncture and moxibustion(A&M) technology is an external treatment method invented by the ancients in the long-term struggle against diseases. It has played an important role in China's medical and health care for thousands of years. It is a bright pearl in the treasure house of Chinese medicine. In 2010, Chinese acupuncture and moxibustion was included in the UNESCO Human Representative List of Intangible Cultural Heritage. Since then, the popularity of A&M is increasing day by day. A&M technology has gradually spread all over the world, and has become the "world acupuncture and moxibustion".

The effectiveness of A&M depends not only on the selection of acupoints based on syndrome differentiation and meridian differentiation, but also on its technical operation, which is directly related to the curative effect of A&M. However, standardization of A&M operation is not only the basis of the development and innovation of A&M therapy, but also one of the important contents of the international communication.

Facing the accelerated pace of "going out" of A&M promoted by the Belt and Road Initiative, facing the continuous development of Chinese medicine education including A&M, and facing the continuous demand of internationalized Chinese medicine and acupuncture talents, we write the book combined the long-term clinical practice of A&M, many years of experience in teaching and bilingual education, and believe that a book focusing on classic and practical clinical A&M technology, with the help of Chinese and English bilingual form, can better promote the popularization and dissemination of Chinese A&M technology in the world.

The book is divided into foundation and application chapters. The foundation part mainly introduces the basic knowledge, operation steps and keys, scope of application and precautions of more than ten kinds of acupuncture techniques, and is equipped with illustrations of operation techniques. The application part mainly introduces some characteristic applications of A&M technology, so as to further reflect the practicability, flexibility, operability and safety of A&M technology. All of the participants in the writing of this book come from universities and medical units, not only members of the World Federation of Acupuncture-Moxibustion Societies(WFAS) but also members of the traditional Chinese medicine acupuncture inheritance base(Wuhan, China) of the World Federation of Acupuncture-Moxibustion Societies(WFAS). Although lack of space, we still pay attention to the integrity of the theory and try to maintain the self-system of A&M.

This book is suitable for all levels of A&M medical workers, scientific research personnel, medical college students and acupuncture enthusiasts at home and abroad. Due to the short time, insufficient writting experience and limited English proficiency, it is inevitable that there might be deficiencies and omissions in the book, and we welcome constructive criticism and guidance from dear readers, for further revision and improvement of this book.

Special thanks to Mr. Unschuld. The English translation of the Huangdi Neijing in this book mainly refers to his translation works.

Contributors

目　录

Contents

Appendix 附 录

Introduction　绪　　论

Acupuncture and moxibustion technique is an important part of acupuncture science, and it is a bridge between the basic theory of acupuncture and moxibustion and clinical treatment. The process of acupuncture and moxibustion treatment of diseases is a specific implementation process of acupuncture method and moxibustion method. Whether the application of acupuncture and moxibustion methods is appropriate directly related to the merit of therapeutic effect. Therefore, acupuncture and moxibustion technique is the basic skill that acupuncturists must master. How to correctly and skillfully master the acupuncture and moxibustion technique becomes the key to learn acupuncture and moxibustion well. Chinese acupuncturists in all the past dynasties have attached great importance to the clinical application of acupuncture and moxibustion and have accumulated rich theoretical knowledge and clinical experience in long-term medical practice, which makes the content of acupuncture and moxibustion constantly enrich and the theory constantly perfect and lays a theoretical and practical foundation for the development and innovation of acupuncture and moxibustion technique.

At present, there are three main categories of acupuncture and moxibustion technique, namely acupuncture method, moxibustion method and cupping method, which all belong to the category of external treatment method of traditional Chinese medicine(TCM).

1. Acupuncture method

Acupuncture method is a method to use different needles in a certain part of the human body, applying different manipulations, or piercing interstices of the flesh, or tapping the skin, or pricking collateral vessel, in order to stimulate the qi of meridians, adjust yin and yang, so as to restore the balance of the body and achieve the purpose of treating diseases. Acupuncture methods are divided into traditional filiform needling method and special needle acupuncture therapy according to different needles.

Traditional filiform needling method is a kind of treatment technique which takes the filiform needle as the carrier, and acts on the acupoints through certain operating techniques and orderly operation process. The basic operation techniques include needle holding, needle insertion, needle manipulation, needle retention and withdrawal of the needle. According to the difference of stimulation sites and methods, it is divided into specific region acupuncture method and unique therapeutical methods of acupoints. Filiform needling method is the basis of all kinds of needling and the basic

针灸技法是针灸医学的重要组成部分，是针灸基础理论与临床治疗之间的桥梁。针灸治疗疾病的过程就是针法与灸法的具体实施过程，针灸技法应用正确与否直接关系到疗效的优劣，故针灸技法是临床医者利用针灸治疗疾病时必须掌握的基本技能，如何正确并熟练地掌握刺灸技法就成为学好针灸的关键。我国历代针灸医家都十分重视针法、灸法的临床运用，不仅在长期的医疗实践中积累了丰富的理论知识和临床经验，且不断充实针灸技法的内容，不断完善其理论，为针灸技法的发展与创新奠定了理论和实践基础。

目前临床针灸技法主要有针法、灸法、罐法三大类，均属中医外治法范畴。

一、针法

针法是利用不同的针具在人体的一定部位，施以不同的手法，或刺入肌腠之间，或叩刺体表皮部，或刺络放血等，以激发经络之气，调整阴阳，使机体恢复平衡，达到治疗疾病的目的。针法依据针具的不同，分为传统毫针刺法和特种针具刺法。

传统毫针刺法是指以毫针为载体，通过一定的操作手法和有序操作流程，作用于腧穴的治疗技术。其基本操作技术包括持针法、进针法、行针法、留针法、出针法等。根据刺激部位与方式的不同，针法又分为特定部位刺法和腧穴特种疗法。毫针刺法是各种针法的基础，是针灸医生必须掌握的基本方法和

methods and operation skills which acupuncturists must master.

Special needle acupuncture therapy refers to the use of acupuncture tools other than filiform needles to act on the meridians, acupoints or specific parts of the human body to prevent and treat diseases, including three-edged needle, dermal needle, intradermal needle, elongated needle, fire needle, spoon needle and superficial needle, etc. This method is generally targeted at specific diseases and syndromes for treatment, and has the characteristics of strong pertinence and definite therapeutic effect.

Specific region acupuncture method refers to the use of acupuncture and other methods to act on relatively independent specific parts of the human body to diagnose and treat systemic diseases, named for that its stimulating parts are different from traditional acupuncture point, including scalp acupuncture, wrist-ankle acupuncture, abdominal acupuncture, tongue acupuncture, facial acupuncture, eye acupuncture, nose acupuncture and so on. It has the characteristics of concentrated acupoints, simple operation and unique curative effect, etc.

Unique therapeutical methods of acupoints refer to the application of various natural and artificial physical factors (electricity, sound, light, heat, magnetism, etc.) and chemical factors (traditional Chinese medicine or Western medicine) on the meridians and acupoints on the basis of traditional acupuncture therapy to prevent and treat diseases, such as electro-acupuncture, acupoint application therapy, acupoint thread-embedding therapy, acupoint injection therapy, acupoint magnet plastering therapy, and acupoint laser therapy.

2. Moxibustion method

Moxibustion method is a method to use various moxibustion materials, such as moxa wool, to burn on or very near the surface of the skin of a certain part or acupoints, so as to achieve the purpose of treating diseases with thermal or medicinal stimulation. Both of moxibustion method and acupuncture method are main contents of acupuncture and moxibustion technique. Despite their own characteristics, they are both applied in specific parts of the human body and given certain stimulation, which can play a benign role in regulating the meridians, or through the transportation of meridians to regulate yin and yang, qi and blood and the function of Zang-Fu, so as to achieve the purpose of prevention and treatment of diseases. There are many kinds of moxibustion method, and each different one has its own advantages. We can not only use them according to the condition of diseases flexibly, but also combine them with acupuncture methods to complement each other. As *Miraculous Pivot—the Official Acupunture* states "if the effect of

操作技能。

特种针具刺法是指利用除毫针以外的针刺工具,作用于人体的经络、腧穴或特定部位,以防治疾病的方法,包括三棱针法、皮肤针法、皮内针法、芒针法、火针法、鍉针法、浮针法等。此类方法一般针对特定病证进行治疗,具有针对性强、疗效确切的特点。

特定部位刺法是指采用针刺等方法作用于人体相对独立的特定部位,以诊断和治疗全身疾病的各种方法,因其刺激部位有别于传统经穴而得名,包括头皮针、腕踝针、腹针、舌针、面针、眼针、鼻针等,具有穴位集中、操作简便、疗效独特等特点。

腧穴特种疗法是指在传统的针灸疗法的基础上,应用自然和人工的各种物理因素(电、声、光、热、磁等)及化学因素(中药、西药)作用于经络、腧穴,以预防和治疗疾病的方法。如电针法、穴位贴敷法、穴位埋线法、穴位注射法、穴位磁疗法、穴位激光照射疗法等。

二、灸法

灸法是借用艾绒等各种施灸材料烧灼、熏熨体表的一定部位或腧穴,以温热或药性的刺激治疗疾病的方法。灸法与针法一样,都是针灸技法的主要内容,两者虽各有特点,但都是在人体的特定部位上施术,给予一定的刺激,这种刺激能够对经络起到良性调整作用,或通过经络的传输,调整人体阴阳、气血、脏腑功能,从而达到防治疾病的目的。灸法的种类很多,每一种灸法各具所长,不仅可根据病情灵活运用,且针法与灸法常配合应用,相互补充,正如《灵枢·官能》论"针所不为,灸之所宜",说明了两者的密切关系。

acupuncture is not significant, try moxibustion", which shows the close relationship between them.

3. Cupping method

Cupping method can be described as a technique that uses cups placed over the skin to create negative pressure inside the cup by different ways of suction like fire, pump or steam, so that the cup could be attached to the acupoints on the surface of body or affected place. Inside the cup, a vacuum or suction force pulls skin upward, leading to local skin expand and break open tiny blood vessels under the skin. Producing a kind of benign stimulation to regulate the function of Zang-Fu, balance yin and yang, unblock meridians, and prevent and control diseases. Cupping method, anciently known as the "horn method" owe to the ancients often used horns as a tool to perform, has a long history, also belongs to the external treatment methods of TCM.

There are three types of cupping method classified by the different ways of suction, including fire cupping, water cupping and suction cupping methods, and the most commonly used clinical method is fire cupping. The application of cupping method is also diversified, including flash-fire cupping, retained cupping, moving cupping, lining-up cupping, needle cupping and so on. The cupping method has a wide scope of adaptation, good and rapid effect, and has the characteristics of easy-to-learn, easy-to-understand, easy-to-promote, economical and practical, safe to use, and less toxic and side effects.

Miraculous Pivot—Nine Needles and Twelve Source said, "Skin, flesh, sinews, and vessels, they all have their respective locations [where they are to be pierced]. As for the diseases, for each exists [a needle] that is appropriate; for each [there is a needle] with a different shape. If each is employed to fulfill its appropriate function, there will be neither repletion nor depletion. To take away from what is insufficient, and to add where there is a surplus, that is termed to aggravate a disease." That is to say, the lesion site of the disease is different, and its condition is different, so that the treatment methods should also be different. Improper treatment may aggravate the condition. Although all kinds of the methods of acupuncture and moxibustion play their role in regulating the body's functional state through the stimulation of meridians and acupoints, they are different from each other in the position of action, the intensity of stimulation, the nature of induction and the principle of curative effect. For example, acupuncture is mainly used for mechanical stimulation, which is suitable for most clinical diseases; moxibustion is mainly used for warm stimulation and medicinal effect, which is mainly suitable for

三、罐法

罐法是一种以罐为工具,利用燃烧、抽吸、蒸汽等方法造成罐内负压,使罐吸附于体表腧穴或患处,使局部皮肤充血产生良性刺激,达到调节脏腑、平衡阴阳、疏通经络、防治疾病的目的的方法。罐法,古称"角法",因古人常使用兽角作为拔罐工具而得名。该法历史悠久,亦属于中医传统外治法范畴。

罐法的吸拔方式有火罐法、水罐法和抽气罐法三种,临床最常用的是火罐法。罐法的运用亦呈多样化,有闪罐法、留罐法、走罐法、排罐法、针罐法等。罐法的适应范围广、疗效好、见效快,且具有易学、易懂、易推广、经济实用、使用安全、毒副作用少等特点。

《灵枢·九针十二原》载:皮肉筋脉,各有所处,病各有所宜,各不同形,各以任其所宜。无实无虚,损不足而益有余,是谓甚病。这是指疾病侵犯人体的部位各不相同,病情各异,治疗方法亦要因之而异,若不问虚实,误犯虚虚实实的错误,就会使病情加剧。尽管各种针灸技法都是通过刺激经络腧穴,发挥其调整机体功能状态的作用,但在作用部位、刺激强度、感应性质和疗效原理等方面又有所不同。如针刺以机械刺激为主,适用于临床大多数病证;艾灸以温热刺激和药性作用为主,主要用于寒证、虚证;三棱针放血刺激性强,作用于浅表血络,适用于青壮年、实热证;而皮肤针叩刺的刺激性较弱,作用于十二皮部,尤宜用于老人、小儿、

cold syndrome and deficiency syndrome; the three-edged needle acts on superficial blood collaterals and is good at bloodletting. It is suitable for young adults and excess heat syndrome; while dermal needle acts on the twelve cutaneous regions and its tapping stimulation is slight, which is especially for the elderly, children and the weak. It can be seen that different methods of acupuncture and moxibustion have their own characteristics in stimulation method, therapeutic effect, indications and acupoint selection formula. In clinical practice, they can be used alone, or according to the actual needs of disease nature, syndrome type, acupoint location, patient's physique and treatment requirements, so as to achieve the best clinical effect.

In a word, acupuncture and moxibustion technique includes dozens of different needles and corresponding treatment techniques with different stimulation methods, stimulation intensity and stimulation sites. Clinical application of each acupuncture technique has its own different operating procedures and implementation procedures. Whether its application is correct or not affects not only its safety and therapeutic effect directly, but also its curative effect level. Fundamentally speaking, the study and application of acupuncture and moxibustion technique is a long-term practice process. In clinical practice, it is an important part of acupuncture treatment to select different acupuncture instruments, carry out different operations, and implement continuous and orderly steps, and treatment process according to the characteristics of diseases.

体弱者。由此可见,不同的针灸技法在刺激方法、治疗作用、主治范围和选穴配方上各有特点,在临床上既可单独应用,也可以根据病证性质、证候类型、腧穴部位、患者体质及治疗要求等实际需要配合应用,以期达到最佳的临床效果。

总之,针灸技法包括几十种不同针具及与之相应的不同的刺激方法、刺激强度、刺激部位的治疗技术。临床应用的每一种针灸技法,都有其各自不同的操作步骤和实施规程。针灸技法应用正确与否,不仅直接影响其安全性和治疗作用,而且与疗效水平有关。从根本上说,针灸技法的学习和应用是一个长期的实践过程,在临床上根据疾病特点选用不同的针灸器具,进行不同的操作,实施连贯有序的步骤和治疗过程,是针灸治疗的重要环节。

Part One　Foundation
基　础　篇

Chapter 1　Filiform Needle Acupuncture

The filiform needle, one of the "nine needles" in ancient China, is a kind of needle with the widest indication in clinic. According to *the Guide to the Acupuncture Classics—Song to Elucidate Mysteries*, the filiform needle acupuncture is the most delicate method to treat diseases with in nine-needle method, and it corresponds to the Big Dipper in the sky and the acupoints in the human body. The filiform needle is suitable for any point all over the body. So, it is a basic technique that must be mastered in clinic of acupuncture and moxibustion.

The basic operation techniques of filiform needles include needle holding, needle insertion, needle manipulation, needle retaining, and needle withdrawing. Each method has strict operating procedures, clear purpose and requirements. Among them, the key techniques such as acupuncture skills, manipulation, measurement, and the arrival of qi are particularly important. Therefore, the filiform needle acupuncture is the basis of all kinds of acupuncture skills, and is the basic method and operation skill that the acupuncturist must master.

Section 1　Basic Knowledge of Filiform Needle

1. Structure of filiform needle

1. 1　The material of filiform needle

Filiform needle is made of metal materials, and stainless steel is the most commonly used material for the advantages of easily keeping straight and smooth, high strength and toughness, resistance of high temperature, rustproof and not easily to be corroded by chemical, so it is widely used in clinic. In addition, other metal needles, such as gold needles and silver needles, are better than stainless steel needles in heat transfer and electrical conductivity, but they are seldom used now in clinic except special need for their disadvantages of weaker strength and toughness, and higher cost than stainless steel needles.

1. 2　The structure of filiform needle

A filiform needle may be divided into five parts: needle tip, needle body, needle root, needle handle and needle tail(Fig. 1-1).

(1) The needle tip is the sharp part of the needle, also called the awn needle.

(2) The needle body is the main part between the needle tip and the needle handle.

第一章　毫　针　法

毫针为古代"九针"之一,是临床应用最为广泛的一种针具。《针经指南·标幽赋》中说"观夫九针之法,毫针最微。七星上应,众穴主持"。这说明精细纤巧的毫针通用于全身任何穴位,应用面很广。因此,毫针法是针灸临床医者必须掌握的基本技术。

毫针的基本操作技术包括毫针的持针法、进针法、行针法、留针法、出针法等针刺方法。每一种方法都有严格的操作规程和明确的目的要求,其中以针刺的式式、手法、量度、得气等关键性技术尤为重要。因此,毫针法是各种针法的基础,是针灸医者必须掌握的基本方法和操作技能。

第一节　毫针的基础知识

一、毫针的结构

(一)制针材料

毫针是用金属制成的,其中最常见的是以不锈钢作为制针材料。不锈钢毫针的针体挺直滑利,具有较高的强度和韧性,耐热、防锈,不易被化学物品等腐蚀,故目前被临床广泛采用。此外,也有用其他金属制作的毫针,如金毫针、银毫针,其传热、导电性能虽优于不锈钢毫针,但针体强度和韧性远不如不锈钢毫针,加之价格昂贵,除特殊需要外,一般临床较少应用。

(二)结构

毫针由针尖、针身、针根、针柄、针尾5个部分构成(图 1-1)。

1. 针尖　针身的尖端锋锐部分,亦称针芒。

2. 针身　针尖至针柄间的主体部分,亦称针体。

（3）The needle root is the demarcation part between the needle body and the needle handle.

（4）The needle handle is the part between the needle root and needle tail, and it is also the part where the doctor hold to operate.

（5）The needle tail is the end of the needle handle.

2. The classification of filiform needle

According to the different composition and shapes of handle and tail of the needle (Fig. 1-2), the filiform needle can be divided into 3 categories.

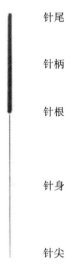

图 1-1　毫针的构成

（1）The ring handle needle, also known as the circle handle needle, that is, a needle whose annular handle is webbed with silver plated or oxidized metal wire.

（2）The flower handle needle, also known as the "Panlong" needle, that is, a needle handle is intertwined with two metal wires in the middle to form a dragon shaped needle.

（3）The flat handle needle, also called the flat head needle, that is, a needle with its handle intertwined with metal wire, and the end without finishing touches.

3. The specifications of filiform needle

The different specifications of filiform needle are mainly distinguished with the diameter and length of the needle body (Tab. 1-1, Tab. 1-2).

3. 针根　针身与针柄分界的部分。

4. 针柄　针根至针尾的部分,也是医者持针操作的部位。

5. 针尾　针柄的末端部分。

二、毫针的分类

根据毫针针柄与针尾的构成和形状不同（图 1-2）,可将其分为以下 3 类。

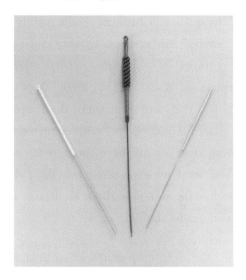

图 1-2　毫针的分类

1. 环柄针　又称圈柄针,即针柄用镀银或经氧化处理的金属丝缠绕成环形针尾的毫针。

2. 花柄针　又称盘龙针,即针柄中间用两根金属丝交叉缠绕成盘龙形的毫针。

3. 平柄针　又称平头针,即针柄用金属丝缠绕,末端不做收尾处理的毫针。

三、毫针的规格

毫针的不同规格,主要以针身的直径和长度区分（表 1-1、表 1-2）。

Tab. 1-1　The thickness specification of filiform needle（表 1-1　毫针的粗细规格表）

No. (号数)	26	27	28	29	30	31	32	33	34	35	36
Diameter/mm(直径/mm)	0.45	0.42	0.38	0.34	0.32	0.30	0.28	0.26	0.24	0.22	0.20

Tab. 1-2　The length of filiform needle（表 1-2　毫针的长短规格表）

Cun(old specification)(寸)	0.5	1.0	1.5	2.0	3.0	4.0	5.0
Length/mm(长度/mm)	15	25	40	50	75	100	125

Filiform needles with thickness of No. 26-30(0. 32-0. 45 mm in diameter)and 1-3 cun(25-75 mm in length)are frequently used in clinic. Short filiform needles are mainly used in the superficial acupoints or shallow puncturing, while long filiform needles are applied for acupoints where muscle is abundant or for deep puncturing. The stimulation intensity of needling is related to the thickness of filiform needles, which should be taken into consideration for the treatment of syndrome differentiation.

4. The quality of filiform needle

The quality of filiform needle mainly depends on the "quality" and "shape" of needles. Quality refers to the advantages and disadvantages of selecting needle materials. According to the provisions of ISO 172118：2014 disposable sterile acupuncture needle and the state standard of the People's Republic of China GB 2024—2016 stipulates in "acupuncture needle", the needle body of stainless steel should be made of 06Cr19Ni10 or other austenitic stainless steel wire specified by GB/T 4240. The material of the needle handle is not unified. If plastic is used, medical nontoxic plastic must be the only choice.

Shape, refers to the shape and modeling of the needle. Greater attention should be paid to following points in the selection of filiform needles.

①The needle tip should be shaped like "pine needle" which is straight, round and unbated, and it should be sharp and highly polished.

②The needle body should be smooth and straight, round and symmetrical, tough and resilient.

③The needle root should be firm, smooth and clean.

④The needle handle should be firmly combined with the needle body. The length and thickness of the needle handle should be moderate, so that the needle holding operation can be easily carried out.

⑤The end of the needle should be normative and tidy.

At present, due to the requirements of the international standard, disposable aseptic filiform needles should be inspected strictly before and after use. For disposable aseptic acupuncture needles, it is necessary to check the packaging and the date of expiration. Choose acupuncture needles in good packaging within the validity period. The needles with the unqualified packaging will be excluded.

临床常用粗细为 26～30 号（0.32～0.45 mm）和长短为 1～3 寸（25～75 mm）的毫针。短毫针主要用于部位浅薄的腧穴或浅刺时，长毫针多用于部位肌肉丰厚的腧穴或深刺时；针刺的刺激强度与毫针的粗细有关，供辨证施治时选用。

四、毫针的质量

衡量毫针的质量，主要看针具的"质"与"形"。质，指制针选料的优劣。根据《ISO 172118：2014 一次性使用无菌针灸针》中华人民共和国国家标准 GB 2024—2016《针灸针》的规定，不锈钢毫针的针体应以 GB/T 4240 中规定的 06Cr19Ni10或其他奥氏体不锈钢丝制成。针柄的材料未做统一规定，如采用塑料，必须用医用无毒塑料。

形，指毫针的形状、造型。在具体选择时应注意以下几点。

（1）针尖要端正不偏，尖中带圆，圆而不钝，形如"松针"，锐利适度，光洁度高。

（2）针身要光滑挺直，圆正匀称，坚韧而富有弹性。

（3）针根要牢固平整，光滑清洁。

（4）针柄要与针身结合牢固，针柄的长短、粗细要适中，便于持针操作。

（5）针尾要规范整洁。

目前按照国际标准的要求，在使用一次性无菌毫针前后，要对其进行严格检查。对于一次性无菌针灸针，要注意检查其包装及有效期。选用在有效期内，包装完好的针灸针。如发现有损坏等不合格品，应予剔除。

Section 2　Preparations Before Filiform Needle Application

1. Postures selection of the patient

An appropriate posture of the patient is significant for correct location of acupoints, manipulation of needling, retention of needling, and in prevention of fainting, sticking, bent and breaking of needle. For some patients with severe diseases, weak constitution, or nervous and afraid of acupuncture, the proper position is particularly important. Generally, the proper posture of the patient should be convenient for correct location of acupoints and needling manipulation of the acupuncturist, and patients feel comfortable for long-time retention of needles.

The common postures in clinical practice are as follows.

(1) Supine body position: it is suitable for acupoints in front part(Fig. 1-3).

(2) Prone body position: it is suitable for acupoints in the back part of the body(Fig. 1-4).

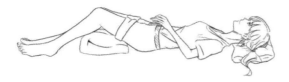

图 1-3　仰卧体位

(3) Lateral recumbent: it is suitable for acupoints on the lateral side of the body(Fig. 1-5).

(4) Sitting on a lazy back: it is suitable for acupoints on head and face, front neck, upper chest, shoulder and arm, leg and knee, ankle, etc(Fig. 1-6).

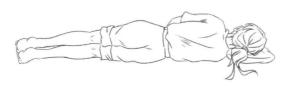

图 1-5　侧卧体位

(5) Sitting in flexion: It is suitable for acupoints on the parietal region and occipital region, hind neck, shoulder and back (Fig. 1-7).

(6) Sitting in lateral flexion: It is suitable for acupoints on the parietal region and temporal region, cheek, lateral side of the neck

第二节　毫针施术前准备

一、体位选择

患者的体位选择合适，对腧穴的正确定位，针刺的施术操作，持久留针以及防止晕针、滞针、弯针甚至折针等针刺意外的发生均具有重要意义。对部分重症和体质虚弱，或精神紧张、畏惧针刺的患者，体位选择尤为重要。指导患者确定针刺时的体位，应以医者能够正确取穴、便于施术，患者感到舒适安稳，并能持久保持为原则。

临床常用体位有以下几种。

1. 仰卧体位　适用于前身部腧穴（图 1-3）。

2. 俯卧体位　适用于后身部腧穴（图 1-4）。

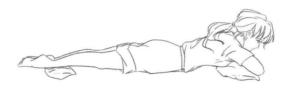

图 1-4　俯卧体位

3. 侧卧体位　适用于侧身部腧穴（图 1-5）。

4. 仰靠坐位　适用于头面、前颈、上胸和肩臂、腿膝、足踝等部腧穴（图 1-6）。

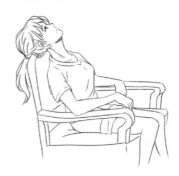

图 1-6　仰靠坐位

5. 俯伏坐位　适用于顶枕、后项和肩背等部腧穴（图 1-7）。

6. 侧伏坐位　适用于顶颞、面颊、颈侧和耳部腧穴（图 1-8）。

and ear(Fig. 1-8).

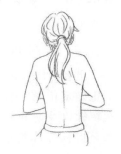

图 1-7　俯伏坐位

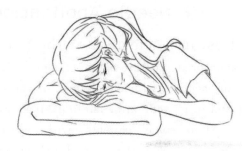

图 1-8　侧伏坐位

2. Palpation and location of acupoints

Before the acupuncture operation, the acupuncturist should locate acupoints according to the location method of the acupoints. The so-called palpating and locating acupoints means that the acupuncturist should use their fingers to touch, press, feel, and find the sensitive points such as soreness, numbness, distension and pain so as to correctly locate acupoints. According to the discussion of "One presses there with the finger, then pierces" in *Miraculous Pivot—miscellaneous diseases*, pressing is the method of palpating acupoints before needling operation.

Dou Hanqing summed up the method of acupoint selection and location in the form of Song in *the Guide to the Acupuncture Classics—Song to Elucidate Mysteries*: "The method of acupoint selection must be appropriate, first of all, it is necessary to examine and then observe the body; or it can be obtained by stretching and bending some parts of the body, or it can be obtained by keeping the body lying flat or upright. On the muscles and bones belong to yang's part, the sunken part is the acupoint, and between the yin and popliteal parts, the artery part is the acupoint. When a certain acupoint is selected, it is necessary to take four points around it, and determine its location according to the mutual relationship between the five points. When choosing a meridian, it is necessary to make clear the location of the two meridians around it, in order to ensure the accurate positioning of the meridian." *Complete Compendium of Acupuncture and Moxibustion* also pointed out, "Where acupoints are pointed out, the hands are used to figure out where they are, according to which, the fingers are used to touch, press, feel, and find." It can be seen that the accuracy of acupoint selection and location is the key to good efficacy of acupuncture.

3. The selection of specifications of filiform needles

Miraculous Pivot—the Official Acupuncture pointed out that each of the nine needles has its own appropriate function. They may be long or short, big or small, and each has its particular application.

二、揣穴与定穴

针刺前,医者需按照腧穴定位方法定准施术的腧穴位置。所谓揣定腧穴,即医者以手指在欲刺腧穴处进行揣摸、按压,寻找酸、麻、胀、痛等敏感点以正确取定腧穴。《灵枢·杂病》中有"按已刺"的论述,其中的"按"就是在针刺施术前进行腧穴揣定的方法。

窦汉卿在《针经指南·标幽赋》中以赋文的形式概括总结了选穴定位的方法:"大抵取穴之法,必有分寸,先审自意,次观肉分;或伸屈而得之,或平直而安定。在阳部筋骨之侧,陷下为真;在阴分郄腘之间,动脉相应。取五穴用一穴而必端,取三经用一经而可正。"《针灸大成》亦指出:"凡点穴,以手揣摸其处……以法取之,按而正之,以大指爪切掐其穴,于中庶得,进退方有准。"可见针灸临床中,选穴定位的准确性是针灸取得良效的关键。

三、毫针规格选择

《灵枢·官针》指出"九针之宜,各有所为,长短大小,各有所施也。不得其用,病弗能移",说明不

However, if one fails to use them adequately, they will be impossible to remove a disease. It shows that different needles have their own characteristics and functions. As far as filiform needle is concerned, the suitable length and thickness should be selected based on the patients' physique, body shape, age, state of illness, place of acupoints, needling manipulation methods and so on.

4. Sterilization

Prior to treatment, the range of sterilization includes needles, practitioners' hands, punctured skin, the treatment environment and so on.

4.1　Needle and appliance sterilization

"One needle-one acupoint-one cotton ball" is suggested and demanded in clinic. Using disposable sterile needles is better to reduce the infection than using repeated needles. The following methods of sterilization are indicated for non-disposable needles, in which the autoclave sterilization is the most effective one.

(1) Autoclave sterilization　Needles should be wrapped up in gauze, and then put in an autoclave at 1.0-1.4 kg/cm^2 pressure and 115-123 ℃ for over 30 minutes.

(2) Immersion disinfection　Soak needles in 75% alcohol liquid for 30-60 minutes, and then remove and wipe off the excess liquid from the needle with a piece of dry cloth. Appliances are also sterilized by being soaked in 2% Lysol solution or 1 : 1000 benzalkonium bromide liquid for 60-120 minutes.

(3) Boiling disinfection　After wrapping needles with gauze, put them in a sterile boiling pot filled with clean water and heat them. Generally, the disinfection can be achieved by boiling for 15-20 minutes after the water is boiling.

4.2　Practitioners' hands disinfection

Before needling, the doctor should wash hands with soap, rinse with tap water, and wipe with 75% alcohol cotton ball. During the needling operation period, the needle body should not be touched directly as much as possible to ensure the needle sterile. That's to say, if the acupuncturist have to touch the needle body in some puncturing techniques, the sterilized dry cotton must be used as a

同针具有其各自的特点和作用。就毫针而言,临床应用时可根据患者的体质、体型、年龄、病情、腧穴部位和刺法等因素,选用长短、粗细规格不同的毫针。

四、消毒

针刺前的消毒范围主要包括针具、医者双手、针刺部位和治疗环境等。

(一)针具、器械消毒

针灸临床提倡"一针一穴一棉球",临床最好使用一次性无菌针,以减少反复使用可能造成的感染。针具的消毒方法很多,首选高压蒸汽灭菌法。

1. 高压蒸汽灭菌法　将针具用布包好,放在密闭的高压蒸汽锅内灭菌。一般在 1.0～1.4 kg/cm^2 的压力、115～123 ℃ 的高温下保持 30 分钟以上,可达到消毒灭菌的要求。

2. 药液浸泡消毒法　将针具放入75%乙醇溶液内浸泡 30～60 分钟,取出用消毒巾或消毒棉球擦干后使用。盛装针具的器械,如针盘、针管、针盒等,可用 2% 来苏尔溶液或1:1000 苯扎溴铵(新洁尔灭)溶液浸泡 60～120 分钟,即可达消毒目的。

3. 煮沸消毒法　将毫针等针具用纱布包扎后,放入盛有清水的消毒煮锅内进行加热。一般在水沸后再煮 15～20 分钟,即可达到消毒目的。

(二)医者双手消毒

在针刺操作之前,医者应按照标准洗手法将手洗刷干净,待手干后再用 75% 乙醇棉球擦拭,方可持针操作。持针施术时,医者应尽量避免手指直接接触针身,如某些刺法需要触及针身时,必须用消毒干

spacer.

4.3 Punctured skin disinfection

The acupoints of the skin must be disinfected with 75% alcohol cotton balls or swabs in a circular manner from the point center to the outside, or first with 2% iodine, and then wiped with 75% alcohol cotton balls or swabs to wipe off the iodine. When wiping, the center point of the puncturing site should be circled outward for disinfection. Keep the disinfected area clean from dirt and contamination to avoid being contaminated again.

4.4 Disinfection of the treatment environment

Disinfection of acupuncture treatment environment, including the washing and drying of mattresses, pillow towels, blankets, mats and other items used on the treatment table on time, as well as regular disinfection and purification of the treatment room to maintain air circulation and clean environment. It is better to use one-person disinfection pad cloth, pad paper and pillow towel.

Section 3   Basic Operation Technology of Filiform Needle

1. Needle grasping method

The method of holding needle means that the acupuncturist holds filiform needle to keep the needle straight and firm for the convenience of needling. There are different methods of holding needles in clinic, but the general principle of holding needles is as *Miraculous Pivot—Nine Needles and Twelve Source* said, "The way to hold the needle, a firm grip is most valuable. "

1.1 Needling hand and pressing hand

As needling treatment, the hand holding the needle to operate is called "needling hand", generally the right hand; the hand to press acupoints and cooperate with needling hand to insert the needle and manipulate the needle is called "pressing hand", generally the left hand.

The needling hand is used to hold and manipulate the needle. During the insertion, the tip of the needle is punctured rapidly through the skin of point with a certain finger force, and then the needling hand exerts the manipulation of rotating, lifting and thrusting, flicking, trembling, scraping, twisting and withdrawing needle. The pressing hand is used to fix the location of acupoints, grip the needle body and keep needle straight to help the insertion of the needle, which can minimize the pain during the insertion and help in adjusting and controlling the needling sensation.

棉球作为间隔物,以确保针身无菌。

(三) 针刺部位消毒

患者针刺部位可用75%乙醇棉球或棉签擦拭消毒;或先用2%碘酊涂擦,再用75%乙醇棉球或棉签擦拭脱碘。擦拭时应从针刺部位的中心点向外绕圈消毒;当针刺部位消毒后,切忌接触污物,应保持洁净,防止再次污染。

(四) 治疗环境消毒

针灸治疗环境的消毒,包括治疗台上用的床垫、枕巾、毛毯、垫席等物品的定时换洗晾晒,以及治疗室的定期消毒净化,保持空气流通,环境卫生洁净等。如采用一人一用的消毒垫布、垫纸、枕巾则更好。

第三节   毫针基本操作技术

一、持针法

持针法是医者握持毫针,保持针身端直坚挺,以便于针刺的方法。临床上持针方法各异,但"持针之道,坚者为宝"(《灵枢·九针十二原》)是持针法的总则。

(一) "刺手"与"押手"

针刺治疗时,执针进行操作的手称为"刺手",一般为右手;配合刺手按压穴位局部,协同刺手进针、行针的手称为"押手",一般为左手。

刺手的作用是握持针具,施行手法操作,进针时运指力于针尖,而使针刺入皮肤,行针时便于左右捻转、上下提插和弹震刮搓以及出针时的手法操作等。押手的作用主要是固定腧穴位置,夹持针身协助刺手进针,使针身有所依附,保持针身垂直,力达针尖以利于进针,减少刺痛和协助调节、控制针感。

Insertion of needle needs coordination of needling hand and pressing hand. Coordination of both hands play a very important role in carrying out basic needling manipulation expertly for acupuncturist. *Miraculous Pivot—Nine Needles and Twelve Source* informed that when inserting the needle, the right hand (needling hand) holds the needle and inserts the needle; the left hand(pressing hand) holds the needle body to prevent it from tilting and bending. *The Seventy—Eight Issue of the Classic of Questioning* informed that the role of pressing hand in acupuncture treatment cannot be ignored. *The Guide to the Acupuncture Classics—Song to Elucidate Mysteries* further elaborated that the left hand pressed hard for many times while the right hand inserted the needle gently and slowly, to disperse the qi so as to relieve pain, which stresses the different applications of needling hand and pressing hand during needling.

1.2　Needle-holding posture

Needle-holding posture likes a posture of holding a brush pen, so it is called "pen holding needle method"(Fig. 1-9). According to the number of fingers used, the holding position and the cooperation of two hands, it can be divided into double-fingered needle-holding method, three-fingered needle-holding method, four-fingered needle-holding method, holding needle body method, and double-handed needle-holding method, among which three-fingered needle-holding method is the most commonly used method.

(1) Double-fingered needle-holding method. The needle handle is held with the finger pulp of thumb and index finger. Or the needle handle is held with the thumb and index finger's radialis fingertip(Fig. 1-10). The method is commonly applied to short filiform needles.

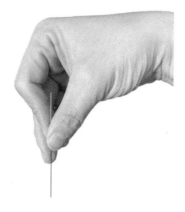

图 1-9　执毛笔式持针法

(2) Three-fingered needle-holding method. The needle handle is held with the finger pulp of thumb, index and middle fingers with the thumb opposite to the others (Fig. 1-11). The method is

在进行针刺操作时,刺手、押手必须协同操作,紧密配合。双手的配合运用对于医者熟练实施毫针基本操作技术具有十分重要的作用。《灵枢·九针十二原》记述:右主推之,左持而御之。《难经·七十八难》说:知为针者信其左,不知为针者信其右。《针经指南·标幽赋》更进一步阐述其义:左手重而多按,欲令气散,右手轻而徐入,不痛之因,强调了针刺过程中对刺手、押手的不同运用。

(二) 持针姿势

持针的姿势,状如执持毛笔,故称为执毛笔式持针法(图 1-9)。根据用指多少、握持部位及双手的配合,可分为二指持针法、三指持针法、四指持针法、持针体法、双手持针法,其中三指持针法临床最为常用。

1. 二指持针法　医者用刺手拇指、食指指腹捏住针柄,或用拇指指腹与食指桡侧指端捏住针柄的握持方法(图 1-10)。一般适用于较短的毫针。

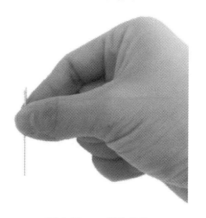

图 1-10　二指持针法

2. 三指持针法　医者用刺手拇指、食指、中指指腹捏持针柄,拇指在内,食指、中指在外,三指协同

commonly applied to various length of needling appliances.

（3）Four-fingered needle-holding method. The needle handle is held with the finger pulp of thumb, index and middle fingers and the leech-finger presses the body (Fig. 1-12). The method is commonly applied to long filiform needles.

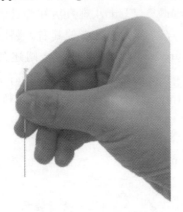

图 1-11　三指持针法

（4）Holding needle body method. The needle shaft is held tightly with the thumb and index finger with a sterilized cotton ball wrapped around the part near the tip(Fig. 1-13). The method is commonly applied to needles with different length.

（5）Double-handed needle-holding method. The needle handle is held with the finger pulp of thumb, index and middle fingers of the needling hand, and the thumb and index finger of the pressing hand with a sterilized cotton ball wrapped around the part near the needle tip(Fig. 1-14). The method is commonly applied to long needles.

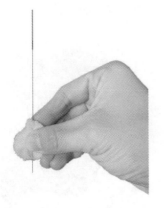

图 1-13　持针体法

2. Needle insertion method

Needle insertion method is the manipulation that acupuncturist uses various ways to insert the needle into the skin. The common methods of needle insertion are as follows.

的握持方法（图 1-11）。适用于各种长度的针具。

3. 四指持针法　医者用刺手拇指、食指、中指指腹捏持针柄，以无名指抵住针身的握持方法（图 1-12）。适用于较长的毫针。

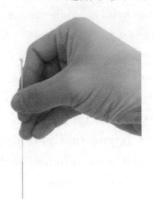

图 1-12　四指持针法

4. 持针体法　医者用拇指、食指拿一消毒干棉球裹夹针体近针尖的部位，并用力捏住的握持方法（图 1-13）。适用于各种长度的针具。

5. 双手持针法　医者用刺手拇指、食指、中指指腹捏持针柄，押手拇指、食指借助无菌干棉球裹夹针身近针尖部分的握持方法（图 1-14）。适用于长针。

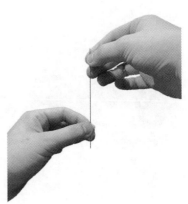

图 1-14　双手持针法

二、进针法

进针法是医者采用各种方法将毫针刺入腧穴皮下的操作方法。常用的进针法有以下几种。

2.1　Inserting the needle with a single hand

Use the right hand thumb and index finger to hold the needle, the middle finger tip is close to the acupoint, and the finger pulps is in the middle of the needle body. When the thumb and index finger are forced down, the middle finger also buckles, and the needle is inserted into the subcutaneous of the acupoint. (Fig. 1-15). This method is commonly applied to short filiform needles.

2.2　Inserting the needle with both hands

（1）Fingernail-pressing needle insertion. It is also called claw-pressing needle insertion. Press on the acupoint-skin with the nail of the thumb or index finger of the pressing hand, hold the needle with the needling hand and keep the needle tip closely against the border of the nail of the pressing hand, and then insert the needle quickly into the skin（Fig. 1-16）. This method is suitable for puncturing with short needles and is also applied to the acupoints close to some important tissue and organs.

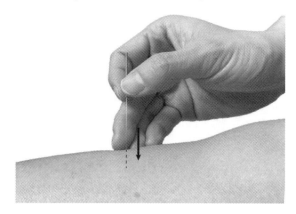

图 1-15　单手进针法

（2）Hand-holding needle insertion. Hold the dried sterilized cotton ball round the needle body with the thumb and index finger of the pressing hand, leaving its tip exposed, fix the needle tip on directly over the selected acupoint, and hold the needle tail with needling hand. Needling hand and pressing hand insert the needle into the acupoint at the same time（Fig. 1-17）. This method is suitable for puncturing with long needles.

（3）Skin-spreading needle insertion. Stretch the skin with the index and middle fingers, or the thumb and index fingers. Hold the needle with needling hand, insert it into the acupoint between the index and middle fingers or the thumb and index fingers of the pressing hand（Fig. 1-18）. This method is suitable for puncturing the acupoints on the areas where the skin is loose.

（4）Pinching needle insertion. Pinch the skin up around the acupoint with the thumb and index finger of the pressing hand, hold the needle with needling hand, and then insert the needle into the

（一）单手进针法

用右手拇指、食指持针,中指端紧靠穴位,指腹抵住针体中部,当拇指、食指向下用力时,中指也随之屈曲,将针刺入腧穴皮下(图1-15)。此法多用于较短的毫针。

（二）双手进针法

1. 指切进针法　该法又称爪切进针法,用押手拇指或食指的指甲切按腧穴皮肤,刺手持针,针尖紧靠押手指甲缘将针迅速刺入(图1-16)。此法适用于短针的进针,亦可用于腧穴局部紧邻重要组织器官者。

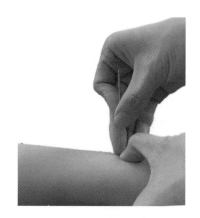

图 1-16　指切进针法

2. 夹持进针法　押手拇指、食指持消毒干棉球,裹于针体下端,露出针尖,使针尖接触腧穴,刺手持针柄,刺手、押手同时用力将针刺入腧穴(图1-17)。此法适用于长针的进针。

3. 舒张进针法　押手食指、中指或拇指、食指将所刺腧穴部位的皮肤撑开绷紧,刺手持针,使针从押手食指、中指或拇指、食指的中间刺入(图1-18)。此法主要用于皮肤松弛部位的腧穴。

4. 提捏进针法　押手拇指、食指将所刺腧穴两旁的皮肤提捏起,刺手持针,从捏起的腧穴上端

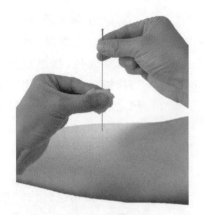

图 1-17 夹持进针法

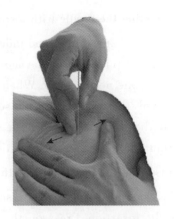

图 1-18 舒张进针法

skin pinched up(Fig. 1-19). This method is suitable for puncturing acupoints on the areas where the muscle and skin are thin.

将针刺入(图 1-19)。此法主要用于皮肉浅薄部位的腧穴。

2.3 Inserting the needle within a guide tube

Put the needle into a needle tube made of glass, plastic or metal which is 4-5 mm shorter than the needle and touch the acupoint skin. Place and press one end of needle tube against the acupoint by pressing hand and hit the needle tail by index finger of needling hand to make the needle tip insert quickly into the skin, and then take the tube off and insert into acupoint(Fig. 1-20). There is also especially-made inserting instrument which installs spring, which is suitable for children and people who fear needles.

(三)管针进针法

将针先插入用玻璃、塑料或金属制成的比针短 4～5 mm 的小针管内,触及腧穴表面皮肤;押手压紧针管,刺手食指对准针柄弹击,使针尖迅速刺入皮肤,然后将针管去掉,再将针刺入穴内(图 1-20)。也有用安装弹簧的特制进针器进针者。此法多用于儿童和惧针者。

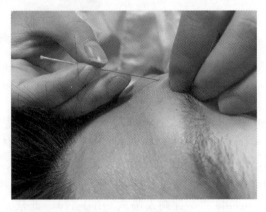

图 1-19 提捏进针法

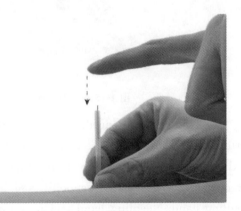

图 1-20 管针进针法

The methods mentioned above may be flexibly adopted according to specific situation, including anatomic features of the area where the acupoint is located, needling depth, manipulation method, the length of needle and so on, in order to be easy to insert, get qi and avoid pain.

以上各种进针法,在临床应用时需根据腧穴所在部位的解剖特点、针刺深度、手法要求以及针具长短等具体情况,以便于进针、易于得气、避免痛感为目的,灵活选用相应的进针法。

3. The angle, direction and depth of needling

In the process of needle insertion and needle manipulation, an appropriate angle, direction and depth of insertion could not only

三、针刺的角度、方向和深度

在进针和行针过程中,合理选择进针角度,适时调整针刺方向,

avoid pain and tissue harm, but also help to gain, maintain or enhance needling sensation to improve therapeutic effects.

控制针刺深度既可以避免进针疼痛和组织损伤,还有助于获得、维持或加强针感,提高疗效。

Needling exerts its therapeutic effects not only depending on the correct location on the surface of the body, but also the angle, direction and depth of insertion. The same acupoint shows obvious different effects on needling sensation and clinical practice due to different angle, direction and depth of insertion.

针刺疗效的取得,不仅取决于腧穴体表定位的准确性,还与恰当的针刺角度、方向、深度的确定密切相关。同一腧穴由于针刺角度、方向与深度的不同,会有不同的针刺感应,临床效应也各不相同。

3.1 The angle of insertion

The angle of insertion refers to included angle formed by the needle and the skin surface as the needle is inserted. The angle of insertion is based on the anatomy of acupoints and the needling therapeutic requirement. Generally, there are three kinds of insertion: perpendicular insertion, oblique insertion, and horizontal insertion(Fig. 1-21).

(一) 针刺角度

针刺角度是指针刺时针身与皮肤表面所形成的夹角。可根据腧穴部位的解剖特点和针刺治疗要求确定。一般分为直刺、斜刺和平刺三种(图 1-21)。

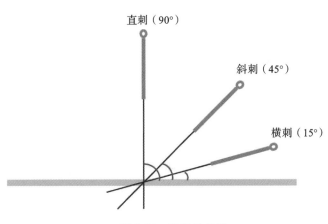

图 1-21 针刺的角度

(1) Perpendicular insertion. In this method, the needle is inserted perpendicularly, forming a 90 degrees angle with the skin surface. Most acupoints on the body can be punctured in this way. The method is suitable for both shallow insertion and deep insertion.

(2) Oblique insertion. The needle is inserted obliquely to form an angle of approximately 45 degrees with the skin surface. This method is suitable for acupoints located at the edge of bone or on the important organs that are not suitable for perpendicular or deep insertion. It is also used when acupoints are close to blood vessel or muscle tendon.

(3) Horizontal insertion. This is also known as transverse insertion, along skin insertion. The needle is inserted horizontally to form a 15 degrees or smaller angles with the skin. This method is commonly used in the places where muscle and skin is thin, such as the acupoints on the head.

1. 直刺 直刺是针身与皮肤表面成 90°角垂直刺入。此法适用于人体大部分腧穴,浅刺与深刺均可。

2. 斜刺 斜刺是针身与皮肤表面成 45°左右角倾斜刺入。此法适用于骨骼边缘或内有重要脏器不宜直刺、深刺的腧穴,如需避开血管、肌腱也可用此法。

3. 平刺 平刺即横刺、沿皮刺,是针身与皮肤表面成 15°左右角或沿皮以更小的角度刺入。此法适用于皮薄肉少部位的腧穴,如头部的腧穴等。

3.2　The direction of insertion

The direction of insertion is the direction the needle tip towards. Generally, it depends on the direction of meridians, the distribution of acupoints and the organizational structure required.

(1) The direction of meridians. According to the requirement of reinforcing and reducing by puncturing confront and follow the direction of meridians, needling should be combined with the direction of meridians. The acupuncturist can puncture following the direction of meridians or confronting the direction of meridians so as to achieve the purpose of reinforcing or reducing acupuncture.

(2) Acupoints. In order to ensure the safety of needling, we should determine the direction of needling according to the anatomical characteristics of the location of acupoints. For example, when needling Yamen (GV15), the needle tip should slowly penetrate into the lower jaw direction, and when needling on Back-shu point, the needle tip should point to the spine.

(3) The needs of disease condition and treatment. In order to achieve "qi extending affected parts", the needle tip should be directed toward the location of pain when needling. For example, Neiguan(PC6), when treating arrhythmia, the needle tip must face upward.

3.3　The depth of insertion

The depth of insertion refers to the depth of the needle body within the skin. It is mainly made according to the anatomy of acupoints and the needling therapeutic requirement. Meanwhile, the patient age, constitution, season and so on need to be considered together.

There is a description of the depth of puncturing at 342 acupoints in Volume Ⅲ of *A-B Classical of Acupuncture and Moxibustion*, which is the basis of most acupuncturists in later generations determining the depth of insertion. With the development of anatomy, the needling depth of acupoints is increasing. But it must be pointed out that the needling depth is based on the disease. It is said in *Plain Question—Treatise on the Essentials of Needling*, "The diseases include [those] at the surface and [others] in the depth; piercing includes shallow [piercing] and deep [piercing]. Always go to the respective structures; never go too far on this way." It should be based on both the needle sensation and the safety.

(1) Location areas. Areas where skin and muscle are thin or important viscera located, shallow puncturing is advisable. Areas where the skin and muscle are thick, deep puncturing is advised.

(二) 针刺方向

针刺方向指针刺时针尖的朝向。一般需根据经脉循行、腧穴分布部位和要求达到的组织结构等情况而定。

1. 依经脉循行定方向　可按照"迎随补泻"的要求,针刺时结合经脉循行方向,或顺经而刺,或逆经而刺,从而达到针刺补泻的目的。

2. 依腧穴定方向　针刺时,为保证针刺的安全,应依据针刺腧穴所在部位的解剖特点确定针刺的方向。如针刺哑门穴时,针尖应朝向下颌方向缓慢刺入;针刺背俞穴时针尖宜指向脊柱。

3. 依病情及治疗需要定方向　为了使"气至病所",在针刺时针尖应朝向病痛部位。例如内关穴,治疗心律失常时,针尖须朝上。

(三) 针刺深度

针刺深度指针身刺入穴位内的深浅度,主要根据腧穴部位的解剖特点和治疗需要确定,同时还要结合患者年龄、体质以及时令等因素综合考虑。

《针灸甲乙经》卷三中有342穴针刺深度的记述,后世医家大多以此为据确定针刺深度。随着解剖学的发展,临床上穴位的刺入深度有增无减。但必须指出,针刺深浅当因病而施,《素问·刺要论》云:病有浮沉,刺有浅深,各至其理,无过其道,应该以既有针感,又能保证安全为基本原则。

1. 依据腧穴部位定深浅　一般肌肉浅薄或内有重要脏器处宜浅刺;肌肉丰厚处宜深刺。即"穴

That is,"shallow points require shallow needling, and deep points require deep needling".

(2) Pathological condition. For patients with a yang syndrome, an exterior syndrome or an acute disease, shallow puncturing is advisable. For those with a yin syndrome, an interior syndrome or a chronic disease, deep puncturing is advisable.

(3) Age. As for the aged, weak and infants with a delicate constitution, deep puncturing is not advisable. For the young and middle-aged with strong constitution, deep puncturing is applicable.

(4) Constitution and body shape. For the patient with a thin physique and weak constitution, shallow puncturing is advisable. Deep puncturing is advised for the patient with excess fat or a strong constitution. Therefore, *Miraculous Pivot—Zhongshi* informs that, before needling operation, we must examine the strength of the patient's constitution and the healthy qi.

(5) Season. Different needling depth can be used in different seasons. Generally speaking, it is suitable for shallow needling in spring and summer and deeper needling in autumn and winter.

(6) Requirements of getting qi and supplementation and draining. After needling, if the superficial part of the acupoint doesn't obtain qi, the needle should be inserted into the deep part to stimulate the qi. If the deep part of the body doesn't get qi, the needle should be lifted into the superficial part to stimulate the qi. Some reinforcing and reducing methods emphasize that needling should from shallow to deep or deep to shallow.

4. Manipulation of needling

Needling manipulation, also known as needling transmission, refers to the operation methods of needling in order to create needling sensation. Furthermore, it refers to adjust the strength of needling sensation or induce the needling sensation transmission along a certain directions called "Xingzhen", also known as "Yunzhen". The manipulation of needling techniques includes fundamental manipulation techniques and supplementary manipulation techniques.

4.1　Fundamental manipulation techniques

Fundamental manipulation techniques include two techniques: lifting and thrusting, and rotating and twirling. These two techniques can be applied respectively or combined together.

(1) Lifting and thrusting method. After inserting to a desired depth, the needle is perpendicularly lifted and thrust in the acupoint. Lifting, means to withdraw the needle from the deep layer to the superficial layer, thrusting, means to insert the needle from

浅则浅刺,穴深则深刺"。

2. 依据病情性质定深浅　阳证、表证、急病宜浅刺;阴证、里证、久病宜深刺。

3. 依据年龄定深浅　年老体弱、气血衰退、小儿娇嫩、稚阴稚阳者,均不宜深刺;中青年、身强体壮者,可适当深刺。

4. 依据体质、体型定深浅　形瘦体弱者,宜浅刺;形盛体强者,可适当深刺。故《灵枢·终始》说:凡刺之法,必察其形气。

5. 依据季节、时令定深浅　不同的季节可采用不同的针刺深度。一般来说,春夏宜刺浅,秋冬宜刺深。

6. 依据得气与补泻要求定深浅　针刺后浅部不得气,宜插针至深部以催气;深部不得气,宜提针至浅部以引气。有些补泻方法强调针刺时先浅后深或先深后浅。

四、行针法

毫针进针后,为了使患者产生针刺感应,或进一步调整针感的强弱,或使针感向某一方向扩散、传导而采取的操作方法,称为"行针",亦称"运针"。行针手法包括基本手法和辅助手法两类。

(一) 基本手法

基本手法包括提插法和捻转法两种,两者既可单独应用,又可配合使用。

1. 提插法　提插法是将针刺入腧穴一定深度后,施以上提下插的操作手法。将针向上引退为提,将针向下刺入为插,如此反复做上

the superficial layer to the deep layer, which is repeatedly preformed as required(Fig. 1-22).

Based on the patients' constitution, pathological condition, location of acupoints and therapeutic purpose, the manipulation of lifting and thrusting may be altered flexibly in the range, layer, frequency and duration of manipulation. During the manipulation, it requires even finger force, general range with 1-3 fen, frequency in 60 times per minute, keeping the needle straight and not changing the angel and direction of insertion. Generally, lifting and thrusting in a large degree and high-frequency may induce a strong stimulation, and in contrast, a small degree and low-frequency lead to a weak stimulation.

(2) Rotating method. After inserting to a desired depth, the needle is rotated clockwise and counter-clockwise continuously and repeatedly(Fig. 1-23).

下纵向运动就构成了提插法(图 1-22)。

提插幅度的大小、层次的变化、频率的快慢和操作时间的长短,应根据患者的体质、病情、腧穴部位和针刺目的等灵活掌握。使用提插法时,指力一定要均匀一致,幅度不宜过大,一般以1～3分为宜,频率不宜过快,每分钟60次左右,保持针身垂直,不改变针刺角度、方向。通常认为行针时提插的幅度大,频率快,刺激量就大;反之,提插的幅度小,频率慢,刺激量就小。

2. 捻转法 捻转法即将针刺入腧穴一定深度后,施以向前向后捻转动作使针在腧穴内反复前后来回旋转的行针手法(图1-23)。

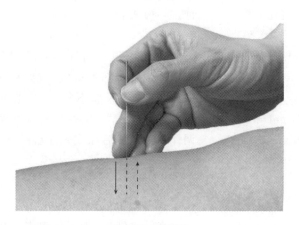

图 1-22 提插法

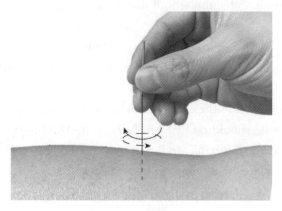

图 1-23 捻转法

The angle, frequency and duration of manipulation are based on the patients' constitution, pathological condition, location of acupoints and therapeutic purpose. During the manipulation, it requires even finger force, general angle with 180 degrees but not rotating clockwise or counter-clockwise alone for it will twine the muscular fibers to cause pain or stuck the needle. Generally, rotating in a large degree and high-frequency may induce a strong stimulation while in a small degree and low frequency lead to a weak stimulation.

捻转角度的大小、频率的快慢、时间的长短等,需根据患者的体质、病情、腧穴部位和针刺目的等具体情况而定。使用捻转法时,指力要均匀,角度要适当,一般应控制在180°左右,不能单向捻针,否则针身易被肌纤维等缠绕,引起局部疼痛和导致滞针而使出针困难。一般认为捻转角度大,频率快,其刺激量就大;捻转角度小,频率慢,其刺激量则小。

4. 2 Supplementary manipulation techniques

Supplementary manipulation techniques are the supplement to the fundamental manipulation techniques, which are conducted to

(二)辅助手法

行针的辅助手法是行针基本手法的补充,是以促使得气、加强

induce arrival of qi, strengthen the needling sensation and activate qi during needling. Clinically, following eight kinds of techniques are commonly applied.

（1）Meridian-massaging method. Acupuncturists slightly press or tap the skin up and down along the course of the channel with the fingers(Fig. 1-24). *Complete Compendium of Acupuncture and Moxibustion* pointed out that if the qi cannot arrive, use the finger to circulate along the meridians and follow it up and down, left and right, so that the qi and blood can flow evenly up and down, qi arrives and it will feel sluggish and tight under the needle, which shows that the method can activate qi and blood, promote the meridian qi and make it easy to obtain qi after insertion. In addition, the massage along meridian method can activate qi in some degree.

针刺感应和行气为目的的操作手法。临床常用的行针辅助手法有以下 8 种。

1. 循法　医者用手指顺着经脉的循行路径,在腧穴的上下部轻柔循按或轻轻弹叩的方法（图1-24）。《针灸大成》指出:凡下针,若气不至,用指于所属部分经络之路,上下左右循之,使气血往来,上下均匀,针下自然气至沉紧。说明此法能推动气血,激发经气,促使针后易于得气。此外,循法还具有一定的行气作用。

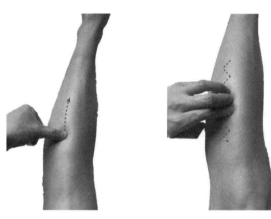

图 1-24　循法

（2）Flicking method. During the retention of needle, flick the tail or handle of the needle lightly, causing it to tremble for the enhancement of the stimulation(Fig. 1-25). *Questions & Answers About Acupuncture and Moxibustion* said, "Gently flick the tail or handle of the needle to make the needle vibrate slightly, so as to enhance the feeling of the needle and help the movement of qi." It shows that this method has the function of hastening and moving qi.

2. 弹法　针刺后在留针过程中,以手指轻弹针尾或针柄,使针体微微振动的方法称为弹法（图1-25）。《针灸问对》载:如气不行,将针轻弹之,使气速行。本法有催气、行气的作用。

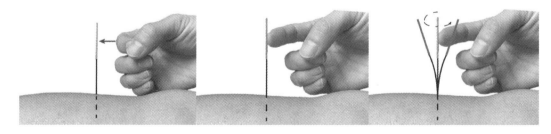

图 1-25　弹法

（3）Scraping method. After the needle is inserted to a desired depth, the thumb or index finger pulps are placed on the tail end and then the thumb, index finger or middle finger scrapes the

3. 刮法　毫针刺入一定深度后,以拇指或食指的指腹抵住针尾,用拇指、食指或中指指甲由下

handle upward or downward. Or the thumb and middle finger keep the needle steady and the handle is scraped by the nail of the index finger upward or downward(Fig. 1-26). This method is applied to promote the meridian qi if fails to obtain qi and strengthen the needling sensation or promote the dispersion of the needling sensation if qi has arrived.

而上或由上而下频频刮动针柄,或者用拇指、中指固定针柄,以食指指尖由上至下刮动针柄的方法称为刮法(图1-26)。本法在针刺不得气时使用可激发经气,如已得气者可以加强针刺感应的传导和扩散。

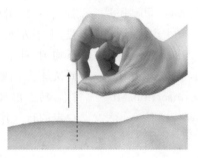
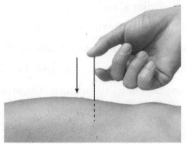

图 1-26　刮法

(4) Shaking method. After the needle is inserted to a required depth, hold the handle of the needle by the needling hand and shake the needle as the movement of sculling. There is a record of "shaking to move qi" in *Questions & Answers About Acupuncture and Moxibustion*, and it is also recorded in *Complete Compendium of Acupuncture and Moxibustion* that shaking the needle, when the needle comes out of three layers and wants to conduct reducing manipulations, the needle should be shaken once in each layer to make the hole open(Fig. 1-27). This method has two kinds: the first one is applied to clear heat when the needle is kept straight and shaken. The second one is applied to promote the dispersion of the needling sensation towards certain path when horizontal and shaken.

4. 摇法　毫针刺入一定深度后,刺手手持针柄,将针轻轻摇动的方法称为摇法(图1-27)。《针灸问对》有"摇以行气"的记载。《针灸大成》亦载有"针摇者:凡出针三部,欲泻之际,每一部摇一次……庶使孔穴开大也"。其法有二:一是直立针身而摇,以泻实清热;二是卧倒针身而摇,使经气向一定方向传导。

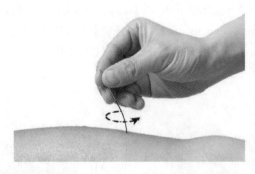
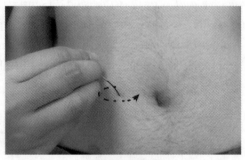

图 1-27　摇法

(5) Flying method. After the needle is inserted at a certain depth, the acupuncturist holds and twirl the needle several times with the thumb and index finger of the needling hand, and then suddenly separate the thumb and index finger from it(Fig. 1-28). *Introduction to Medicine* recorded, "Twists the needle with the thumb and forefinger, rubs three times continuously. The

5. 飞法　毫针刺入一定深度后,医者用刺手拇指、食指持针,细细捻搓数次,然后张开两指,一搓一放,反复数次,状如飞鸟展翅,故称飞法(图1-28)。《医学入门》载:"以大指次指捻针,连搓三下,如手

movement of the fingers looks like the birds' wing waving, so calls it flying method. " This method is often used to hasten qi, move qi and strengthen needling sensation, and commonly used in the places where muscle is thick.

颤之状,谓之飞。"本法的作用在于催气、行气,并使针刺感应增强,适用于肌肉丰厚部位的腧穴。

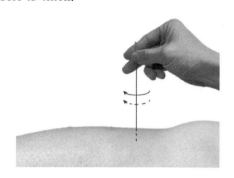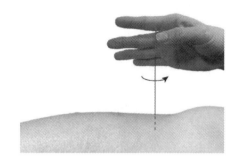

图 1-28　飞法

（6）Trembling method. After the needle is inserted to an appropriate depth, hold the needle hand with thumb and index finger of the needling hand and apply quick lift-thrust or twirl method in a small amplitude and a high frequency to cause vibration (Fig. 1-29). This method is suitable for promoting the arrival of qi and strengthening the needling sensation.

（7）Twisting method. After the needle is inserted to an appropriate depth, the acupuncturist twists the needle handle repeatedly, such as rubbing the thread, so that the muscle fibers could be properly wound the needle body (Fig. 1-30). *Questions & Answers About Acupuncture and Moxibustion* said, "After inserting the needle, rub the needle inside or outside, as if rubbing the line, do not turn too tight, it will make the muscle fiber entangle the needle and make it difficult for the needle to insert and retreat. " This method is suitable for promoting the arrival of qi and strengthening the needling sensation.

6. 震颤法　毫针刺入一定深度后,医者刺手拇指、食指夹持针柄,用小幅度、快频率的提插、捻转手法,使针身轻微震颤的方法称为震颤法（图 1-29）。本法可促使针下得气,增强针刺感应。

7. 搓法　毫针刺入一定深度后,医者持针柄反复做单向捻转,如搓线状,使肌纤维适度地缠绕针体的方法（图 1-30）。《针灸问对》说:"搓,下针之后,将针或内或外,如搓线之状。勿转太紧,令人肥肉缠针,难以进退。"本法有催气、加强针感的作用。

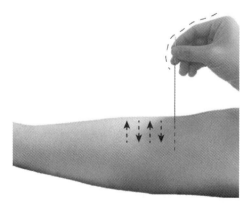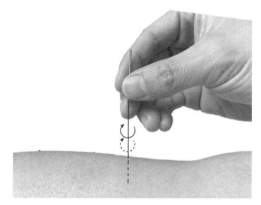

图 1-29　震颤法　　　　　图 1-30　搓法

（8）Pressing method. After qi arrives, the acupuncturist uses the pressing hand to press the upper or lower part of the acupoints to control the direction of the needle sensation (Fig. 1-31). As is

8. 按法　针刺得气后,医者用押手按压所刺腧穴的上方或下方,以控制针感走向的方法（图

explained in *Questions & Answers About Acupuncture and Moxibustion*, "During needling manipulation, when open the upper qi while close the lower qi, qi will up; when open the lower qi while close the upper qi, qi will down. When piercing acupoints on the hands and feet, if you want to make the qi up, you need to use your fingers to suppress qi in the lower areas; if you want to make qi down, you need to use your fingers to suppress qi in the upper parts." This method has the function of activating qi.

1-31)。《针灸问对》中的"行针之时,开其上气,闭其下气,气必上行;开其下气,闭其上气,气必下行。如刺手足,欲使气上行,以指下抑之;欲使气下行,以指上抑之"即是此法。本法具有行气的作用。

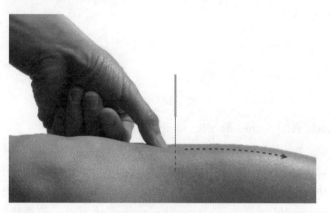

图 1-31 按法

5. Needle retention methods

After the needle is inserted into the acupoints and the manipulation is completed, the needle is retained in the acupoints, namely needle retention. The purpose of retaining needles is to strengthen the function of needling and facilitate the continuous application of needle manipulation. In general, as long as the qi is arrived and proper reinforcing or reducing manipulation is applied, the needle can be removed or retained for 10-30 minutes. But for some special diseases and syndromes, such as acute abdominal pain, tetanus, opisthotonus, cold and intractable pain or spasmodic diseases, the needle retention time can be appropriately extended, sometimes up to several hours, so as to intermittently perform the manipulation in the process of needle retention to enhance and consolidate the curative effect. The needle retention method can be divided into static needle retention method and dynamic needle retention method. Whether or not to retain a needle in clinical practice and which method to retain the needle should be flexibly selected depend on the nature of the patient's disease and physical condition.

（1）Static needle retention method. The needle is inserted into the acupoint and keep for a period of time without any needling manipulation. It is said in *Treatise on Lihe Zhenxie of Plain Questions* that, "[Hold the needle] calmly and let it remain [inserted] for long to keep the qi arrive. As if one was waiting for someone of noble rank; one does not know whether [he will come

五、留针法

将针刺入腧穴并施行手法后,使针留置穴内称为留针。留针的目的是加强针刺的作用和便于继续行针施术。一般病证只要针下得气而施以适当的补泻手法后,即可出针或留针10～30分钟。但对一些特殊病证,如急性腹痛,破伤风,角弓反张,寒性、顽固性疼痛或痉挛性病证,可适当延长留针时间,有时留针可达数小时,以便在留针过程中做间歇性行针,以增强、巩固疗效。留针方法可分为静留针法和动留针法两种,临床中留针与否及选用何种留针方法要根据患者的疾病性质和身体状况而灵活选用。

1. 静留针法　将针刺入穴位内,静置一段时间,其间不施行任何针刺手法的留针方法。《素问·离合真邪论》载:静以久留,以气至为故,如待所贵,不知日暮。即是此法。静留针法,又可根据病证情

during] daytime or in the evening. " According to the different conditions of diseases and syndromes, short-term and long-term static needle retention methods can be adopted, respectively. Short-term static needle retention method, meaning needle retaining for 10-30 minutes, is commonly used in clinic; the method of long-term static needle retention, which could be replaced by intradermal needle nowadays, can be used for several hours or even dozens of hours.

（2）Dynamic needle retention method. During the period of retaining needles, the method of intermittently performing needling operation and applying needling manipulation is adopted. According to the patient's condition and the length of needle retention time, the needle can be manipulated every 5-10 minutes. This method helps to maintain or enhance the needling sensation.

During the needle retention period, acupuncturists should pay close attention to the complexion and expression of patients to prevent needle syncope. In addition, when retaining the needle, pay attention to make the patient's posture comfortable and stable, and keep the patient warm in winter.

6. Method for withdrawing the needle

Withdrawing the needle also known as the out of the needle. After the manipulation or needle retention reaches the predetermined acupuncture purpose and treatment requirements, the needle can be removed. *Rhythm of Golden Needle* contained, "Withdrawing the needle gradually, if withdrawing the needle in a hurry to give an injection, it is easy to hurt qi. " *Yijing Xiaoxue* also said, "Out of the needle can not be fierce, must be done three or four times, slowly turn out, there is no blood, if fierce out bleeding can be seen. " The *Compendium of Acupuncture and Moxibustion* also said, "When you hold the needle and want to withdraw it out, you will feel light and smooth and the qi under the needle is slow and not heavy. Then you can twist the needle with your fingers like pulling out the tail of a tiger. " It is suggested that the withdrawal of the needle should be operated flexibly according to the deficiency and excess of the disease, the condition and constitution, the depth of the needle insertion and the characteristics of the acupoints, so as not to affect the curative effect, or even cause adverse consequences such as bleeding, hematoma, and the remaining feeling after needling.

While withdrawing the needle, presses the skin around the acupoint with sterilized dry cotton ball gently, and then slightly twists the needle. When feels loose, retracts the needle to the subcutaneous slowly, and then quickly withdraws the needle, and then presses the needle hole with the sterilized dry cotton ball for a

况的不同，分别采取短时间静留针法和长时间静留针法。短时间静留针法，即留针10～30分钟，临床常用；长时间静留针法，可留针几小时，甚至几十小时，现多以皮内针埋藏的方式代替。

2. 动留针法　在留针期间，间歇进行行针操作、施以针刺手法的方法。可根据患者病情和留针时间的长短，每隔5～10分钟行针一次。该方法有助于保持或加强针感。

在留针期间，要密切注意患者的面色和表情，以防晕针。此外，在留针时注意保持患者姿势舒适、平稳，冬季注意保暖。

六、出针法

出针，又称起针、退针。在施行针刺手法或留针达到预定针刺目的和治疗要求后，即可出针。《金针赋》载："出针贵缓，太急伤气。"《医经小学》也载："出针不可猛出，必须作三四次，徐徐转而出之则无血，若猛出必见血也。"《针灸大成》亦云："凡持针欲出之时，待针下气缓不沉紧，便觉轻滑，用指捻针，如拔虎尾之状也。"这些均说明出针应根据患者病证虚实、体质强弱、针刺深浅和腧穴特点等具体情况灵活操作，以免影响疗效，甚或引起出血、血肿、针刺后遗感等不良后果。

出针时，医者先以押手持消毒干棉球轻轻按压于针刺部位，刺手持针做轻微的提捻动作，感觉针下松动后，将针缓慢退至皮下，再将针迅速退出，然后用消毒干棉球按

moment. If the depth of the needle is shallow and there is no tight feeling under the needle, the needle can be withdrawn quickly.

The sequencing of needle withdraw is very crucial. Generally speaking, the needle should be withdrawn in the up-down and inside-out order. After the needle out, it is supposed to observe whether there is bleeding, especially parts easy to bleed, such as the scalp and orbit. After withdrawing the needle, use the dry cotton ball to press the acupoint for a moment to avoid bleeding or hematoma. And check whether the number of needles is right, and manage the post-needling sensation in time. Advise the patient to have a rest, and leave after his/her breath is even and his/her mood is stable.

Section 4　Reinforcing and Reducing Methods of Needling

Reinforcing and reducing methods of needling, the core content in the filiform needle acupuncture, are one of the important link in acupuncture therapy. The theory of reinforcing and reducing methods of needling originated from *Huangdi Neijing*. For example, *Miraculous Pivot—Meridians* said: "If the [evil] qi abound, they are to be drained. If the [proper qi] are depleted, they are to be supplemented. In the case of heat, [the needle is to be inserted and withdrawn] quickly. In the case of cold it may remain [inserted] for a while. If an indentation forms, [when the vessel is squeezed, that fails to level again when the finger is withdrawn] then it is to be cauterized. "*Miraculous Pivot—Nine Needles and Twelve Source* said: "To meet the requirements of treating depletion and repletion, the nine needles are the most wonderful. When the time has come to supplement [proper qi] or drain [evil qi], this is done with the needles. "*Miraculous Pivot—Zhongshi* said: "The way of all piercings aims at regulating the qi, and then [the treatment] is to end. "

1. The concept of reinforcing and reducing methods of needling

Reinforcing and reducing methods of needling refer to the methods that on the basis of getting qi, using appropriate needling techniques to invigorate the body's healthy qi or eliminate the pathogenic factors, thereby regulating the functions of body's Zang-Fu and Meridians-Collaterals, promoting the balance of yin and yang and renewing body's health.

The theory of traditional Chinese medicine holds that maintaining the dynamic balance of yin and yang is the basic condition for normal life. Clinical practice indicates that the balance of yin and yang is bound up with healthy energy-evil struggle. *Plain Questions—Theory of Tong Ping Xu Shi* said, "When evil qi

压针孔片刻。如刺针深度较浅，针下无紧涩感，也可迅速将针退出。

出针应当重视先后顺序，一般而言，出针应按"先上后下、先内后外"的顺序进行。出针后应注意观察有无出血，尤其是头皮、眼眶等易出血的部位，出针后应用干棉球按压片刻，以免出血或血肿。出针后还要核对针数是否有遗漏，并及时处理针刺后遗感，嘱患者稍休息，待患者气息调匀、情绪稳定后方可离去。

第四节　针刺补泻

针刺补泻是针刺治病的重要环节之一，是毫针刺法的核心内容。针刺补泻理论的建立源于《黄帝内经》，如《灵枢·经脉》说："盛则泻之，虚则补之，热则疾之，寒则留之，陷下则灸之。"《灵枢·九针十二原》言："虚实之要，九针最妙，补泻之时，以针为之。"《灵枢·终始》说："凡刺之道，气调而止。"

一、针刺补泻概念

针刺补泻是指在针刺得气的基础上，采用适当的针刺手法补益正气或疏散病邪，从而调节人体脏腑经络功能，促使阴阳平衡，恢复健康的针刺方法。

中医理论认为"阴平阳秘，精神乃治"。临床实践表明，阴阳平衡与邪正盛衰变化关系密切，《素问·通评虚实论》曰："邪气盛则实，精气夺则虚。"针灸调节阴阳平

abounds, then [this is] repletion. When the essence qi is lost, then [this is] depletion. " Acupuncture regulates the balance of yin and yang by reinforcing the deficiency and reducing the excess. "Reinforcing the deficiency and reducing the excess" is achieved by specific acupuncture techniques. The one which can invigorate the body's healthy qi and strengthen weak physiological function is called "reinforcing method"; the one which can eliminate the pathogenic factors and harmonize hyperactive physiological function is called "reducing method".

2. The principle of reinforcing and reducing methods of needling

(1) Reinforcing the deficiency and reducing the excess. *Miraculous Pivot—Nine Needles and Twelve Source* said, "Whenever the needles are used, what is depleted [of proper qi], it must be replenished. What is full [of evil qi], it must be drained. What has accumulated over an extended period of time, that is to be discarded. Where evil has been victorious, it is to be depleted. " *Miraculous Pivot—Meridians* said, "If the [evil] qi abound, they are to be drained. If the [proper qi] are depleted, they are to be supplemented. In the case of heat, [the needle is to be inserted and withdrawn] quickly. In the case of cold it may remain [inserted] for a while. If an indentation forms, [when the vessel is squeezed, that fails to level again when the finger is withdrawn,] then it is to be cauterized. When [the qi] neither abound nor are depleted, then [the disease] is to be removed from the [respective] conduit. " It is illustrated that reinforcing deficiency and reducing excess is the fundamental principle of reinforcing and reducing methods of acupuncture, meanwhile explaining that reinforcing and reducing methods of acupuncture must be realized by concrete acupuncture techniques.

(2) The sequence of reinforcing and reducing methods. When the deficiency and excess are mixed, we should pay attention to prioritize the healthy qi deficiency and the pathogenic factors excess. As the pathogenic factors excess and the healthy qi is deficient, but the healthy qi is still capable of defending, or when reinforcing deficiency will worsen the condition on the contrary, we should reduce first and reinforce later. As the pathogenic factors excess and the healthy qi is deficient, and it is mainly about the healthy qi deficiency, or when reducing excess is more harmful to healthy qi because healthy qi is too weak, we should reinforce first and reduce later. *Miraculous Pivot—Xieqi Zangfu Bingxing* said, "If one supplements and drains contrary to the requirements, then the disease will become even more severe. "

When the deficiency and excess are phase tilting, yin and yang

衡通过"补虚泻实"以实现。"补虚泻实"通过特定的针刺操作手法完成。其中能鼓舞人体正气,使低下的机能状态恢复正常的针刺手法,即为"补法";能疏散病邪,使亢进的机能状态恢复正常的针刺手法,即为"泻法"。

二、针刺补泻原则

1. 补虚泻实　《灵枢·九针十二原》说"凡用针者,虚则实之,满则泄之,宛陈则除之,邪胜则虚之",《灵枢·经脉》则说"盛则泻之,虚则补之,热则疾之,寒则留之,陷下则灸之,不盛不虚以经取之",揭示了针灸补泻的基本原则就是补虚泻实,同时也说明了针灸补泻一定是通过具体的针刺操作手法来实现的。

2. 补泻先后　虚实夹杂时,应注意分清正虚与邪实的主次。如邪盛正虚,但正气尚能耐攻,或同时兼顾补虚反会助邪的病证,当先泻后补;正虚邪实,以正虚为主,或因正气过于虚弱,泻法更亦伤正的情况下,应先补而后泻。《灵枢·邪气脏腑病形》曰:"补泻反,则病益笃。"

虚实相倾、阴阳相移时,更应

are transforming, more attention should be paid to the sequence of reinforcing and reducing. *Miraculous Pivot—Zhongshi* said, "When the yin [qi] abound while the yang [qi] are in a state of depletion, the yang [qi] are to be supplemented first, and then the yin [qi] are to be drained to achieve harmony. When the yin [qi] are in a state of depletion while the yang [qi] abound, the yin [qi] are to be supplemented first, and then the yang [qi] are to be drained to achieve harmony." And it illustrates that protecting healthy qi first and eliminating pathogenic factors later are the fundamental points to deal with complex situations.

(3) Moderate reinforcing and reducing methods. *Miraculous Pivot—Genjie* said, "If both the qi forming one's physical appearance and the qi of disease are insufficient, in this case the yin and the yang qi are all insufficient. When they all are insufficient, such a condition must not be pierced. If one were to pierce, the insufficiency would be aggravated." It shows that the application of reinforcing and reducing methods of needling has a certain range of adaptation. In the case of deficiency of yin essence, yang qi and blood, reinforcing and reducing methods of needling should not be used, but drug therapy should be the main method.

3. The basis of reinforcing and reducing methods of needling

Miraculous Pivot—Xiao Zhen Jie said, "In the case of abundant [qi], it is not advisable to supplement … in the case of qi depletion, it is not advisable to drain." *Miraculous Pivot—Xieqi Zangfu Bingxing* said, "If one supplements and drains contrary to the requirements, then the disease will become even more severe." *The Seventy-Third Issues of the Classic of Questioning* said, "Those who should use the complementary method cannot use the reducing method, and those who should use the reinforcing method cannot use the complementary method." *The Eighty-First Issues of the Classic of Questioning* said, "The excessiveness cannot be supplemented, and the deficiency cannot be reduced. If reduce insufficiency and (or) reinforce excessiveness, the disease will get worse." These discussions all show that the correct application of reinforcing and reducing manipulation is the key for clinical efficacy, and the correct application of reinforcing and reducing manipulation must seek the basis from clinical practice.

(1) Identify the deficiency and excess. Before treatment, we must make a correct diagnosis through synthesis of the four diagnostic methods, and identify the deficiency and excess, as the basis of reinforcing and reducing methods of needling. *Miraculous Pivot—Genjie* said, "It is essential to examine the diseases

该注意补泻的先后。《灵枢·终始》曰："阴盛而阳虚，先补其阳，后泻其阴而和之；阴虚而阳盛，先补其阴，后泻其阳而和之。"这说明先保正气，后祛邪气，是处理复杂情况的根本所在。

3. 适度补泻　《灵枢·根结》说："形气不足，病气不足，此阴阳气俱不足也，不可刺之，刺之则重不足，重不足则阴阳俱竭。"这说明针刺补泻具有一定的适用范围，在人体阴精阳气、形体气血俱虚的情况下，不宜采用针刺补泻，而应以药物治疗为主。

三、针刺补泻依据

《灵枢·小针解》说："气盛不可补也……气虚不可泻也。"《灵枢·邪气脏腑病形》言："补泻反，则病益笃。"《难经·七十三难》说："补者不可为泻，泻者不可为补。"《难经·八十一难》说："无虚虚实实，损不足而益有余。"这些论述均说明补泻手法的正确应用是临床有效的关键，而正确应用补泻手法又必须从临床寻求依据。

1. 辨别虚实　施治前必须通过四诊合参对病证做出正确的判断，辨明虚实，作为针刺补泻的依据。《灵枢·根结》云："必审五脏变化之病，五脉之应，经络之实虚，

associated with changes in the five long-term depots, and how the five [movements in the] vessels correspond to them, whether the conduits and network [vessels] have a repletion or depletion, and whether the skin is soft or rough. Only then does one remove the [evil qi]." The changes of deficiency and excess in human diseases can be manifested in Zang-Fu organs, meridians, pulse conditions, skin and many other aspects. As *Plain Questions—Tiaojing Lun* said, "The spirit, qi, blood, body and will all have excess or deficiency." In the face of such a complex situation, we should synthesize the information obtained from the four diagnostic methods, and according to *Miraculous Pivot—Tongtian*, "It is advisable to carefully examine their yin and yang [conduits], and to find out whether there are evil or proper [qi], to take into regard their appearance and demeanor, and to check whether there is a surplus or an insufficiency. When [the qi] abound, then they are to be drained. A depletion is to be supplemented. If there is neither an abundance nor a depletion, the [disease] is to be removed from the conduits."

Huangdi Neijing emphasized that different changes of pulse conditions should be regarded as the basis for determining the actual situation of disease and syndrome and the reinforcing and reducing method of needling. *Miraculous Pivot—Nine Needles and Twelve Source* said, "Whenever one is about to employ the needle, it is essential to first inspect the vessels, to see whether the qi are tense or relaxed. And it is only then that a therapy may begin." *Miraculous Pivot—Meridian* said, "The conduit vessels are usually invisible. Whether they are in a condition of depletion and repletion, that can be known from [the movement of the qi at] the qi openings."

(2) Examine meridians and collaterals. In the clinical application of acupuncture in reinforcing and reducing methods of needling, the acupuncturist should pay attention to examine the situation of the deficiency and excess of meridians and collaterals on the basis of syndrome differentiation of yin and yang of Zang-Fu organs' qi and blood. *Miraculous Pivot—Cijie Zhenxie* said, "When using the needles, it is imperative to check whether meridians and collaterals are insufficient or excess. One presses the finger [into the vessels] and follows their course. Once squeezes [the skin] and pulls it up. One checks which movements correspond, and then removes [the evil qi] by moving them downward." It shows that the phenomenon of deficiency and excess of meridians and collaterals can be distinguished by palpating, pressing the body surface and sensation under the needle. All the manifestations of paralysis, cold sensation, depression, emaciation,

皮之柔粗,而后取之。"人体疾病的虚实变化可表现在脏腑、经脉、脉象、皮肤等诸多方面,正如《素问·调经论》所言:"神有余有不足,气有余有不足,血有余有不足,形有余有不足,志有余有不足。"面对这些复杂情况,应综合四诊得到的信息,并按照《灵枢·通天》所云:"谨诊其阴阳,视其邪正,安容仪,审有余不足,盛则泻之,虚则补之,不盛不虚,以经取之。"

《黄帝内经》更强调要将脉象的不同变化,作为确定病证虚实、针刺补泻的依据。譬如《灵枢·九针十二原》云:"凡将用针,必先诊脉,视气之剧易,乃可以治也。"《灵枢·经脉》又云:"经脉者常不可见也,其虚实也,以气口知之。"

2. 审察经络　临床应用针刺补泻手法,还要在脏腑气血阴阳辨证的基础上,注重审察经络的虚实情况。《灵枢·刺节真邪》说:"用针者,必先察其经络之实虚,切而循之,按而弹之,视其应动者,乃后取之而下之。"这说明经络的虚实现象,可以从切循、按弹和针下感应加以辨别。凡表现麻痹、厥冷、陷下、瘦弱、针下空虚和感觉迟钝等现象为经脉之虚证;表现疼痛、红肿、硬结、肥大、针下紧涩和感觉过敏等现象为经脉之实证。

emptiness under the needle and insensibility are the deficiency of meridians. Manifestations of pain, redness, induration, hypertrophy, tight needles and sensory hypersensitivity are the excess of meridians.

The examination of meridians and collaterals also means in the process of acupuncture, carefully observing the state of qi and blood, and the activity of healthy qi and evil qi; and then implementing reinforcing and reducing according to the situation of the deficiency and excess of meridians and collaterals. *Miraculous Pivot—Xiao Zhen Jie* said, "The unrefined [practitioner] guarding the trigger is concerned with guarding the four extremities, and they know nothing of the coming and going of blood and qi, and of proper and evil [qi]. The outstanding [practitioner] guarding the inner mechanism knows how to guard the qi. Those who arrive must not be confronted is [to say] that in the case of abundant [qi] it is not advisable to supplement. Those who go away must not be pursued is [to say] that in the case of qi depletion it is not advisable to drain."

(3) Examine the configuration and spirit. *Miraculous Pivot—Zhongshi* emphasized that "All patterns of piercing require an examination of [the patient's] physical appearance and qi." *Miraculous Pivot—Benshen* said, "All norms of piercing [require one] to first of all consider the spirit as the foundation... The fact is that those who apply the needles, they observe a patient's condition to get to know whether his essence, spirit, hun soul and po soul are still present or have been lost, and whether he is subjected to a gain or loss. If all five [long-term depots] are harmed, the needles will be unable to achieve a cure." It not only explains the dialectical relationship between body and spirit, but also emphasizes the important role of grasping configuration and spirit in clinical implementation of reinforcing and reducing method.

Miraculous Pivot—Shou Yao Gang Rou said, "In a person's life there is hardness and softness, weakness and strength, shortness and length, and yin and yang." That is to say, the observation before treatment should also include the physical constitution, as well as the observation of the strength of physical constitution and the rise and fall of spirit. *Miraculous Pivot—Tongtian* said: "For sure, there are major yin type persons and minor yin type persons, major yang type persons and minor yang type persons, and there are persons with harmonious, even shares of yin and yang. All these five types of persons, their attitudes are different, and their sinews and bones, their qi and blood are not alike either." This divides the individual physical differences into "

审察经络还在于在针刺过程中,细心体察指下气血正邪活动的状态,然后根据经气的虚实情况施行补泻。《灵枢·小针解》曰:"粗守关者,守四肢而不知血气正邪之往来也。上守机者,知守气也……其来不可逢者,气盛不可补也。其往不可追者,气虚不可泻也。"

3. 审察形神 《灵枢·终始》曰:"凡刺之法,必察其形气。"《灵枢·本神》说:"凡刺之法,先必本于神……是故用针者,察观病人之态,以知精、神、魂、魄之存亡,得失之意,五者以伤,针不可以治之也。"这既说明了形神的辨证关系,又强调了形神的把握对临床补泻的重要作用。

《灵枢·寿夭刚柔》曰:"人之生也,有刚有柔,有弱有强,有短有长,有阴有阳。"即施治前的观察也应包含对患者素有体质的观察,以及形态强弱、神气盛衰。《灵枢·通天》曰:"盖有太阴之人,少阴之人,太阳之人,少阳之人,阴阳和平之人。凡五人者,其态不同,其筋骨气血各不等。"这将个体的体质差异分为"五态",并指出古之善用针艾者,视人五态乃治之,盛者泻之,虚者补之。在临床上虽然不能

five states",and points out that those in antiquity who knew well how to use needles and moxa,they took into regard the five attitudes of man,and then cured them. Where [the qi] abounded, they drained them. Where they were depleted,they supplemented them." Although we can not mechanically adhere to the "five states" in clinical practice,we must understand the strength of the patient's normal constitution and the attributes of yin and yang as a reference and basis for treatment.

4. The factors affecting the needling reactions of reinforcing and reducing

(1) The functional state of patients. The decisive factor affecting the needling effect is the functional state of the body. When the functional state of the body is low and deficiency syndrome occurs,needling can strengthen the body resistance and tonify deficiency syndrome. When the body's functional state is hyperfunction,or excess heat and pathogen closure are positive, needling can play a role in clearing away heat,opening and closing, eliminating pathogen excess. For example, needling can relieve spasm and pain when gastrointestinal hyperfunction causes spasm and pain;needling can promote gastrointestinal peristalsis,eliminate abdominal distension and stimulate appetite when gastrointestinal function is inhibited and leads to abdominal distension.

(2) Therapeutic properties of acupoints. The clinical function of acupoints not only has universality,but also has certain relative specificity. Acupoints such as Guanyuan (CV4), Qihai (CV6), Mingmen(GV4) and Gaohuang(BL43) can inspire healthy qi of human body, promote vigorous function, have strengthening function and are suitable for reinforcing deficiency. Acupoints such as Shuigou(GV26),Weizhong(BL40),the twelve Jing-well points, and Shixuan (EX-UE11) can dispel pathogenic factors, inhibit hyperfunction of human body, have the function of dispelling pathogenic factors,and are suitable for reducing the excess. When applying needling to reinforcing deficiency and reducing the excess, we should combine the relative specificity of acupoint action,which is helpful to obtain better needling effect of reinforcement and reduction.

(3) Needling techniques. The functional state of patients and the choice of acupoints with special functions are the basic conditions that affect the reinforcing and reducing effect. Needle manipulation is the means to stimulate and promote the exertion of the functional characteristics of acupoints and improve the body reaction state,and the key factor to achieve the reinforcing and reducing effect. It is also the reflection of clinical treatment

机械地拘守"五态"来施行治法,但必须了解患者平素体质的强弱及阴阳属性,将其作为施治的参考和依据。

四、针刺补泻的影响因素

1. 机体功能状态　影响针刺作用效应的决定因素是机体的功能状态。当机体功能状态低下而呈虚证时,针刺可以起到扶正补虚的作用;当机体功能状态亢进,或实热、邪闭而呈实证时,针刺可以起到清热启闭、祛邪泻实的作用。如胃肠功能亢进而痉挛疼痛时,针刺可解痉止痛;胃肠功能抑制而腹胀纳呆时,针刺可促进胃肠蠕动,消除腹胀,增进食欲。

2. 腧穴相对特异性　腧穴的临床主治功用不仅具有普遍性,还具有一定的相对特异性。如关元、气海、命门、膏肓等腧穴,能鼓舞人体正气,促使功能旺盛,具有强壮作用,适用于补虚。如水沟、委中、十二井、十宣等腧穴,能疏散病邪,抑制人体功能亢进,具有祛邪作用,适用于泻实。当施行针刺补泻时,结合腧穴作用的相对特异性,有助于取得更好的针刺补泻效果。

3. 针刺手法　机体的功能状态以及具有特殊作用腧穴的选择,是影响补泻效果的基础条件,针刺手法是激发、促进腧穴功能特性发挥,改善机体反应状态的手段,是取得补泻效果的关键因素,是临床治疗过程的体现。

process.

At the same time, the selection of needles with different specifications, and the choice of puncture angle, direction and depth will also have some influence on the effect of reinforcing and reducing of needling.

同时,不同规格针具的选用以及刺入角度、方向与深度的选择也会对针刺补泻效果产生一定的影响。

Chapter 2　Moxibustion

Section 1　Basic Knowledge of Moxibustion

Moxibustion is a form of external treatment method that mainly ignites the moxa sticks or moxa cones made of Chinese mugwort leaves and burns or fumigates the acupoints of affected area, and adjusts the functions of meridians and viscera by stimulating acupoints through its warm stimulation and pharmacological effects of argy wormwood leaves, so as to achieve the purpose of disease prevention and treatment.

All moxibustion methods with argy wormwood leaves as the main moxibustion material belong to moxa therapy. Moxibustion is widely used in clinic. According to different operation modes, it can be divided into moxa-cone moxibustion, moxa stick moxibustion, warming needle moxibustion, moxa burner moxibustion and so on (Fig. 2-1). Moxa-cone moxibustion and moxa stick moxibustion are the main parts of moxa therapy, which are commonly used in clinical practice. Moxa-cone moxibustion can be divided into direct moxibustion and indirect moxibustion according to whether the moxa cone is directly burned on the skin. Direct moxibustion can be divided into purulent moxibustion (scarring moxibustion) and non-purulent moxibustion (non-scarring moxibustion) according to the size of moxa cone, the degree of moxibustion and whether there is burn or purulent after moxibustion. Purulent moxibustion is not easy to be accepted by most patients because of severe burns and local scar formation, so in this chapter non-purulent moxibustion will be mainly introduced. Moxa stick moxibustion can be divided into suspension moxibustion and pressing moxibustion according to different operation methods. Suspension moxibustion also includes three commonly used clinical methods: mild-warm moxibustion, sparrow-pecking moxibustion and circling moxibustion.

Because moxibustion can produce warm stimulation on acupoints or specific areas, it is generally believed that moxibustion has the function of warming and tonifying, and is good at treating deficiency cold syndrome and prevention and healthcare. According to *Huangdi Neijing*, a disease that may not be treated by acupuncture, may be treated by moxibustion. *Introduction to Medicine* said that moxibustion is suggested when a disease fails to respond to acupuncture and medicine. It shows that moxibustion has a wide range of clinical treatment, and moxibustion can promote and achieve better result on many diseases, especially when

第二章　艾　灸　法

第一节　艾灸法的基础知识

艾灸法是指点燃用艾叶加工制作的艾条或艾炷后在穴位或患处进行烧灼或熏熨，借其温热性及艾叶的药理作用，通过刺激腧穴来调整经络与脏腑的功能，以达到防病治病目的的一种外治方法。

凡以艾叶为主要施灸材料的方法均属于艾灸法。艾灸法临床应用广泛，依据操作方式的不同，可分为艾炷灸、艾条灸、温针灸、温灸器灸等（图 2-1）。艾炷灸和艾条灸是艾灸法的主体部分，临床较为常用。在使用艾炷灸时，根据艾炷是否直接置于穴位皮肤上燃灼分为直接灸和间接灸两种方法。直接灸根据使用艾炷的大小、施灸程度不同、灸后有无烧伤化脓，又分为化脓灸（瘢痕灸）和非化脓灸（无瘢痕灸）。前者因灼伤较重，局部易形成瘢痕，大多数患者不易接受，故本章主要介绍非化脓灸。艾条灸根据操作术式不同分为悬起灸和实按灸，悬起灸又包括温和灸、雀啄灸、回旋灸三种临床常用方法。

由于艾灸法能对穴位或患处产生温热性的刺激，所以一般认为其具有温补作用，擅长治疗虚寒病证和预防保健。《黄帝内经》云"针所不为，灸之所宜"，《医学入门》曰"凡药之不及，针之不到，必须灸之"，说明艾灸法的临床治疗范围十分广泛，许多疾病在用针刺或用药后无效或疗效不明显的情况下，用艾灸法往往能取得较好效果。

acupuncture and traditional Chinese herbs used is ineffective or the effect is not obvious. For example, in the clinical treatment of rheumatic arthritis, rheumatic myositis, rheumatoid arthritis, periarthritis of shoulder joint, chronic bronchitis, and bronchial asthma, the simple use of moxibustion or combined with acupuncture has a significant effect. At the same time, moxibustion operation is relatively simple, easy for patients to master and operate on their own, which is conducive to the popularization in family healthcare and treatment of common diseases.

如临床治疗风湿性关节炎、风湿性肌纤维炎、类风湿性关节炎、肩周炎、慢性支气管炎、支气管哮喘等疾病时，单纯采用灸法或配合针法均有显著的疗效。同时，艾灸法操作相对简便，患者容易掌握而能自行操作，有利于其在家庭保健和常见病治疗中的普及。

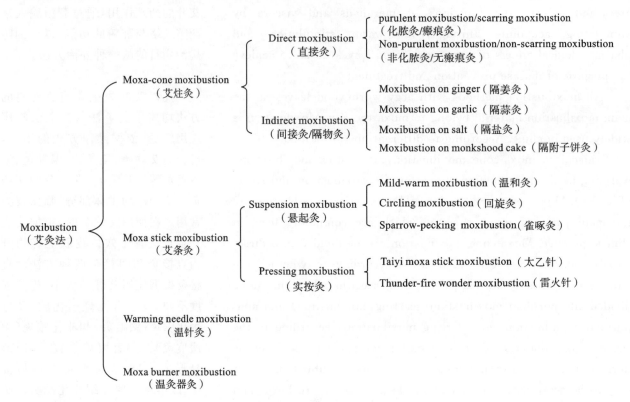

图 2-1　常用艾灸法分类

Section 2　Basic Operation of Moxibustion

1. Moxibustion with seed-sized moxa cone

Moxibustion with seed-sized moxa cone, also known as non-purulent moxibustion, or non-scarring moxibustion, is a moxibustion treatment method in which the skin is warm and hot, that is, the local skin at acupoints is red or slightly burned, without purulent or scarring after moxibustion. Before moxibustion treatment, a small amount of petroleum jelly was applied on patient's skin of selected point to enhance adhesion. And place a small moxa cone shaped like wheat grains with the height and bottom diameter of 0.3 cm on the acupoints, and then light and burn it. The burning moxa is pinched out or taken away by the therapist before it is half burned, as well as when the patient feels a

第二节　艾灸法的基本操作

一、麦粒灸

麦粒灸又称为非化脓灸、无瘢痕灸，是以皮肤达到温烫为主，即穴位局部皮肤出现红晕或轻微烫伤，灸后不化脓、不留瘢痕的灸治方法。施灸时，先将施灸部位涂以少量凡士林，然后将炷高和炷底直径均为 0.3 cm、状如麦粒的小艾炷放在穴位上，并将其点燃，当艾炷燃至一半左右，患者感到皮肤发烫或灼痛时，即用镊子将艾炷移去或压灭，更换新艾炷再灸。一般每穴

burning discomfort, and the moxa cone is replaced by a new one to continue moxibustion. Generally, the moxibustion on an acupoint requires repetition of this process 3-7 moxa cones until local skin in the area being treated become rosy. This method has a wide range of indications, and can be applied to common diseases. It is easy to be accepted by patients because of its less pain during treatment and without suppuration or scar.

[Operation key points] Select a small moxa cone; incompletely burn out; immediately and skillfully replace moxa cone when there is burning pain to prevent scalding.

2. Indirect moxibustion

Indirect moxibustion is a method of moxibustion with material insulation between moxa cone and skin. Ginger-partitioned moxibustion, salt-partitioned moxibustion, garlic-partitioned moxibustion and monkshood cake-partitioned moxibustion are commonly used in clinical practice.

(1) Moxibustion on ginger. Fresh ginger is cut into slices, each about 0.3 cm thick, punched several needle holes and placed on the acupoints/areas selected. The moxa cone is then placed on the top of the ginger slice where it is ignited and burned(Fig. 2-2). When the patient feels the heat is intolerable, the ginger slice can be raised off the skin for a moment, and replaced on the same area to continue moxibustion. When the cone has burned completely, and the ash is removed, it is replaced with another one and the procedure is repeated until the local skin in the area being treated become rosy, generally 5-7 moxa cones per point. This method can be used to treat cold cough, abdominal pain, diarrhea, wind-cold-dampness arthralgia, dysmenorrhea, facial palsy and so on, especially suitable for cold syndrome.

灸 3～7 壮，以局部皮肤出现红晕为度。本法适应证广泛，一般常见病均可应用，因其灸时痛苦小，且灸后不化脓、不留瘢痕，易为患者接受。

【操作要点】选用小艾炷；勿待艾炷燃尽；有灼痛感时即刻更换艾炷；动作需连贯，防止烫伤。

二、隔物灸

隔物灸是指在艾炷与皮肤之间衬隔某种物品而施灸的一种方法。临床常用的有隔姜灸、隔盐灸、隔蒜灸、隔附子饼灸四种。

1. 隔姜灸　切取厚约 0.3 cm 生姜 1 片。在其中心处用针穿刺数孔，上置艾炷放在穴位上，用火点燃施灸（图 2-2），如患者感觉灼热不可忍受，可将姜片向上提起，稍待片刻，重新放下再灸，艾炷燃尽后另换一炷依前法再灸，直到局部皮肤潮红为止。一般每穴灸 5～7 壮。本法可根据病情反复施灸，风寒咳嗽、腹痛、泄泻、风寒湿痹、痛经、颜面神经麻痹等均可应用，尤宜用于寒证。

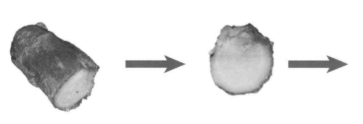
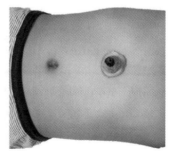

图 2-2　隔姜灸

[Operation key points] Select medium or large moxa cone; ginger should be fresh; grasp the number of moxa cones and temperature of moxibustion to prevent scalding.

(2) Moxibustion on salt. This method is also known as Shenque(CV8) moxibustion, as it is only done on the umbilicus. First, the umbilicus is filled with pure dry edible salt to the level of

【操作要点】选择中或大艾炷；所隔生姜宜新鲜；掌握施灸壮数和温度，防止烫伤。

2. 隔盐灸　又称神阙灸，仅用于脐窝部施灸，取干燥纯净的食盐末适量，将脐窝填平，上置艾炷，

the skin, followed by placing a moxa cone on the top of the salt; it is then ignited and burnt (Fig. 2-3). When consumed, the ash is removed, and it is replaced with another until all the cones required have been consumed. This method is effective in case of abdominal pain, vomiting and diarrhea, pain around umbilicus, hernia, and dysentery. In addition, moxibustion on salt has the function to restore to yang to save from collapse, such as symptoms of excessive sweating, peripheral coldness and undetectable pulse. Continuous moxibution with large-sized moxa cones is applied until the patient's vital signs are steady. That is, his/her sweating stops, pulse can be palpated and the extremities have become warm.

用火点燃施灸(图 2-3)。如患者感到灼痛时即用镊子夹去残炷,另换一炷再灸,灸满规定的壮数为止。该疗法适用于腹痛、上吐下泻、脐周痛、疝气、痢疾等疾病。此外,隔盐灸还有回阴救逆的作用,用于治疗大汗淋漓、四肢厥冷和脉微弱等症,此时可用大艾炷持续施灸,直至汗止、脉复、四肢转温。

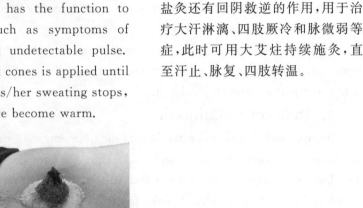

图 2-3 隔盐灸

[Operation key points] Select medium or large moxa cones; grasp the number of moxa cones and temperature of moxibustion; salt is easy to explode in case of fire, placing ginger slice on the top of salt can prevent abdominal scald.

【操作要点】选择中或大艾炷;掌握施灸壮数和温度;食盐遇火易爆,以姜片间隔食盐,可防止腹部烫伤。

(3) Moxibustion on garlic. The garlic clove is cut into slices, each about 0.3 cm thick, punch several needle holes at the center, put it on the acupoints/areas selected and moxa cones are ignited and burned on the top of the garlic slice(Fig. 2-4). Renew the moxa cone when the patient feels it scorching. After burning 4-5 moxa cones replace a new garlic slice. The garlic mud also can be applied to the affected area and place a ignited moxa cone on it. 7 moxa cones per point until the local skin in the area being treated become rosy. This method can be to scrofula, pulmonary tuberculosis, the early stages of skin ulcers or scabies, poisonous insect bite, etc.

3. 隔蒜灸 用独头蒜或较大蒜瓣横切成 0.3 cm 厚的蒜片,中心处用针穿刺数孔,置于穴位或患处皮肤上,再将艾炷置于蒜瓣上,用火点燃施灸(图 2-4)。当患者感到灼痛时,另换一炷再灸,每灸 4~5 壮可换一新蒜片。也可将大蒜捣烂如泥,敷于患处,上置艾炷点燃施灸。每穴每次宜灸足 7 壮,以灸处泛红为度。该疗法适用于瘰疬、肺结核、皮肤溃疡和疮疖早期阶段,以及毒虫咬伤等。

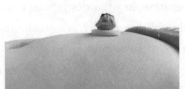

图 2-4 隔蒜灸

[Operation key points] Select medium or large moxa cones; fresh single head garlic should be used; grasp the number of moxa cones and temperature of moxibustion to prevent local blistering and scalding.

(4) Moxibustion on monkshood cake. A cake of monkshood is approximately 1-2 cm in diameter and 0. 3-0. 5 cm in thickness, and it is made of monkshood powder mixed with yellow rice wine. It is punched with several needle holes at the center. Place on the acupoints or affected areas where moxa cones are placed on top of it to be ignited and burnt. Renew the moxa cone when the patient feels it scorching. Generally, 5-10 moxa cones per acupoint until the local skin in the area being treated become rosy(Fig. 2-5). Since pungent in flavor, extremely hot in nature, monkshood cake moxibustion has the function of warming kidney and supplementing yang. Thus it is often adopted to treat various yang-deficiency diseases, such as impotence, premature ejaculation, infertility, dysmenorrhea, amenorrhea by declination of the Mingmen (vital gate) fire, and the Guanyuan(CV4) and Mingmen(GV4) points are suitable and effective to be used.

【操作要点】选择中或大艾炷；宜用新鲜的独头大蒜；掌握施灸壮数和温度，防止局部起疱与烫伤。

4. 隔附子饼灸　将生附子研为细末，用黄酒调和制饼，直径1～2 cm，厚0.3～0.5 cm，中心处用针穿刺数孔。上置艾炷并放于穴位或患处，点燃施灸，当患者感到灼痛时另换一炷再灸，一般每穴灸5～10壮，灸至皮肤出现红晕为度（图2-5）。附子辛温大热，有温肾益阳的作用，多用来治疗各种阳虚病证，如命门之火不足导致的阳痿、早泄、不孕症、痛经、闭经等，常灸关元、命门等穴。

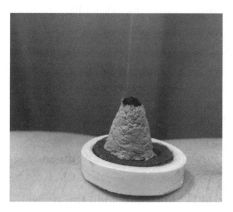

图2-5　隔附子饼灸

[Operation key points] Select medium or large moxa cones; grasp the number of moxa cones and temperature of moxibustion to prevent scalding.

【操作要点】选择中或大艾炷；掌握施灸壮数和温度；防止烫伤。

3. Suspension moxibustion

Suspension moxibustion is a kind of moxibustion method in which the ignited moxa stick is holding over the selected site during the treatment. The end of the moxa stick should not make contact with the skin, in generally, the moxa fire is 2-3 cm away from the skin, moxibustion for 10-15 minutes, until the skin become warm and red without burning pain. Suspension moxibustion can be divided into mild-warm moxibustion, circling moxibustion and sparrow-pecking moxibustion.

(1) Mild-warm moxibustion. One end of a moxa stick is ignited and during the treatment, the practitioner holds the stick and aims

三、悬起灸

悬起灸是将点燃的艾条悬于施灸部位之上的一种灸法。一般艾火距皮肤2～3 cm，灸10～15分钟，以灸至皮肤温热红晕，而又不致烧伤皮肤为度。悬起灸又分为温和灸、回旋灸和雀啄灸。

1. 温和灸　将艾条的一端点燃，对准应灸的腧穴或患处，距离

the ignited end of the stick to the selected acupoints or treated area to do moxibustion. The distance between the end of the stick and the skin should be 2-3 cm. The intention here is to bring warmth to the treatment area, so the patient should not feel any burning sensations. Generally, moxibustion at each acupoint for 10-15 minutes until the skin become rosy (Fig. 2-6). The practitioners should place their index and middle fingers on the sides of the affected area to feel the heat, so that they can determine and adjust the appropriate distance between the end of the stick and the patient's skin, and master the moxibustion time to avoid burning for patients who have delayed sensory perception or children.

[Operation key points] The distance and position are relatively fixed; master the time and temperature of moxibustion; prevent burns.

(2) Circling moxibustion. One end of a moxa stick is ignited and held over an acupoint/affected area. When using this method, maintain a parallel distance of 2-3 cm above the skin, but the position is not fixed. It is evenly moved left and right or circularly repeatedly, to bring mild warmth to the local place, but not burning. Generally, for 10-15 minutes until the skin becomes slightly red(Fig. 2-7).

[Operation key points] The distance is fixed but the position is not fixed; master the time and temperature of moxibustion; prevent burns.

(3) Sparrow-pecking moxibustion. Sparrow-pecking moxibustion is done by holding the ignited end of a moxa stick about 3 cm over the acupoint or the affected area during the treatment. With this method, the distance between the ignited end of a moxa stick and the patient's skin is not fixed. Instead, as its name indicates, it is moved up and down over the area like a pecking bird(Fig. 2-8).

皮肤 2～3 cm 进行熏烤,以患者局部有温热感而无灼痛为宜,一般每穴灸 10～15 分钟,至皮肤出现红晕为度(图 2-6)。如遇到局部知觉减退的患者及小儿,医者可将食指、中指置于施灸部位两侧,这样可以通过医者的手指来测知患者局部受热程度,以便随时调节施灸距离,掌握施灸时间,防止烫伤。

【操作要点】距离与位置相对固定;掌握施灸时间与温度;防止烫伤。

2. 回旋灸　将艾条的一端点燃,对准应灸部位,与皮肤表面始终保持 2～3 cm 的平行距离,均匀地向左右移动或反复旋转进行灸治,以患者局部有温热感而无灼痛为宜,一般施灸 10～15 分钟,至皮肤红晕为度(图 2-7)。

【操作要点】距离固定但位置不固定;掌握施灸时间与温度;防止烫伤。

3. 雀啄灸　将点燃的艾条置于腧穴或患处上方约 3 cm 高处,施灸时,艾条点燃的一端与施灸部位的皮肤并不固定在一定的距离,而是像鸟雀啄食一样,将艾条一上一下、忽远忽近地移动(图 2-8)。

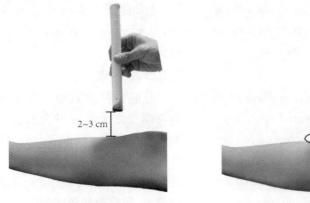

图 2-6　温和灸　　　　图 2-7　回旋灸

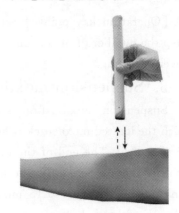

图 2-8　雀啄灸

[Operation key points] Operate moxa stick up and down like a pecking bird; master the time and temperature of moxibustion; prevent burns.

【操作要点】一上一下如鸟雀啄食;掌握施灸时间与温度;防止烫伤。

Section 3　The Precautions of Moxibustion

Moxibustion has functions as follows. Warm meridians and free collateral vessels, dissipate cold and eliminate pathogenic factors; promote qi and activate blood circulation, disperse abscesses and nodules, reinforce deficiency and cultivate root, restore yang to save from collapse; prevention and healthcare, prolong life. Moxibustion has a wide range of applications. It can not only treat the diseases of meridians and the exterior part of the body, but also treat the diseases of viscera; and it can not only treat many chronic diseases, but also treat some acute and critical diseases. Moxibustion can be used in the treatment and adjuvant treatment of the vast majority of clinical diseases, especially for wind-cold-dampness arthralgia, cold-phlegm cough and asthma, and various diseases caused by viscera deficiency and cold, or by deficiency fo Yuanyang. However, no matter what kind of disease moxibustion is used for, we must make a detailed investigation and careful diagnosis. According to the patient's age and constitution, we should choose the appropriate acupoints and moxibustion methods, and master the appropriate moxibustion quantity, so as to achieve the desired effect.

At the same time, attention should be paid to the following matters.

(1) Position. Moxibustion position should not only make the patient comfortable, but also be convenient for the doctor to operate. Try to take the lying position, and pay attention to preventing the occurrence of faint. Generally, moxibustion is not suitable for hunger, over satiety and extreme fatigue.

(2) Sequence. Generally, we should start moxibustion from the upper part of the body, to the lower part; first the back and waist, then the abdomen; first the head, then the limbs.

(3) The position of forbidden moxibustion and cautious moxibustion. Scarring moxibustion is prohibited on the face and head, areas close to large blood vessels and joint tendon. For pregnant women, scarring moxibustion is forbidden in the lumbosacral region and the lower abdomen, and other moxibustion methods should not be too much. For comatose patients with numbness and insensitive limbs, do not moxibustion too much to avoid burns.

(4) Deal wtih vesiculation. The small bubble can be absorbed, and the large one should be pierced with a disinfectant needle to release the liquid, apply a disinfectant gauze, and fix it with adhesive tape.

第三节　艾灸法的注意事项

艾灸法具有温通经络、驱寒散邪，行气活血、消肿散结，补虚培本、回阳固脱，预防保健、益寿延年的作用。艾灸法的适用范围非常广泛，它既可以治疗经络、体表的病证，也可以治疗脏腑的病证；既可以治疗许多慢性病证，也可以治疗一些急性、危重病证。艾灸法可应用于临床上绝大多数病证的治疗及辅助治疗，尤其对风寒湿痹、寒痰咳喘，以及脏腑虚寒、元阳虚损引起的各种病证，疗效较好。但艾灸法无论用于何种疾病，都必须详查病情，细心诊断，根据患者的年龄和体质，选择合适的穴位和施灸方法，掌握适当的灸量，以达到预期的效果。

同时，艾灸时需注意以下事项。

1. 施灸体位　施灸体位既要使患者舒适，也要便于医者操作，尽量采取卧位，注意防止晕灸的发生。一般空腹、过饱、极度疲劳时不宜施灸。

2. 施灸顺序　一般是先灸上部，后灸下部；先灸背、腰部，后灸腹部；先灸头部，后灸四肢。

3. 禁灸与慎灸的部位　颜面部、心区、体表大血管部和关节肌腱部不可用瘢痕灸。妊娠期妇女腰骶部和小腹部禁用瘢痕灸，其他灸法也不宜灸量过重。对昏迷、肢体麻木不仁及感觉迟钝的患者，勿灸过量，以避免烧伤。

4. 灸疱的处理　灸疱小者可自行吸收，灸疱大者可用消毒针穿破，放出液体，敷以消毒纱布，用胶布固定即可。

(5) Environment and fire prevention. In the process of moxibustion,good ventilation should be maintained in the room to prevent clothing and bed sheets from being damaged by the fire. After moxibustion,the moxa fire must be put out completely to prevent the fire hazard.

Appendix:Governor Vessel moxibustion

Governor Vessel moxibustion is a new type of indirect moxibustion,which is based on inheriting the traditional method of moxibustion on ginger. Its moxa cone is large with sufficient firepower. The treatment time is long,and the application area is wide and involve multiple acupoints. Its moxibustion temperature and quantity are enhanced,and its effect is beyond the reach of ordinary moxibustion. Because governor vessel moxibustion is often performed on the Governor Vessel on the back and waist like a long snake,so called "spreading moxibustion" and "long-snake moxibustion".

During the operation,first mash 300-600 g ginger into mud, squeeze part of the juice,and make the ginger mud into a rectangular separated moxibustion cake with a 1. 5 cm thickness and 4 cm width,which can cover the length from Dazhui(GV14) to Yaoshu(GV2). Then take a proper amount of moxa to make a long,triangular moxa cone with 4 cm height,so that the bottom width of moxa cone is slightly narrower than the width of moxibustion cake,and the length is slightly shorter than the length of moxibustion cake. Ask the patient to lie prostrate position, translate the moxibustion cake to the operation area, seal the surrounding area with cotton lint paper, and then place the long moxa cone in the center of the cake and light the moxibustion at the upper(dip a small amount of alcohol into the cotton swab and evenly apply it to the upper corner of moxa stick to support the combustion)(Fig. 2-9). When the patient has a burning sensation or is intolerable, the doctor takes off the burnt down moxa, and replaces the moxa cone. Every time performed for 3 moxa cones and 3-6 times as a course of treatment.

5. 环境与防火　施灸过程中,室内宜保持良好的通风,严防艾火烧坏衣服、床单等。施灸完毕,必须把艾火彻底熄灭,以防火灾。

【附:督灸】督灸是在继承传统隔姜灸法的基础上变化而来,是一种新型艾炷间接灸法。其艾炷大、火力足、灸治时间较长,在灸温、灸量上都有所增强,而且施灸面广,施灸部位可涉及多个腧穴,功效非一般灸法所及。因督灸常选在背腰部施治如长蛇状,故也被称为"铺灸""长蛇灸"。

操作时,先将 300～600 g 生姜捣烂如泥,挤去部分汁液,将姜泥做成厚约 1. 5 cm、宽约 4 cm,长度能覆盖督脉大椎穴至腰俞穴的长方形隔灸饼。再取适量艾绒做成高约 4 cm,横截面为三角形的大艾炷,使艾炷的底宽略窄于隔灸饼的宽度,长度略短于隔灸饼的长度。令患者取俯卧位,将隔灸饼平移至施术部位上,可用棉皮纸将周围封固,然后将该长条艾炷置于隔灸饼中央并在上端点燃施灸(可用棉签蘸取少量酒精均匀涂滴于艾炷上角以助燃)(图 2-9)。待患者有灼热感或难以忍受时,医者取下燃尽的艾绒,保留隔灸饼,更换艾炷续灸。每次施灸 3 壮,3～6 次为一疗程。

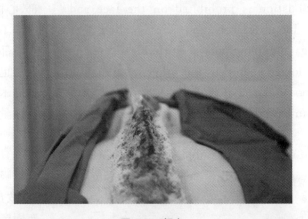

图 2-9　督灸

According to traditional Chinese medicine, the Governor Vessel govern all the yang meridians, it is called the "sea of yang meridians". Governor Vessel moxibustion can be used to treat diseases caused by wind, cold and dampness, or yang deficiency and cold coagulation, such as cervical spondylosis, lumbago, arthralgia syndrome, rheumatic arthritis, ankylosing spondylitis, menstrual pain, and postpartum pain. For local qi stagnation and blood stasis, it can also be applied locally to warm meridians and dredge collaterals, activate blood circulation and relieve pain.

中医学认为，督脉总督六阳经，为"阳脉之海"。铺灸于督脉处，可用于治疗风、寒、湿邪侵袭，或阳虚寒凝所致的疾病，如颈椎病、腰痛、痹证、风湿性关节炎、强直性脊柱炎、经行身痛、产后身痛等。对局部气滞血瘀者，也可于局部施灸而温经通络，活血止痛。

Chapter 3　Cupping

1. Basic knowledge of cupping

Cupping is a kind of method which uses cup as suction devices, to create negative pressure in the cup via the use of combustion, suction, steam and other methods, so that makes the cup absorb on the acupoints or a certain part of the affected area on the body surface, causes local skin congestion and blood stasis to produce benign stimulation, and achieves the purpose of regulating viscera, balancing yin and yang, dredging meridians and collaterals, to prevent and treating diseases.

The types of cups have developed from the early horn cups, bamboo cups, ceramic cups to glass cups, metal cups, plastic cups and rubber cups. Subsequently, there are a series of new style cups, such as magnetic therapy cups, infrared cups, and laser cups. Glass cup are transparent in texture and skin reactions can be observed and controlled at any time, which is beneficial to master the degree of blood stasis and regulate the treatment time. Therefore, the glass cup is the most commonly used cup in clinic.

Cupping method can cause local tissue congestion, resulting in smooth and expedite of qi and blood. Therefore, it has the functions of moving qi to relieve pain, dispersing abscesses and nodules, dispelling wind and cold, and clearing heat and drawing out toxin. Studies have shown that cupping with the effect of mechanical stimulation and warming, which can promote blood circulation and metabolism, regulate the function of nervous system, muscles and joints, ease the body pain, improve the whole functional status of the body.

Cupping with far-ranging adaptation scope, especially for all kinds of pain, soft tissue injury, acute or chronic inflammation, the wind cold dampness of Bi syndrome, and various diseases caused by viscera dysfunction and meridian occlusion. In the meanwhile, the clinical application of cupping has developed from the early treatment of ulcers to the treatment of more than 100 diseases including internal medicine, surgery, gynecology, pediatrics, dermatology, and so on.

2. Basic operation of cupping

2.1　Cup-sucking methods

Flash-fire method is one of the most important methods that create the suction in the glass cups. Its principle is to use part of the oxygen in the cup to be consumed during combustion, and to

第三章　拔　罐　法

一、拔罐法的基础知识

拔罐法是一种以罐为工具,利用燃烧、抽吸、蒸汽等方法造成罐内负压,使罐吸附于体表腧穴或患处的一定部位,使局部皮肤充血、瘀血产生良性刺激,达到调节脏腑、平衡阴阳、疏通经络以防治疾病的方法。

罐具种类从早期的角罐、竹罐、陶瓷罐发展到玻璃罐、金属罐、塑料罐、橡胶罐,并相继出现了磁疗罐、红外线罐、激光罐等新型罐具。基于玻璃罐具有质地透明,可随时观察罐内皮肤瘀血的程度,以便掌握治疗时间的优点,因而玻璃罐是目前临床使用较多的罐具。

拔罐后,局部组织充血,致使经络气血通畅,发挥行气止痛、消肿散结、祛风散寒、清热拔毒等功效。现代研究表明拔罐法的机械刺激作用和温热作用,可以促进血液循环和新陈代谢,从而调节神经系统功能,调节肌肉及关节活动,缓解机体疼痛,改善机体整体功能状态。

拔罐法的适应范围非常广泛,尤其对于各种疼痛类疾病、软组织损伤、急慢性炎症、风寒湿痹证,以及脏腑功能失调、经脉闭阻不通所引起的各种病证均有较好的疗效。同时,拔罐法的临床运用已从早期的疮疡发展到包括内科、外科、妇科、儿科、皮肤科等100多种疾病的治疗。

二、拔罐法的基本操作

(一)吸拔方式

玻璃罐的吸拔方式主要是闪火法。其原理是利用燃烧消耗罐中部分氧气,并借火焰的热力使罐

expand the gas in the cup by the heat of the flame to remove part of the air in the cup, forming a negative pressure(that is, the pressure in the cup is lower than the outside atmospheric pressure), thereby adsorbing the cup to the skin.

When flash-flame cupping, the doctors ignite a 95% alcohol-soaked cotton ball held with tweezers or hemostat, holds the cup body in the other hand with the mouth of the can facing down, and immediately put the flame into the cup and circle the flame inside it 2 to 3 times, and then withdraw it, and quickly place the cup onto the skin. At this time, the negative pressure in the cup make it possible for the skin to be absorbed. This method is suitable for all parts of the human body and is most commonly used in clinic. It can be used to retained cupping, successive flash cupping, moving cupping and lining-up cupping.

[Operation key points] The tweezers or hemostat should be tilted slightly. Cotton balls should be dipped in less alcohol and should not stick to the cup mouth. Moving quickly to avoid scalding the skin.

The suction force is related to the size and depth of the cup, the temperature and manner of the fire in the cup, the timing and speed of cup-sucking, and the amount of air enter the cup when cupping. If the cup is deep and large, the fire flame is strong, the temperature of the cup is high, the speed of cup-sucking is fast, and the air inside is less, then the suction force is large, otherwise it is small, which can be flexibly controlled according to the clinical treatment needs.

2.2　Cup-retaining time

Retaining time usually last 5 to 15 minutes, can be one-time daily or every other day for 1 time, 5 to 10 times a course of treatment, the interval between two courses may be 3 to 5 days(or until the cup-blackspot disappear).

2.3　Cup-lifting methods

Cup lifting is also known as cup opening, which is the method of taking off the sucked and pulled cups.

When lifting the cup, the doctor holds the bottom of the cup body with one hand and tilts it slightly, and presses the skin on the edge of the cup mouth with the thumb or index finger of the other hand to create a gap between the cup mouth and the skin to let air in, and then the cup can be removed. Do not drag or stretch the cup by improper force when lifting, so as to avoid skin injury and pain.

2.4　Degree of cupping

The degree of cupping depends on the suction and the cup-

内的气体膨胀而排出罐内部分空气，形成负压（即罐内气压低于外面大气压），借以将罐吸附于施术部位的皮肤上。

操作时一手用镊子或止血钳夹住 95% 酒精棉球，另一手握罐体，罐口朝下，将棉球点燃后立即伸入罐内摇晃数圈随即退出，迅速将罐扣于应拔部位，此时罐内已成负压即可吸住。此法适用于人体各部位，可拔留罐、闪罐、走罐、排罐等，临床最为常用。

【操作要点】镊子或止血钳稍倾斜；棉球蘸酒精宜少，且不能沾到罐口；动作迅速，以免烫伤皮肤。

吸拔力的大小与罐具的大小和深度、罐内燃火的温度和方式、扣罐的时机与速度、扣罐时空气再次进入罐内的多少等因素有关。如罐具深而且大，在火力旺时扣罐，罐内热度高，扣罐动作快，下扣时空气再次进入罐内少，罐的吸拔力大，反之则小，临床上可根据治疗需要灵活掌握。

（二）留罐时间

留罐时间一般为 5～15 分钟，可每日 1 次或隔日 1 次，5～10 次为 1 个疗程，2 个疗程之间应间隔 3～5 日（或等拔罐斑痕消失）。

（三）起罐法

起罐又名启罐，即将吸拔牢固的罐具取下的方法。

起罐时，医者一手握住罐体腰底部稍倾斜，另一手拇指或食指按压罐口边缘的皮肤，使罐口与皮肤之间产生空隙，空气进入罐内即可将罐取下。不可生硬拉拔，以免拉伤皮肤，产生疼痛。

（四）拔罐的程度

拔罐的程度决定于罐吸拔的

retaining time. In general, slight suction force and short retaining time of cupping makes the local skin reddish; strong suction force and long-time cupping makes the local skin appear fuchsia (ecchymosis). How to control the degree of cupping depends on the needs of the disease. Treatment as warming yang to tonify qi, warming meridians to dispel cold can be used with local flush and congestion with cupping (congestion cupping). Treatment as invigorate the circulation of blood to remove blood stasis, relieve swelling and pain can be used with local fuchsia and ecchymosis with cupping(blood stasis cupping). Do not blindly pursue with the local stasis, in order to avoid the local damage after repeated excessive cupping.

2.5　Postoperative treatment

After lifting the cup, a sterile cotton ball should be used to gently wipe the local part. If the man who is operated cupping feels slightly painful and itchy on the cup-spot, do not scratch it, and it will subside within a few days. If blister appears after lifting the cup, it can be absorbed naturally as long as they are not bruised. If the blister is too big, it can be pierced from the bottom with a disposable sterile needle. After the blister fluid is released, cover it with a sterile dressing. If bleeding, the spot should be wiped off with a sterile cotton ball. If the skin is damaged, it should be routinely sterilized and covered with a sterile dressing. If cupping is used to treat sore carbuncle, pus and blood should be wiped off after cupping, and the sore should be treated routinely.

3.　Applications of cupping

3.1　Flash-cupping method

Flash-cupping method is to use flash-fire method to draw the cup at the place where it should be pulled out, then take it off, suck it out, and then take it off again and again until the local skin is flushed or the bottom of the cup is hot. The action should be rapid and accurate. If necessary, the cup can be left after successive flash cupping(Fig. 3-1). It is suitable for patients with muscle relaxation that may lead to loose adsorption or difficult to retain cup. It is also suitable for patients with local skin numbness and deficiency syndrome of hypofunction.

[Operation key points] Move quickly and accurately; repeated action of drawing and pulling; during operation, the temperature should be acceptable to the patients.

3.2　Retaining cupping method

The method of retaining cupping is also called the method of sitting cupping. It is to leave the cupping on the skin for a certain

力度和留罐的时间。一般情况下，罐吸拔力度轻、留罐时间短，拔罐后局部皮肤可出现潮红；罐吸拔力度重、留罐时间长，拔罐后局部皮肤可出现紫红色（瘀斑色）。拔罐的程度取决于病情的需要，一般来说，温阳益气、温经散寒可采用局部潮红充血的拔罐法（充血罐），活血化瘀、消肿止痛可采用局部紫红瘀斑的拔罐法（瘀血罐）。但需注意，不可一味追求拔罐后局部出现瘀斑，以免反复过重拔罐引起的局部损伤。

（五）施术后的处理

起罐后应用消毒棉球轻拭吸拔局部，若罐斑处微觉痛痒，不可搔抓，数日内自可消退。起罐后如果出现水疱，只要不擦破，可任其自然吸收。若水疱过大，可用一次性消毒针从疱底刺破，放出水液后，再用消毒敷料覆盖。若出血应用消毒棉球拭净，若皮肤破损应常规消毒，并用无菌敷料覆盖其上。若用拔罐治疗疮痈，起罐后应拭净脓血，并常规处理疮口。

三、拔罐法的应用
（一）闪罐法

闪罐法是用闪火法将罐吸拔于应拔部位，随即取下，再吸拔，再取下，反复吸拔至局部皮肤潮红，或罐体底部发热为度，动作要迅速而准确，必要时也可在闪罐后留罐（图3-1）。本法适用于肌肉较松弛，吸拔不紧或留罐有困难之处，以及局部皮肤麻木或功能减退的虚证患者。

【操作要点】动作要快而准；反复吸拔；温热度以患者舒适能接受为度。

（二）留罐法

留罐法又名坐罐法，是将吸拔在皮肤上的罐具留置一定时间，使

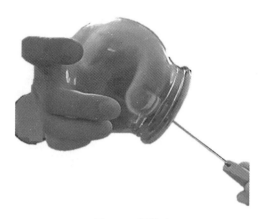

图 3-1　闪罐法

period of time until the shallow skin and muscles become reddish, even subcutaneous blood stasis is prunosus, and then remove it. Generally, the time of retaining the cup is 5 to 15 minutes. If the cup is large and has strong suction, the time should be reduced appropriately. This method is mainly used for deep tissue damage, neck-shoulder and lumbocrural pain, arthropathy, and various clinical diseases.

〔Operation key points〕 The time of cupping can be determined by the reaction and constitution of patients. For the elderly, children and those with obvious skin reaction, it is not advisable to keep the cup for a long time as well as in hot summer to avoid blistering and damaging the skin.

3.3　Moving cupping method

Spread some lubricant (commonly used medical Vaseline, medical glycerin, liquid paraffin or moisturizing cream, etc.) to patient's skin, warm water or liquid medicine can also be used, and grease can also be applied on the cup mouth. After using the flash-fire method to absorb the cup, immediately hold the cup by hand, push and pull the cup repeatedly along a certain route with a little force until the skin of the cup walking part is purplish red (Fig. 3-2). When pushing the cup, the pressure should be adjusted according to patients' constitution and condition. If the negative pressure is too large or the suction force is too heavy and the speed is too fast, patients often have unbearable pain and easily strain the skin; if the negative pressure is too small, the suction force is insufficient, the cup is easy to fall off, and the treatment effect is poor. This method is suitable for places with thick muscles in large areas, such as the waist, back and thighs.

〔Operation key points〕 The movement should be gentle, and the force should be uniform, steady and slow. The cups should be moved and slid immediately after suction and pulling. The negative

皮肤局部潮红，甚或皮下瘀血呈紫红色后，再将罐具取下。留罐时间一般为 5～15 分钟，罐大且吸力强的应适当缩短留罐时间。此法多用于深部组织损伤、颈肩腰腿痛、关节病变以及临床各科多种疾病。

【操作要点】留罐时间视患者体质与拔罐反应而定。老人与儿童、肌肤反应明显者以及炎热夏季之时留罐时间均不宜过长，以免起疱伤及皮肤。

（三）走罐法

先于施罐部位涂上润滑剂，如医用凡士林、医用甘油、液体石蜡或润肤霜等，也可用温水或药液，同时还可将罐口涂上油脂；使用闪火法将罐吸住后，立即用手握住罐体，略用力将罐沿着一定路线反复推拉，至走罐部位皮肤紫红为度（图 3-2）。推罐时着力在罐口，用力均匀，防止罐漏气脱落，且需根据患者体质与病情调节负压大小及走罐快慢与轻重。若负压过大或用力过重、速度过快，患者往往疼痛难忍，且易拉伤皮肤；负压过小，吸拔力不足，罐容易脱落，治疗效果较差。该法适用于病变范围较广、肌肉丰厚而平整的部位，如腰背部、大腿处等。

【操作要点】动作轻柔、用力均匀、平稳、缓慢；吸拔后应立即走罐；罐内负压大小以推拉顺利为宜。

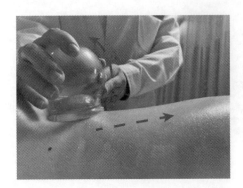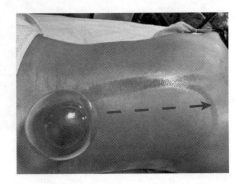

图 3-2　走罐法

pressure in the cup should be adjusted based on the patient's condition to keep the cups pushed and pulled smoothly.

3.4　Lining-up cupping method

Use many cups for cupping along meridians or muscles groups for treatment,and line up multiple cans along with the position of meridian course or the surface of any muscle bundle,known as lining-up cupping.

[Operation key points] The distance between cups should not be too close,so as to prevent the cups from straining the skin to produce pain or falling off due to mutual extrusion between cups.

3.5　Needle cupping method

Needle cupping method is a therapeutic method combining cupping with needling. It is suitable for heat syndrome,excess syndrome,blood stasis syndrome and certain dermatopathy conditions. According to the different use of needle,this method is divided into the following three types.

(1) Needle-retaining cupping. When the filiform needle is punctured and retained,cupping should be carried out with the needle as the center. At the end of the treatment,the cup should be started first and then the needle should be taken out. The negative pressure inside the can will increase the depth of the needle body inserted,which can cause the pneumothorax,so this method should not be used for chest and backside(Fig. 3-3).

（四）排罐法

沿某一经脉循行路线或某一肌束的体表位置,按照顺序排列成行吸拔多个罐具,称为排罐法。

【操作要点】罐具之间的距离不宜太近,以免罐具牵拉皮肤产生疼痛,或因罐具间互相挤压而脱落。

（五）针罐法

针罐法是拔罐与针刺相结合的一种治疗方法,适用于热证、实证、瘀血证及某些皮肤病证。根据针具使用的不同分为如下 3 种。

1. 留针拔罐　在毫针针刺留针时,以针为中心拔罐,留置规定时间后,先起罐再出针。此法不宜用于胸背部,因罐内负压易加深针刺深度,从而容易引起气胸(图 3-3)。

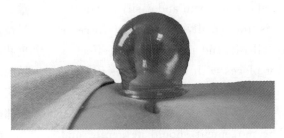

图 3-3　留针拔罐

[Operation key points] Move quickly;do cupping with a needle

【操作要点】动作迅速;以针

retained in the center of the cup;control the depth of needling;the cup should not be kept for too long.

（2）Needle-withdrawing cupping. Attach a cup on the position after withdrawing the filiform needle immediately,remove the cup at the end of the treatment,and wipe the cupping position with a sterilized cotton balls.

（3）Bloodletting and cupping. Prick the acupoints or affected part of patient's body with dermal needle,three-edged needle or rude filiform needle to induce bleeding,and then cupping and retain the cup on the area. Wipe the bloodstain with sterilized cotton ball after lifting the cup,and paste the sterilized dressing or band aid on the pricking part if necessary.

［Operation key points］Pay attention to disinfection and prevent infection;the scope of bloodletting should be appropriate; the amount of bleeding should not be large.

4. Precautions of cupping

4.1　Contraindications

（1）Patients with high fever,convulsions or/and spasms.

（2）Patients with acute severe disease, chronic systemic debilitating or/and contagious disease.

（3）Patients with bleeding diseases, such as leukemia, thrombocytopenic purpura,and hemophilia.

（4）Patients with severe emphysema should not have negative pressure suction on the back and chest;patients with heart failure; apex area of heart,body surface aortic pulsation,varicose veins.

（5）Fracture patients before completely healed;acute joint, ligament,and tendon injury.

（6）The orifice of the eye,ear,nose,etc. The skin has ulcers and ruptures;an unknown lump.

（7）Infants and young children, and the lumbosacral and abdomen,front and rear vulva, and breast of pregnant women should not be cupping.

（8）Patients with tuberculosis, malignant tumor, or/and scrofula,should not be cupping on hernia.

（9）Too hungry, drunk, too full, too tired people are not suitable for cupping. Those who cannot cooperate with treatment for mental disorders, psychotic episodes, manic restlessness, tetanus,rabies,etc. are not suitable for cupping.

4.2　Precautions

（1）The choice of cupping site. Generally choose the site with

为中心拔罐;控制针刺深度;留罐时间不宜过长。

2. 出针拔罐　在毫针针刺出针后,立即于该部位拔罐,留置规定时间后起罐,起罐后再用消毒棉球将拔罐处擦净。

3. 刺络拔罐　用皮肤针、三棱针或粗毫针等,先在腧穴或患处点刺出血,再局部施以拔罐、留罐。起罐后用消毒棉球擦净血迹,必要时用消毒敷料或创可贴贴敷。

【操作要点】注意消毒,预防感染;放血范围需适当;出血量不宜多。

四、拔罐法的注意事项

（一）禁忌证

（1）高热、抽搐和痉挛发作者。

（2）急性严重疾病、慢性全身虚弱性疾病及接触性传染病。

（3）有出血倾向的患者如白血病、血小板减少性紫癜、血友病等。

（4）有严重肺气肿患者的背部及胸部不宜负压吸拔;心力衰竭患者;心尖区、体表大动脉搏动处、静脉曲张处。

（5）骨折患者在未完全愈合前;急性关节、韧带、肌腱严重损伤者。

（6）眼耳口鼻等五官孔窍处;皮肤有溃疡、破裂处;局部原因不明的肿块。

（7）婴幼儿,孕妇的腰骶及腹部、前后阴、乳房部不宜拔罐。

（8）肺结核、恶性肿瘤、瘰疬者,疝气之处不宜拔罐。

（9）过饥、醉酒、过饱、过度疲劳者均不宜拔罐;因患精神失常、精神病发作期、狂躁不安、破伤风、狂犬病等不能配合者不宜拔罐。

（二）注意事项

（1）拔罐部位的选择。一般

full muscle, full subcutaneous tissue and less hair.

(2) The choice of body position. The patient should be in a comfortable position, and the cupping area should be relaxed to stretch and flabby. When cupping, ask the patient not to move the body position, so as to avoid the cups falling off.

(3) For the elderly, children, and those who are weak in constitution and receive cupping treatment for the first time, fewer cups and short retention of cupping should be adopted, and it is better to lie down. Cupping should be done with great care for pregnant women and infants.

(4) When using the needle-retaining cupping, we should choose the large cupping apparatus and the filiform needle with short needle handle, so as to avoid the cup apparatus touching the needle handle and causing damage such as broken needle.

(5) The doctor should be skilled in cupping technique, and the action should be light, fast, stable and accurate. The alcohol cotton ball used for fire should not absorb too much alcohol, so as to avoid dripping on the skin during cupping and causing burns. In case of burns, they should be treated as surgical burns.

(6) During cupping, if the patient has symptoms such as dizziness, chest tightness, nausea, weakness of the limbs, cold sweat dripping, even unconsciousness, the processing method is immediately remove the cup, put the patient in a head-lower feet-higher position, give him/her a warm and sweet drink, or pinch Shuigou(GV 26). Pay attention to the changes of patient's blood pressure and heart rate, if it is serious, patient needs to be treated as syncope.

宜选择肌肉丰满、皮下组织充实及毛发较少的部位。

（2）体位的选择。患者体位应舒适，局部宜舒展、松弛。拔罐时嘱患者勿移动体位，以免罐具脱落。

（3）老年、儿童、体质虚弱及初次接受治疗，易发生意外反应的患者，拔罐数量宜少，留罐时间宜短，以卧位为宜。妊娠妇女及婴幼儿慎用拔罐方法。

（4）留针拔罐时，选择罐具宜大，毫针针柄宜短，以免吸拔时罐具碰触针柄而造成折针等损伤。

（5）拔罐手法要熟练，动作要轻、快、稳、准。用于燃火的酒精棉球，不可吸含酒精过多，以免拔罐时滴落到皮肤上造成烧烫伤。若不慎出现烧烫伤，应按外科烧烫伤处理。

（6）拔罐过程中若患者出现头晕、胸闷、恶心欲呕、肢体发软、冷汗淋漓，甚者瞬间意识丧失等晕罐现象，处理方法是立即起罐，使患者呈头低脚高卧位，必要时可饮用温开水或温糖水，或掐水沟穴等。密切注意其血压、心率变化，严重时按晕厥处理。

Chapter 4　Scrapping Therapy

1.　Basic knowledge of scraping

Scrapping is one of the traditional natural therapies in China. It is based on the theory of traditional Chinese medicine, to dredge the meridians, promote blood circulation, and remove blood stasis by scrapping corresponding part of skin with ox horn, jade, etc. Scrapping shows immediate effect in high blood pressure, heatstroke, and muscle soreness and pain caused by bi syndrome and other causes via the effect of expanding capillaries, increasing sweat gland secretion, and promoting blood circulation. Often scrapping could adjust the meridian qi, relieve fatigue, and increase the immune function.

2.　Operation method of scraping

2.1　Scrapping tools/instruments

Scraping plate, the main tool of scrapping, can be used in all parts of the body. The common scrapping plates are made of buffalo horn and jade products. Both of them have the function of promoting circulation of qi and blood, dredging the meridian, and with non-toxic side effects. Besides, there are scrapping plates made of shell, wood products and smooth-edged fresh bamboo plate, porcelain pieces, small spoon, coins or ramie and other appliances.

In terms of shape, the scrapping plate has the fishlike shape, rectangle, triangle and the deformation of these shapes. No matter what shape the scrapping plate takes, it is best to choose one with inconsistent thickness in both sides, so that the thick side can be used as daily health care, and the thin side can be used for physiotherapy.

2.2　Scrapping methods

(1) Plate holding. The operator holds the scraping plate with the hand. The bottom edge of the scraping plate lies on the palm of the hand. The thumb and the other four fingers are naturally bent on the two sides of the scraping plate, respectively.

(2) Scrapping method. Applying the scraping oil on the operating part. The operator holds the scraping plate and squeezes it with a certain force until the scratch marks appear. When scrapping, in addition to applying a certain amount of pressure to the scrapping direction, the operation parts should also be pressed down. Downward pressure varies from person to person. The strength is determined by the patient's condition and endurance. The operator should scrap with uniform velocity, the smoothly

第四章　刮　痧　法

一、刮痧法的基础知识

刮痧法是中国传统的自然疗法之一，它以中医皮部理论为基础，用牛角、玉石等在皮肤相应部位刮拭，以达到疏通经络、活血化瘀之目的。刮痧可以扩张毛细血管，增加汗腺分泌，促进血液循环，对于风寒痹证等所致的高血压、中暑、肌肉酸疼都有立竿见影之效。经常刮痧，可起到调节经气，解除疲劳，增强免疫功能的作用。

二、刮痧的基本操作

（一）刮痧工具

刮痧板是刮痧的主要工具，可在人体各部位使用。常见的刮痧板材料为水牛角和玉制品，两者均有行气活血、疏通经络之功，且无毒副作用。此外，还有以贝壳、木制品以及边缘光滑的嫩竹板、瓷器片、小汤匙、硬币，或苎麻等制成的刮痧用具。

从形状上来说，刮痧板有鱼形、长方形、三角形以及这几种形状的变形。不管什么形状的刮痧板，最好选择两边厚薄不一致的，厚的一边可以作为日常保健用，薄的一边可以作为理疗用。

（二）刮痧方法

1.　持板方法　用手握住刮痧板，刮痧板的底边横靠在手掌心部位，拇指与另外四根手指自然弯曲，分别放在刮痧板的两侧。

2.　刮拭方法　在操作部位涂上刮痧油后，操作者手持刮痧板，在施术部位按一定的力度刮拭，直至皮肤出现痧痕为止。刮痧时，除了向刮拭的方向用力施加一定的压力外，还要将刮拭部位向下按压。向下的按压力因人而异，力度大小根据患者体质、病情及承受能

strength every time, and do not change suddenly.

The operator should also pay attention to point, line and surface combination during scraping, which is a characteristic of scraping. The so-called point is actually the acupoint; the line is the meridian; the surface is the part of the scraping plate that touches the skin, about 1 cun wide. The method of scraping with point-line-surface combination is to strengthen the stimulation of main points while dredging the meridians, and to master a certain wiper width, which can improve the therapeutic effect.

2.3　Common scrapping methods

(1) Surface-scrapping. It is applied to flat areas of the body.

(2) Angle-scraping. It is applied to the smaller parts or ditch of the body, or nest, concave parts. Scrapping plate is tilted 45 degrees to the skin.

(3) Point-pressing method. When using this method, a corner of the scrapping plate is 90 degrees to the skin of operating part, which is lifted gradually from light to heavy. It is suitable for the hollow part without bones.

(4) Flap method. Use the five fingers or on one end of the scraping plate to pat the points of the body surface. Before slapping, first apply the scrapping oil on the skin, and this method commonly used on the limbs, especially the elbow and popliteal fossa.

(5) Rubbing method. When using this method, a corner of the scraping board is pressed on the skin at an angle of 20 degrees to do a gentle massage movement. This technique is often used in the acupoints that have a strong effect on Zang-Fu organs, as well as the pain points in the back neck, back, waist and holographic acupoints.

In addition, there are special scrapping methods, including pinching scrapping method, picking scrapping method and scrapping blood letting method. Pinching scrapping method can be divided into three kinds including pulling scraping, clamping scraping and grasping scraping. scrapping blood letting method can be divided into two kinds: purging blood and pricking method.

3. Clinical application of scrapping

Scrapping has the effects of dredging meridians, promoting blood circulation to remove blood stasis, clearing heat and resuscitation, smoothing circulation of healthy qi, removing dirty and turbidity, eliminating toxin, and so on, so it has a wide clinical application range. It can be used for internal medicine, external

力决定。每次刮拭应保持速度均匀、力度平稳，不要忽轻忽重。

刮拭时还应注意点、线、面结合，这是刮痧的一个特点。所谓点就是指穴位；线就是指经脉；面即指刮痧板边缘接触皮肤的部分，约有 1 寸宽。点线面结合的刮拭方法，是在疏通经脉的同时，加强重点穴位的刺激，并掌握一定的刮拭宽度，其可以提高治疗效果。

（三）常用刮痧法

1. 面刮法　适用于人体比较平坦的部位。

2. 角刮法　多用于人体面积较小的部位或沟、窝、凹陷部位，刮痧板与刮痧皮肤成 45°角倾斜。

3. 点按法　刮痧板的一角与操作部位成 90°角，由轻到重逐渐加力抬起，适用于人体无骨骼的凹陷部位。

4. 拍打法　用刮痧板一端的平面或五指合拢的手掌拍打体表部位的经络腧穴。拍打前一定要在相应部位先涂上刮痧油，多用在四肢，特别是肘窝和腘窝处。

5. 揉按法　用刮痧板的一角，成 20°角倾斜按压在操作部位上，做柔和的旋转运动，这种手法常用于对脏腑有强壮作用的穴位，以及后颈、背、腰部和全息穴区中的痛点。

此外还有特殊刮痧法，包括撮痧法、挑痧法和放痧法 3 种，其中撮痧法又分扯痧法、夹痧法和抓痧法 3 种；放痧法又分泻血法和点刺法 2 种。

三、刮痧法的应用

刮痧法具有疏通经络、活血化瘀、开窍泄热、通达阳气、泻下秽浊、排除毒素等作用，临床应用范围较广，可用于内科、外科、妇科、儿科、五官科等病证，还可用于强

medicine, gynecology, pediatrics, facial features and other diseases, and can also be used to strengthen physical health, loss weight, beauty, etc. In particular, it has an immediate effect on acute "Sha disease" caused by excess heat or damp, or pain and acid distension caused by blockage of qi or stagnation of meridians and collaterals.

(1) Sha disease. Most of Sha disease occur in summer and autumn, with sudden symptom of eupyrexia, coldness of body, dizziness, nausea, vomiting, chest and abdominal distension or pain, and even vomiting and diarrhea. Scrapping from top to bottom on both sides of the spine of the back, add the points like Taiyang(EX-HN5) and Yintang(GV29) when unconsciousness.

(2) Heat stroke. Scrapping from top to bottom on both sides of the spine gently. The exterior syndrome affected by summer-heat, take the patient neck(bilateral) to scraping. Interior syndrome affected by summer-heat, take the back to scrape, and matched with the chest, neck and other places to scrape.

(3) At the beginning of damp-warm syndrome. With symptoms of cold, anorexia, tiredness, low fever and so on, scrapping top-down of the back, combined in popliteal fossa, neck and elbow fossa with ramie oil scraping.

(4) The cold. Cut ginger and scallion 10 g each, mix well, and then wrap them in cloth, dip them in hot wine, use it to scrape the forehead and the Taiyang(EX-HN5) firstly, and then scrape both sides of the spine. It can also be combined with scraping the elbow and popliteal fossa. If there is vomiting or nausea, the chest should be scraped.

(5) Fever and cough. Smooth scraping the downward of to the neck and 4th lumbar vertebra, at the same time scraping the elbow, Quchi(LI11). If the cough obvious, then scrap the chest.

(6) Laryngalgia due to wind-heat. Scrap the 7th cervical vertebra and the 7th thoracic vertebra(dip in salt water), and screw up the lateral muscles of anterior neck (sternocleidomastoid muscles) about 50 times.

(7) Vomiting. Smooth scraping both sides of the spine from top to down, finally to the waist. For abdominal pain, scraping both sides of the spine, it can also be applied to the chest and abdomen.

(8) Infantile malnutrition. Scraping from Changqiang(GV1) to Dazhui(GV14) point. For vomiting and diarrhea caused by food injury, scraping both sides of the spine; for chest tightness or/and abdominal distension severe pain, scraping chest and abdomen.

4. Precautions of scrapping

4.1 Preoperative precautions

(1) The scrapping should expose the skin. When scraping, the

身健体、减肥、美容等。尤其对实热或湿热引起的急性"痧证"，或因气机闭阻、经络瘀滞所致的疼痛、酸胀类病证，其有立竿见影的功效。

1. 痧证　多发于夏秋两季，微热形寒，头昏、恶心、呕吐、胸腹或胀或痛，甚则上吐下泻，多起病突然，取背部脊柱两侧自上而下刮治，如见神昏可加用印堂穴、太阳穴。

2. 中暑　取脊柱两侧自上而下轻轻顺刮，逐渐加重。伤暑表证，取患者颈部痧筋（颈项双侧）刮治。伤暑里证，取背部刮治，并配用胸部、颈部等处刮治。

3. 湿温初起　见感冒、厌食、倦怠、低热等症，取背部自上而下顺刮，并配用苎麻蘸油在腘窝、后颈、肘窝部擦刮。

4. 感冒　取生姜、葱白各 10 g，切碎、混匀后用布包，以之蘸取热酒先刮擦前额、太阳穴，然后刮背部脊柱两侧，也可配合刮肘窝、腘窝。如有呕恶者加刮胸部。

5. 发热咳嗽　取颈部向下至第 4 腰椎处顺刮，同时刮治肘部、曲池穴。如咳嗽明显，再刮治胸部。

6. 风热喉痛　取第 7 颈椎至第 7 胸椎两旁（蘸盐水）刮治，并配用拧提颈部前两侧肌肉（胸锁乳突肌）约 50 次。

7. 呕吐　取脊柱两旁自上而下至腰部顺刮。腹痛时，取背部脊柱旁两侧刮治；也可同时刮治胸腹部。

8. 疳积　取长强穴至大椎穴处刮治。伤食所致呕吐、腹泻，取脊椎两侧顺刮；如胸闷、腹胀剧痛，可在胸腹部刮治。

四、刮痧法的注意事项

（一）术前注意事项

（1）刮痧法须暴露皮肤，且刮

interstices open and release. Therefore, it is necessary to select the treatment place with fresh air circulation before scrapping and pay attention to keep warm, in case that pathogenic wind and cold, evil qi enter patient's body and cause new diseases. In summer, do not scrape in the place where there is a draft.

（2）The performer's hands should be disinfected. Scrapping tools should also be strictly disinfected to prevent cross infection. Before scraping, the scrapping tools should be carefully checked to avoid scratching the skin.

（3）Do not perform scraping treatment when the patient is hungry, too full or excessive strain to prevent dizzy.

4.2　Precautions during scraping

（1）The scraping strength should be applied evenly to the extent that the patient can tolerate until the appearance of Sha. For infants and the elderly, the scraping technique should be gentle.

（2）Do not blindly pursue the Sha and use excessive strength or prolong the scraping time. In general, there is a lot of Sha caused by blood stasis, excess syndrome and heat syndromes; Sha are rare in deficiency syndrome and cold syndrome.

（3）During scraping, in case of dizzy, fatigue, dazzle, pale face, nausea vomiting, sweating, palpitation, coolness of extremities or drop of blood pressure, coma, we should immediately stop scrapping, comfort patients, let them lie flat, pay attention to keep them warm, and ask them to drink some warm water or sugar water, generally they will recover.

4.3　Postoperative precautions

（1）Scrapping makes the patient's interstices open to dispel the evil qi, which will consume the body fluid, so after scraping, the patient should drink a cup of warm water and have a rest.

（2）Generally about 3 hours after the scraping, it is suggested to take a bath when the skin pores are closed and restored to their original state to avoid the invasion of wind and cold.

痧时皮肤汗孔开泄，如遇风寒之邪，邪气可从开泄的毛孔入里，引发新的疾病。故刮痧前要选择空气流通的治疗场所，注意保暖，夏季不可在有过堂风的地方刮痧。

（2）施术者的双手要消毒。刮痧工具也要严格消毒，防止交叉感染。刮拭前须仔细检查刮痧工具，以免刮伤皮肤。

（3）勿在患者过饥、过饱及过度紧张的情况下进行刮痧治疗，以防晕刮。

（二）术中注意事项

（1）刮拭手法要用力均匀，以患者能忍受为度，达到出痧为止。对于婴幼儿及老年人，刮拭手法用力宜轻。

（2）不可一味追求出痧而用重手法或延长刮痧时间。一般情况下，血瘀之证出痧多；实证、热证出痧多；虚证、寒证出痧少。

（3）刮拭过程中，如遇患者晕刮，出现精神疲惫、头晕目眩、面色苍白、恶心欲吐，出冷汗、心慌、四肢发凉或血压下降、神志昏迷时，应立即停止刮痧，抚慰患者勿紧张，让其平卧，注意保暖，饮温开水或糖水，一般即可恢复。

（三）术后注意事项

（1）刮痧治疗使汗孔开泄，邪气外排，要消耗体内津液，故刮痧后应饮温水一杯，休息片刻。

（2）刮痧治疗后，为避免风寒之邪侵袭，须待皮肤毛孔闭合恢复原状后，方可洗浴，一般 3 小时左右。

Chapter 5　Auricular Acupuncture

Auricular acupuncture refers to the use of filiform needles or other needles to stimulate specific parts of the ear to prevent, diagnose and treat systemic diseases. It has wide treatment range, convenient operation, and has certain significance to the prevention and treatment of disease.

Auricular diagnosis and treatment of diseases has a long history, which was recorded as early as the Spring and Autumn period and the Warring States period. In the Chapter of *Miraculous Pivot—Five Evils*, it said, "When evil [qi] are in the liver, then [the patient] will feel pain in the upper flanks... One chooses the greenish-blue vessels in the ears to eliminate the pulling [pain]." "The ears are deaf with [the patient] hearing nothing, one chooses the center of the ears [to remove the disease]", recorded in the Chapter of *Miraculous Pivot—Jue-disease*. In Tang Dynasty, *Important Formulas Worth a Thousand Gold Pieces* recorded that Ear Center (HX_1) can be used to treat jaundice, cold and heat pestilence and other diseases. Later, the related narratives of diagnosing diseases with auricle, stimulating auricle with acupuncture, massage, medicine, moxibustion, warm ironing and other methods to prevent and treat diseases are scattered in the medical books of past dynasties, which laid a theoretical foundation for the formation and development of auricular acupuncture. In the late 1950s, a French physician Dr P. Nogier M. D. , put forward 42 auricular points and an inversed auricular point diagram looked like an embryon, which greatly influenced Chinese scholars and promoted the popularization and development of auricular acupuncture therapy in China to a certain extent. In order to promote the development and research of auricular point application, the General Administration of Quality Supervision, Inspection and Quarantine of the People's Republic of China and the National Standardization Administration of the People's Republic of China first promulgated in 1992 and then revised and implemented the National Standard of the People's Republic of China GB/T 13734—1992/2008 "*Nomenclature and Location of Auricular Points*" in 2008.

So far, more than 200 kinds of diseases have been treated by auricular acupuncture, involving internal, external, women, children, facial features, skin, bone injury and other clinical departments; It not only has good curative effect on some functional diseases, allergic diseases and inflammatory diseases, but

第五章　耳　针　法

耳针法是指采用毫针或其他针具刺激耳部特定部位,以预防、诊断和治疗全身疾病的一种方法。耳针治疗范围较广,操作方法简单易行,对于疾病的预防和诊治具有一定的意义。

耳针治病之法历史悠久,早在春秋战国时期即有记载,如《灵枢·五邪》云:"邪在肝,则两胁中痛……取耳间青脉以去其掣。"《灵枢·厥病》云:"耳聋无闻,取耳中。"唐朝《备急千金要方》中有取耳中穴治疗黄疸、寒暑疫毒等病的记载。其后,以耳郭诊断疾病,以针刺、按摩、塞药、艾灸、温熨等方法刺激耳郭以防治疾病等有关叙述更是散见于历代医书之中,为耳针的形成和发展奠定了理论基础。20世纪50年代,法国医学博士诺基尔(P. Nogier)提出42个耳穴点和形如胚胎倒影的耳穴图,对我国学者影响很大,在一定程度上推动了耳针疗法在我国的普及和发展。为促进耳穴应用的发展与研究,国家质量监督检验检疫总局和国家标准化管理委员会于1992年首次颁布并于2008年修订和实施了中华人民共和国国家标准 GB/T 13734—1992/2008《耳穴名称与定位》。

迄今为止,可采用耳针疗法治疗的疾病种类已达200余种,涉及内、外、妇、儿、五官、皮肤、骨伤等临床各科;它不仅对某些功能性病变、变态反应性疾病、炎症性疾病有较

also has certain curative effect on some organic diseases and some difficult and miscellaneous diseases.

1. Stimulus area of auricular acupuncture

The stimulating part of the ear acupuncture is the auricular point（AAP）, a special part where the surface of the auricle communicates with the body's viscera, channels and collaterals, tissues and limbs. The auricular point is not only the response point of disease, but also the stimulus part for disease prevention and treatment.

1.1　The anatomy of the surface of the auricle

（1）The front of the auricle

（Fig. 5-1）

Ear lobe：The lowest part of the auricle devoid of cartilage.

Anterior groove of ear lobe：The groove between the ear lobe and the cheek.

Helix：The prominent, curved, and free rim of the auricle.

Crus of helix：The transverse ridge of the helix that continues posteriorly into the ear cavity.

Spine of the helix crus：The bulge between the helix and the crus of helix.

Notch of the helix crus：The cartilaginous prominence between the helix and the crus of helix.

Helix tubercle：The small prominence located on the posterior-superior portion of the helix.

Cauda helicis：The inferior part of the helix at the junction of the helix and the ear lobe.

Helix-lobe notch：The depression between the helix and the posterior rim of the ear lobe.

Anterior groove of the helix：The groove formed by the connection between the helix and the cheek.

（Fig. 5-2）

Antihelix：The "Y" shape prominence, roughly opposite the helix, formed by the body of antihelix, the superior antihelix crus, and the inferior antihelix crus.

Body of antihelix：The principal, rough and vertical part of the antihelix.

Superior antihelix crus：The superior branch of the bifurcation of the antihelix.

Inferior antihelix crus：The inferior branch of the bifurcation of the antihelix.

Antihelix-antitragus notch：The depression between the antihelix and the antitragus.

好的疗效，对部分器质性病变以及某些疑难杂症也具有一定疗效。

一、耳针刺激部位

耳针刺激部位即为耳穴，是耳郭表面与人体脏腑经络、组织器官、躯干四肢相互沟通的特殊部位。耳穴既是疾病的反应点，也是防治疾病的刺激点。

（一）耳郭表面解剖

1. 耳郭正面

（以下见图 5-1）

耳垂：耳郭下部无软骨的部分。

耳垂前沟：耳垂与面部之间的浅沟。

耳轮：耳郭外侧边缘的卷曲部分。

耳轮脚：耳轮深入耳甲的部分。

耳轮脚棘：耳轮脚和耳轮之间的隆起。

耳轮脚切迹：耳轮脚棘前方的凹陷处。

耳轮结节：耳轮外上方的膨大部分。

耳轮尾：耳轮向下移行于耳垂的部分。

轮垂切迹：耳轮和耳垂后缘之间的凹陷处。

耳轮前沟：耳轮与面部之间的浅沟。

（以下见图 5-2）

对耳轮：与耳轮相对呈"Y"字形的隆起部，由对耳轮体、对耳轮上脚和对耳轮下脚三部分组成。

对耳轮体：对耳轮下部呈上下走向的主体部分。

对耳轮上脚：对耳轮向上分支的部分。

对耳轮下脚：对耳轮向前分支的部分。

轮屏切迹：对耳轮与对耳屏之间的凹陷处。

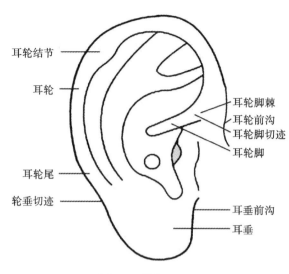

图 5-1　耳郭正面 1

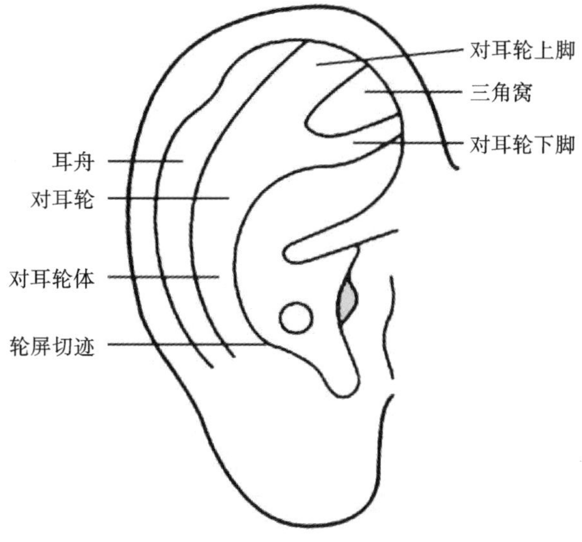

图 5-2　耳郭正面 2

Scapha：The curved depression between the helix and the antihelix；the scaphoid fossa.

Triangular fossa：The triangular depression bordered by the two antihelix crus and the helix.

(Fig. 5-3)

Concha：The hollow area borders the orifice of the external auditory meatus. It is bordered by the helix and the antihelix，the tragus，and the antitragus；it is composed of the cymba conchae and the cavum conchae.

Cymba concha：The part of the concha superior to the crus of helix.

Cavum concha：The part of the concha inferior to the crus of helix.

Tragus：The curved cartilaginous flap projecting lateral to the external auditory meatus.

Supratragic notch：The depression between the tragus and the lower border of the crus of helix.

Apex of the upper tragus：The superior prominence on the free rim of tragus.

Apex of the lower tragus：The inferior prominence on the free rim of tragus.

Anterior groove of the tragus：The shallow groove between the tragus and the cheek.

Antitragus：The flap opposite the tragus and superior to the ear lobe.

Intertragic notch：The depression between the tragus and the antitragus.

External acoustic pore：The foramen anterior to the cavum conchae.

耳舟：耳轮与对耳轮之间的凹沟。

三角窝：对耳轮上、下脚与相应耳轮之间的三角形凹窝。

（以下见图 5-3）

耳甲部分：部分耳轮和对耳轮、对耳屏、耳屏及外耳门之间的凹窝。由耳甲艇、耳甲腔两部分组成。

耳甲艇：耳轮脚以上的耳甲部。

耳甲腔：耳轮脚以下的耳甲部。

耳屏：耳郭前方呈瓣状的隆起。

屏上切迹：耳屏与耳轮之间的凹陷处。

上屏尖：耳屏游离缘上隆起部。

下屏尖：耳屏游离缘下隆起部。

耳屏前沟：耳屏与面部之间的浅沟。

对耳屏：耳垂上方，与耳屏相对的瓣状隆起。

屏间切迹：耳屏和对耳屏之间的凹陷处。

外耳门：耳甲腔前方的孔窍。

（2）Posterior surface of the auricle(Fig. 5-4)

Back of the helix：The flat area on the posteromedial surface of the auricle formed by the helix.

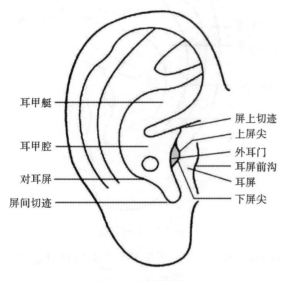

图 5-3　耳郭正面 3

Back of the helix cauda：The flat area on the posteromedial surface of the auricle formed by the cauda helicis.

Back of the ear lobe：The flat area on the posteromedial surface of the ear lobe.

Eminence of the scapha：The eminence formed by the scapha on the posteromedial surface of the auricle.

Eminence of the triangular fossa：The eminence formed by the triangular fossa on the posteromedial surface of the auricle.

Eminence of the cymba conchae：The eminence formed by the cymba concha on the posteromedial surface of the auricle.

Eminence of the cavum conchae：The eminence formed by the cavum concha on the posteromedial surface of the auricle.

Groove of the superior antihelix crus：The depression formed by the superior antihelix crus on the posteromedial surface of the auricle.

Groove of the inferior antihelix crus：The depression formed by the inferior antihelix crus on the posteromedial surface of the auricle.

Groove of the antihelix：The depression formed by the antihelix on the posteromedial surface of the auricle.

Groove of crus of helix：The depression formed by the crus of helix on the posteromedial surface of the auricle.

Groove of the antitragus：The depression formed by the antitragus on the posteromedial surface of the auricle.

（3）Ear root(Fig. 5-4)

Upper ear root：The highest part of the auricular attachment to

2. 耳郭背面（图 5-4）

耳轮背面：耳轮背部的平坦部分。

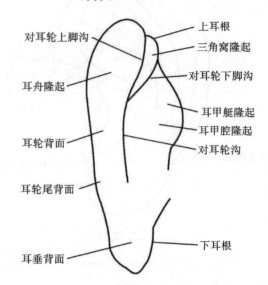

图 5-4　耳郭背面及耳根

耳轮尾背面：耳轮尾背部的平坦部分。

耳垂背面：耳垂背部的平坦部分。

耳舟隆起：耳舟在耳背呈现的隆起。

三角窝隆起：三角窝在耳背呈现的隆起。

耳甲艇隆起：耳甲艇在耳背呈现的隆起。

耳甲腔隆起：耳甲腔在耳背呈现的隆起。

对耳轮上脚沟：对耳轮上脚在耳背呈现的凹沟。

对耳轮下脚沟：对耳轮下脚在耳背呈现的凹沟。

对耳轮沟：对耳轮体在耳背呈现的凹沟。

耳轮脚沟：耳轮脚在耳背呈现的凹沟。

对耳屏沟：对耳屏在耳背呈现的凹沟。

3. 耳根（图 5-4）

上耳根：耳郭与头部相连的最

the scalp.

Lower ear root: The lowest part of the auricular attachment where the ear lobe attaches to the cheek.

1.2 The distribution of auricular points

The distribution of auricular points on the surface of auricle is similar to that of fetus in uterus (head down, buttock up) (Fig. 5-5).

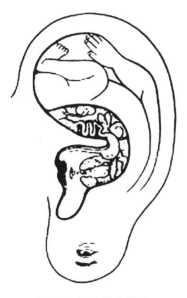

图 5-5 耳穴分布规律

There exists some regularity in the distribution of auricular points. They are based on the upside-down fetus distribution theory, which is explained below. Points related to the portions of the head are located on the ear lobe. Points related to the upper limbs are located on the scapha. Points related to the trunk and lower limbs are located on the body of the antihelix and the superior and inferior antihelix crus. Points related to the internal organs are located on the cavum and cymba conchae, while points related to the organs in the abdomen are located on the cymba concha; these particular points are related to the organs in the chest which are located on the cavum concha. Points related to the spine and trunk are located in the antihelix. Points related to the pelvic cavity are located in the triangular fossa. Points related to the digestive tract are distributed around the crus of helix. Points related to the urinary tract are located at the junction of the inferior antihelix crus and the cymba concha.

2. Operation methods of auricular acupuncture

2.1 Preparation before operation

According to the principle of auricular acupoint selection or method of auricular acupoint detection to select auricular points.

According to the different operations, use iodophor or 75%

上处。

下耳根：耳郭与头部相连的最下处。

（二）耳穴分布规律

耳穴在耳郭表面的分布状态形似倒置在子宫内的胎儿（头部朝下，臀部朝上）（图 5-5）。

其分布规律：与头面相应的穴位分布在耳垂；与上肢相应的穴位分布在耳舟；与躯干相应的穴位分布在对耳轮体部；与下肢相应的穴位分布在对耳轮上、下脚；与腹腔脏器相应的穴位分布在耳甲艇；与胸腔脏器相应的穴位分布在耳甲腔；与盆腔脏器相应的穴位分布在三角窝；与消化道相应的穴位分布在耳轮脚周围等。

二、耳针操作技术

（一）操作前准备

1. 选穴　根据耳穴选穴原则或采用耳穴探测法进行选穴组方。

2. 消毒　根据操作方法用碘

alcohol to disinfect auricular cavity.

2. 2　Stimulus measures

（1）Filiform needle method.

The No. 28-30(0. 5-1. 0 cun) filiform needle were commonly advised.

When puncturing,the doctor should fix the auricle by pressing hand and prick into auricular point quickly with filiform needle by needling hand. The direction of acupuncture should be flexible according to the position of auricular acupoint. The depth of acupuncture should be 0. 1-0. 3 cm. Acupuncture treatment and time of needle retention should be considered according to the patient's condition, constitution and tolerance. Generally, retain needle for 15 to 30 minutes,and manipulate the needle 1 to 2 times during retention. Fix the eardrum with one hand and withdraw the needle by the other hand. Apply sterile cotton ball to press the needle hole.

Precautions:Same as filiform needle acupuncture.

（2）Electric acupuncture method.

The No. 28-30(0. 5-1. 0 cun) filiform needle and G6805 electro acupuncture apparatus were advised.

When puncturing,the doctor should fix the auricle by pressing hand and prick into auricular point quickly with filiform needle by needling hand. After arrival of qi,connect the electro acupuncture apparatus,choose density wave,adjust intensity appropriately,and set time for 15-20 minutes. As treatment completed,remove the wire first,hold the auricle firmly by hand,withdraw the needle quickly,and then press the needle hole with a sterile cotton ball for a moment.

Precautions:Same as electronic acupuncture therapy.

（3）The needle-embedding method.

Thumbtack intradermal needle was advised.

When puncturing,the doctor should fix the auricle by pressing hand and prick into auricular point quickly with needle by needling hand,and then secure with tape and press moderately. The needle could be remained for 1-3 days. During needle retention,the doctor should advise the patient to press the needle 2-3 times a day. As treatment completed,tear off the tape to remove the needle and disinfect it again. Two sides of auricular points alternately embedded the needle,when necessary,with the use of both sides of auricular points.

Precautions:Same as the intradermal acupuncture.

伏或 75％酒精消毒耳穴。

（二）刺激方法

1. 毫针刺法

针具选择：选用 28～30 号粗细的 0.5～1 寸长的毫针。

操作方法：进针时，押手固定耳郭，刺手持针速刺进针；针刺方向视耳穴所在部位灵活掌握，针刺深度宜 0.1～0.3 cm，以不穿透对侧皮肤为度；多用捻转、刮法或震颤法行针，刺激强度视患者病情、体质和敏感性等因素综合决定；得气以热、胀、痛，或局部充血红润多见；一般留针 15～30 分钟，可间歇行针 1～2 次。疼痛性或慢性疾病留针时间可适当延长；出针时，押手托住耳背，刺手持针速出，同时用消毒干棉球按压针孔片刻。

注意事项：同毫针法。

2. 电针法

针具选择：选用 28～30 号粗细的 0.5～1 寸长的毫针；G6805型电针仪。

操作方法：押手固定耳郭，刺手持针速刺进针；得气后连接电针仪，多选用疏密波、适宜强度，刺激 15～20 分钟；起针时，先取下导线，押手固定耳郭，刺手持针速出，并用消毒干棉球压迫针孔片刻。

注意事项：同电针法。

3. 埋针法

针具选择：揿针型皮内针为宜。

操作方法：押手固定耳郭并绷紧欲埋针处皮肤，刺手用镊子夹住皮内针针柄，速刺（压）入所选穴位皮内，再用胶布固定并适度按压，可留置 1～3 日，其间可嘱患者每日自行按压 2～3 次；起针时轻轻撕下胶布即可将针一并取出，并再次消毒。两耳穴交替埋针，必要时双耳穴同用。

注意事项：同皮内针法。

（4）Auricular points plaster therapy.

This method is pressing auricular point with the seed of cowherb,magnetic bead or magnetic sheet,etc. The seed is affixed to the selected auricular point with the appropriate size of adhesive cloth,and the auricular point is rubbed properly until the local redness or thermal distension appear is appropriate. Remain it for 2 to 4 days,during treatment advising patients to press it 2 to 3 times a day by himself.

Precautions：

①The tape should be prevented from being wet or contaminated,so as not to cause skin inflammation.

②If the patient is allergic to the tape,or red miliary papules and itching occur locally in the auricular points during the treatment process,it is advisable to use other methods.

③When pregnant women choose this method,the stimulation should be light,and those with abortion tendency should be cautious.

④When using medical magnetic disks,the precautions are the same as magnetic therapy.

（5）Warming moxibustion.

Moxa stick,moxibustion stick,common rush,and joss stick can be used.

Take common rush moxibustion as an example. The doctor should hold a common rush with its front exposed for 1-2 cm,dip it in sesame oil and ignite it,aim at the auricular points and burn them quickly. It is advised 1-2 points at a time,alternating the two ears. The operation of moxa stick and joss stick is similar,that is,after moxa stick is ignited,moxibustion should be carried out 1-2 cm away from the auricular point,and it is suitable for local redness or thermal distension,and continuous moxibustion should be carried out for 3-5 minutes.

Precautions：Same as moxibustion.

（6）Bloodletting.

Choose three-edged needle or thick filiform needle.

Before acupuncture,the doctor should massage around the selected points to the center to make the blood gather；after routine disinfection,pressing hand fix the auricle,prick the points to bleed by needling hand；generally,2-3 points at a time,take 3-5 times as a course of treatment.

4. 压籽法

压籽选择：压籽又称压豆或埋豆，以王不留行籽、磁珠、磁片等为主，或以油菜籽、小绿豆、莱菔子等表面光滑、硬度适宜、直径在 2 mm 左右的球状物为宜，使用前用沸水烫洗后晒干备用。

操作方法：将所选压豆贴于 0.5 cm×0.5 cm 大小的透气胶布中间，医者用镊子将其夹持，敷贴于所选耳穴并适当按揉，以耳穴发热、胀痛为宜；可留置 2～4 日，其间可嘱患者每日自行按压 2～3 次。

注意事项：

（1）使用中应防止胶布潮湿或污染，以免引起皮肤炎症。

（2）个别患者胶布过敏，局部出现红色粟粒样丘疹并伴有痒感，宜改用他法。

（3）孕妇选用本法时刺激宜轻，有流产倾向者慎用。

（4）使用医用磁片的注意事项同磁疗法。

5. 温灸法

灸具选择：艾条、灸棒、灯心草、线香等。

操作方法：以灯心草灸为例，医者手持灯心草，前端露出 1～2 cm，浸蘸香油后点燃，对准耳穴迅速点烫，每次 1～2 穴，两耳交替；艾条或灸棒、线香等灸法操作类似，即将艾条等物点燃后，距欲灸耳穴 1～2 cm 处施灸，以局部红晕或患者有热胀感为宜，持续施灸 3～5 分钟。

注意事项：同艾灸法。

6. 刺血法

针具选择：三棱针、粗毫针。

操作方法：针刺前在欲点刺部位的周围向中心处推揉，使血液聚集；常规消毒后，押手固定耳郭，刺手持针点刺出血；一般点刺 2～3 穴，3～5 次为一个疗程。

Precautions: Same as the three-edged acupuncture.

(7) Massage method.

It mainly includes whole ear massage, hand rubbing of the ear wheel and pinching of the earlobe, etc. The whole ear massage is to massage the front and back sides of the auricle with the palms of both hands in turn until the auricle is congested and hot; the hand massage of the ear wheel is to hold an empty fist with both hands, and massage along the external ear wheel up and down with the thumb and fingers until the ear wheel is congested and hot; pinching of the earlobe is to lift and knead the earlobe with both hands from light to heavy. The massage time should be 15-20 minutes, as the degree of congestive and hot in both ears.

(8) TCM cutting therapy.

Using a surgical blade or a scalpel.

After routine disinfection of the corresponding auricular points or varicose blood vessels, the auricle was fixed by pressing hand, and the hand-held surgical blade or scalpel was used for slight cutting, with local bleeding as the degree. Finally, the sterilized dry cotton ball was used to compress the cutting site for a moment; generally, 2-3 points were cut at a time, take 3-5 times as a course of treatment.

Precautions: Same as the three-edged acupuncture.

(9) Acupuncture point injection therapy.

Use 1 mL syringe and No. 26 injection needle.

After routine disinfection of the selected auricular point, the auricle was fixed by pressing hand, and the medicine selected according to the condition was slowly pushed into the skin at auricular point or subcutaneous 0. 1-0. 3 mL with a syringe. The auricle may have reactions such as redness, heat, swelling and pain. After the injection, press the local part with a sterile dry cotton ball for a moment. Generally, 2-3 points at a time, take 3-5 times as is a course of treatment.

Precautions: Same as acupoint injection.

3. Clinical application of auricular acupuncture

3.1　Auxiliary diagnosis

The occurrence of human diseases, often in the corresponding parts of the auricle appear different pathological reaction (positive reaction), such as changes of skin color and morphology (deformation, discoloration, desquamation and papules), decrease of local pain threshold and decrease of ear resistance. The above changes can be judged by the following examination methods, combined with clinical symptoms and signs, so as to play the role on

注意事项：同三棱针法。

7. 按摩法

操作方法：主要包括全耳按摩、手摩耳轮和提捏耳垂。全耳按摩，是用两手掌心依次按摩耳郭前后两侧至耳郭充血发热为止；手摩耳轮，是两手握空拳，以拇指、食指沿着外耳轮上下来回按摩至耳轮充血发热为止；提捏耳垂，是用两手由轻到重提捏耳垂。按摩时间以 15～20 分钟为宜，两耳充血发热为度。

8. 割治法

针具选择：手术刀片或手术刀。

操作方法：在相应耳穴或曲张的血管处常规消毒后，押手固定耳郭，刺手持手术刀片或手术刀进行轻微的切割，以局部出血为度，最后用消毒干棉球压迫割治部位片刻；一般割治 2～3 穴，3～5 次为一个疗程。

注意事项：同三棱针法。

9. 穴位注射法

针具选择：1 mL 注射器和 26 号注射针头。

操作方法：在所选耳穴处常规消毒后，押手固定耳郭，刺手持注射器将按照病情所选用的药物缓慢推入耳穴皮内或皮下 0.1～0.3 mL，耳郭可有红、热、胀、痛等反应；注射完毕用消毒干棉球按压局部片刻，一般注射 2～3 穴，3～5 次为一个疗程。

注意事项：同穴位注射法。

三、耳针临床应用

（一）辅助诊断

人体疾病的发生，往往会在耳郭的相应部位出现不同的病理反应（阳性反应），如皮肤色泽、形态改变（变形、变色、脱屑、丘疹），局部痛阈降低，耳穴电阻下降等。以上改变可以借助下列检查方法加以判定，结合临床症状、体征，从而

auxiliary diagnosis.

(1) Common methods of auricular point examination.

①Inspection and observation. Under natural light, the skin of auricle is observed with naked eye or magnifier for signs of discoloration and deformation, such as desquamation, papule, induration, hyperemia, and changes of blood vessel shape and color, so as to determine the relationship between the region and viscera.

②Determination of pain sensitive point. Around the whole ear or around the disease-related auricular points, use the spring probe and other tools to touch and press the auricular points with uniform pressure. When touching a certain point area, the patient has reactions such as wheezing pain, dodging, frowning and blinking, it can be determined as pain sensitive point.

③Skin resistance measurement. Special instruments such as auricular point detector are used to measure skin resistance, potential, capacitance and other changes according to the usage; the instrument will display its abnormality in the form of buzzer or pointer, indicating abnormal changes such as decreased resistance and increased conductivity in a certain point area.

(2) Precautions.

①When the multi-acupoint area is sensitive, pay attention to the relationship and difference between them. The occurrence of any disease is the result of the joint action of multiple factors, and the internal correlation and influence between related viscera, tissues and organs are bound to occur, which may be manifested in auricular points. Therefore, we should pay attention to the primary and secondary relationship and correlation between sensitive acupoints.

②The difference between pain sensitivity, deformation and discoloration and normal reaction. In order to avoid false positive, we can use the method of combining pressure with observation to determine the nature of pain sensitive points. In addition, pigmentation, wart nevus, frostbite and scar on the auricle should also be distinguished from disease-related deformation and discoloration.

③In the observation, it is necessary to observe comprehensively, orderly and without omission; the point pressure degree is uniform and consistent, and the point pressure position should be the center point of the acupoint area; pay attention to the difference between different degrees of pain sensitive points.

3.2　Clinical application

(1) Scope of application.

①Various painful diseases: such as migraine, trigeminal

起到辅助诊断的作用。

1. 常用耳穴检查方法

（1）望诊观察法：在自然光线下，肉眼或借助放大镜观察耳郭皮肤有无变色、变形等征象，如脱屑、丘疹、硬结、充血，以及血管形状、颜色的改变等，以确定所在区域与脏腑的关系。

（2）痛敏点测定法：围绕全耳或在与疾病相关耳穴的周围，用弹簧探棒等工具以均匀的压力触压耳穴，当触压某穴区时患者出现呼痛、躲闪、皱眉或眨眼等反应，即可确定为痛敏点。

（3）皮肤电阻测定法：用特制仪器如耳穴探测仪等，依照使用方法测定皮肤电阻、电位、电容等的变化；仪器会以蜂鸣或指针等形式显示其异常，提示某穴区有电阻降低、导电增加等异常改变。

2. 注意事项

（1）多穴区敏感时，注意其之间的联系与区别。任何疾病的发生都是多因素共同作用的结果，相关脏腑、组织、器官之间必然会产生内在的关联与影响，且均可能在耳穴上有所表现。因此，要注意敏感穴区之间的主次关系和关联度。

（2）痛敏以及变形、变色与正常反应的区别。点压刺激健康人耳郭也可有不同程度的反应，可采用看压结合的方法综合判定痛敏点的性质，以避免假阳性。此外，耳郭上的色素沉着、疣痣、冻疮、瘢痕等也要与疾病相关的变形、变色相区分。

（3）在观察中要做到全面望诊，有顺序，无遗漏；点压力度均匀一致，点压位置以穴区中心点为宜；注意不同程度痛敏点之间的差异。

（二）临床应用

1. 适应范围

（1）各种疼痛性病证：如偏头

neuralgia, intercostal neuralgia and other neuropathic pain; sprain, contusion, stiff neck and other traumatic pain; various surgical wound pain; biliary colic, renal colic, angina pectoris, stomachache and other visceral pain syndrome.

②Various inflammatory diseases: such as acute conjunctivitis, periodontitis, pharyngitis, tonsillitis, cholecystitis, mumps, bronchitis, rheumatoid arthritis, and facial neuritis.

③Dysfunctional disorders: such as cardiac neurosis, arrhythmia, hypertension, hyperhidrosis, vertigo, gastrointestinal neurosis, irregular menstruation, enuresis, neurasthenia, and hysteria.

④Allergic and allergic diseases: such as allergic rhinitis, bronchial asthma, allergic colitis, urticaria, and allergic purpura.

⑤Endocrine and metabolic diseases: such as simple obesity, diabetes, hyperthyroidism or hypothyroidism, and menopausal syndrome.

⑥Others: such as anesthesia for surgery, prevention of cold, carsickness and seasickness, smoking cessation, detoxification, beauty, anti-aging, disease prevention and health care.

(2) Principle of acupoint selection and prescription.

①Acupoint selection based on syndrome differentiation. According to the theory of viscera and meridians in TCM, the relevant auricular points were selected. For example, for skin diseases, the lung acupoint should be selected according to the theory of "the lung dominates the skin and hair"; for red eyes, the liver acupoint should be selected according to the theory of "the liver opens its orifices to the eyes"; for fracture patients, the kidney acupoint should be selected according to the theory of "the kidney dominates the bone".

②Acupoint selection according to symptoms. According to the theory of TCM, acupoints can be selected according to symptoms, for example, Ear Center (HX1) is corresponding to diaphragm, so HX1 can be used to treat hiccup and to treat blood syndrome and skin diseases due to its function of clearing heat and cooling blood. What's more, auricular points can also be selected according to the physiological and pathological knowledge of modern medicine. For example, to treat irregular menstruation by Endocrine (CO18), to treat neurasthenia by Subcortex (AT4).

③Acupoint selection according to the corresponding positions. The auricular points corresponding to viscera and organs were selected directly. For example, Eye (LO5), Anterior Intertragic

痛、三叉神经痛、肋间神经痛等神经性疼痛；扭伤、挫伤、落枕等外伤性疼痛；各种外科手术所产生的切口痛；胆绞痛、肾绞痛、心绞痛、胃痛等内脏痛证。

(2) 各种炎症性病证：如急性结膜炎、牙周炎、咽喉炎、扁桃体炎、胆囊炎、腮腺炎、支气管炎、风湿性关节炎、面神经炎等。

(3) 功能紊乱性病证：如心脏神经官能症、心律不齐、高血压、多汗症、眩晕症、胃肠神经官能症、月经不调、遗尿、神经衰弱、癔病等。

(4) 过敏与变态反应性疾病：如过敏性鼻炎、支气管哮喘、过敏性结肠炎、荨麻疹、过敏性紫癜等。

(5) 内分泌代谢性疾病：如单纯性肥胖症、糖尿病、甲状腺功能亢进或低下、绝经期综合征等。

(6) 其他：如用于手术麻醉、预防感冒、晕车、晕船、戒烟、戒毒、美容、延缓衰老、防病保健等。

2. 选穴组方原则

(1) 辨证取穴：根据中医的脏腑、经络学说辨证选用相关耳穴。如皮肤病，按"肺主皮毛"的理论，选用肺穴；目赤肿痛，按"肝开窍于目"的理论，选用肝穴；骨折的患者，按照"肾主骨"的理论选取肾穴。

(2) 对症取穴：可根据中医理论对症取穴，如耳中穴与膈相应，可以治疗呃逆，又可凉血清热，用于治疗血证和皮肤病；也可根据现代医学的生理病理知识对症选用有关耳穴，如月经不调选内分泌穴，神经衰弱选皮质下穴等。

(3) 对应取穴：直接选取发病脏腑器官对应的耳穴。如眼病选眼穴及屏间前、屏间后穴；胃病取

Notch(TG21) and Posterior Intertragicus (AT11) are selected for eye diseases；Stomach(CO4) are selected for stomach diseases；Endocrine(CO18) are selected for gynecopathy.

④Empirical acupoint selection. Clinicians flexibly select acupoints according to their own experience. Such as External Genitals(HX4) can be treated the low back and leg pain.

3.3　Prescription example

①Stomachache：Main points such as Stomach(CO4), spleen (CO13), Sympathetic nerve (AH6a) and Shenmen (TF4). Combination of points such as pancreas and Gallbladder(CO11) and Liver(CO12).

②Headache：Main points such as Occiput (AT3), Temple (AT2), Forehead (AT1) and Subcortex(AT4). Combination of points such as Sympathetic Nerve(AH6a) and Shenmen(TF4).

③Dysmenorrhea：Main points such as internal genitals(TF2), Endocrine(CO18) and Shenmen(TF4). Combination of points such as Liver(CO12),Kidney(CO10),Subcortex(AT4) and Sympathetic Nerve(AH6a).

④Insomnia：Main points such as Shenmen (TF4), Endocrine (CO18), Heart (CO15), and Subcortex (AT4). Combination of points such as Stomach (CO4), Spleen (CO13), Liver (CO12), Kidney(CO10)and Pancreas and Gallbladder(CO11).

⑤Asthma：Main points such as Lung(CO14),Adrenal Gland (TG2p) and Sympathetic Nerve (AH6a). Combination of points such as Shenmen (TF4), Endocrine (CO18), Trachea (CO16), Kidney(CO10)and Large Intestine(CO7).

⑥Urticaria：Main points such as Lung(CO14),Adrenal Gland (TG2p), Windstream (SF11, 2i) and Ear Center (HX1). Combination of points such as Shenmen(TF4),Spleen(CO13) and Liver(CO12).

⑦Acne：Main points such as Ear Apex(XH6,7i),Endocrine (CO18),Lung(CO14),Spleen(CO13),Adrenal Gland(TG2p) and Cheek(LO5.6i). Combination of points such as Heart(CO15), Large Intestine(CO7) and Shenmen(TF4).

⑧Vertigo of inner ear：Main points such as Internal Ear (LO6), External Ear (TG1u), Kidney (CO10) and Brain Stem (AT3,4i). Combination of points such as Occiput(AT3),Subcortex (AT4),Shenmen(TF4) and Triple Energizer(CO17).

⑨Myopia：Main points such as Eye (LO5), Liver (CO12), Spleen(CO13) and Kidney(CO10). Combination of points such as Anterior Intertragic Notch (TG21) and Posterior Intertragicus (AT11).

⑩Quitting smoking：Main points such as Shenmen (TF4), Lung(CO14),Stomach(CO4) and Mouth(CO1). Combination of

胃穴；妇女经带疾病取内分泌穴。

（4）经验取穴：临床医者结合自身经验灵活选穴。如外生殖器穴可以治疗腰腿痛。

3. 处方示例

（1）胃痛。主穴：胃、脾、交感、神门。配穴：胰胆、肝。

（2）头痛。主穴：枕、颞、额、皮质下。配穴：神门、交感。

（3）痛经。主穴：内生殖器、内分泌、神门。配穴：肝、肾、皮质下、交感。

（4）失眠。主穴：神门、内分泌、心、皮质下。配穴：胃、脾、肝、肾、胰胆。

（5）哮喘。主穴：肺、肾上腺、交感。配穴：神门、内分泌、气管、肾、大肠。

（6）荨麻疹。主穴：肺、肾上腺、风溪、耳中。配穴：神门、脾、肝。

（7）痤疮。主穴：耳尖、内分泌、肺、脾、肾上腺、面颊。配穴：心、大肠、神门。

（8）内耳眩晕症。主穴：内耳、外耳、肾、脑干。配穴：枕、皮质下、神门、三焦。

（9）近视眼。主穴：眼、肝、脾、肾。配穴：屏间前、屏间后。

（10）戒烟。主穴：神门、肺、胃、口。配穴：皮质下、内分泌。

points such as Subcortex(AT4) and Endocrine(CO18).

3.4　Precautions

①Strictly disinfect to prevent infection; the needle embedding method should not be kept for too long.

②Auricular points are used alternately on both sides.

③Acupuncture syncope reaction may also occur in auricular acupuncture treatment, which should be prevented and treated in time.

④Pregnant women with a history of habitual abortion should be banned from acupuncture.

⑤Acupuncture is not suitable for patients with severe organic diseases or high anemia, and strong stimulation is not suitable for the elderly and weak patients with hypertension.

⑥Auricular points pricking method is forbidden in patients with coagulation disorder.

⑦Auricular acupuncture is not allowed for patients with abscess, ulceration or frostbite.

⑧During the needle retention period of auricular points plaster therapy and auricular intradermal needle therapy, the occurrence of allergic, shedding or contamination of adhesive tape should be prevented.

⑨For the disease of dyskinesia, the combination of exercise acupuncture is helpful to improve the curative effect.

⑩When auricular bloodletting is performed, the doctor should avoid contacting the patient's blood as much as possible.

4.　Principle of auricular acupuncture

4.1　The relationship between the meridians and viscera

Ear is closely related to meridians. *The Moxibustion Canon of Eleven Meridians of Yin-Yang System* unearthed from Mawangdui tomb refers to the "ear pulse" associated with upper limbs, eyes, cheeks and throat. In *Huangdi Neijing*, it not only developed ear pulse into Sanjiao Meridian of Hand-Shaoyang, but also recorded the relationship between ear and meridians, divergent meridians and meridian musculature in detail. In the circulation of twelve meridians, some enter the ear directly, and some distribute around the auricle. For example, the small intestine meridian of Hand-Taiyang, the Sanjiao meridian of Hand-Shaoyang and the gallbladder meridian of Foot-Shaoyang and their musculature enter into the ear, or circulate in front of or behind the ear, respectively; the stomach meridian of Foot-Yangming and the bladder meridian of Foot-Taiyang respectively go up in front of the ear and reach the

4. 注意事项

（1）严格消毒，防止感染；埋针法不宜留置过久。

（2）耳穴多左右两侧交替使用。

（3）耳针治疗亦可发生晕针，应注意预防并及时处理。

（4）有习惯性流产史的孕妇应禁针。

（5）患有严重器质性病变和伴有高度贫血者不宜针刺，对年老体弱的高血压患者不宜行强刺激法。

（6）凝血机制障碍患者禁用耳穴刺血法。

（7）脓肿、破损、冻疮局部的耳穴禁用耳针。

（8）耳穴压丸、耳穴埋针留置期间应防止胶布过敏、脱落或污染等情况的发生。

（9）对运动障碍性疾病，结合运动针法有助于提高疗效。

（10）耳穴放血割治时，医者应尽量避免接触患者血液。

四、耳针作用原理

（一）耳与经脉脏腑的关系

耳与经脉有着密切的关系。马王堆帛书《阴阳十一脉灸经》提及与上肢、眼、颊、咽喉相联系的"耳脉"。《黄帝内经》中，不仅将"耳脉"发展成了手少阳三焦经，而且对耳与经脉、经别、经筋的关系均有详细的记载。在十二经脉循行中，有的经脉直接入耳中，有的分布在耳郭周围。如手太阳小肠经、手少阳三焦经、足少阳胆经等经脉、经筋分别入耳中，或循耳之前后；足阳明胃经、足太阳膀胱经则分别上耳前，至耳上角；手阳明大肠经之别络入耳合于宗脉。六

upper corner of the ear; the collaterals of Hand-Yangming enters the ear and connect with the converging meridians. Although the six yin meridians do not directly contact the auricle, they can reach the ear with the help of the combination of divergent meridians and yang meridians. Therefore, the twelve meridians are directly or indirectly ascending to the ear. As *Miraculous Pivot—Oral Question* said, "The ears are where the stem vessels come together." *Miraculous Pivot—Form of Evil Qi and Zangfu Disease* also said, "[Humans have] twelve conduit vessels and 365 network [vessels]. Their blood and qi all rise into the face and move into the empty orifices. The essence yang qi rise and move into the eyes where they enable the eyesight. The remaining qi move into the ears where they enable hearing." Therefore, stimulating the auricular points can dredge the meridians, activate qi and blood, and harmonize the pulse.

The relationship between ear and viscera is very close, and its discussion is scattered in the medical classics of the past dynasties. The earliest records are found in *Huangdi Neijing* and *Classic of Questioning*. Such as *Plain Questions—Jin Kui Zhen Yan Lun* contained, "The south; red color. Having entered it communicates with the heart; it opens an orifice in the ears. It stores essence in the heart." *Miraculous Pivot—Maidu* said, "The qi of the kidneys pass through the ears. When the [qi of the] kidneys are in harmony, then the ears can hear the five tones." Another example is *Plain Questions—Yu Ji Zhen Zang Lun* which said, "When the movement of spleen is inadequate, then this let a person's nine orifices become impassable." *Plain Questions—Zang Qi Fa Shi Lun* contained, "In the case of a liver disease... In the case of depletion, the ears cannot hear anything. If qi moves contrary [to its regular course], when the head aches, the ears are deaf, [or the hearing is] not clear." It is said in *the Fortieth Question* of the *Classic of Questioning*—, "the lung dominates the sound, so the sound is heard." Since then, the relationship between the ear and the viscera has been discussed in more detail in the medical works of the past dynasties, such as *Invaluable Prescriptions for Ready Reference* said, "The heart qi flowing through the tongue... pass through the ears." According to the *Standards of Diagnosis and Treatment*, "Kidney is the master of ear, and heart is the guest of ear." In *Lizheng Massage Essentials*, the back of the ear is further divided into five parts: heart, liver, spleen, lung and kidney. It says, "The ear bead belongs to the kidney, the ear wheel belongs to the spleen, the ear wheel belongs to the heart, its skin and muscle belongs to the lung, and the back of the ear belongs to the liver." It shows that ear and viscera are closely related in physiology and pathology.

条阴经虽不直接联系耳郭,但均可借助经别与阳经相合而达于耳。因此十二经脉均直接或间接上行到达于耳。故《灵枢·口问》曰:"耳者,宗脉之所聚也。"《灵枢·邪气脏腑病形》亦云:"十二经脉,三百六十五络,其血气皆上于面而走空窍。其精阳气上走于目而为睛,其别气走于耳而为听。"所以刺激耳郭上的穴位,具有疏通经络、行气活血、调和百脉的作用。

耳与五脏六腑的关系十分密切,其论述散见于历代医典。最早的记载始见于《黄帝内经》和《难经》,如《素问·金匮真言论》所载:"南方赤色,入通于心,开窍于耳,藏精于心。"《灵枢·脉度》所载:"肾气通于耳,肾和则耳能闻五音矣。"又如《素问·玉机真藏论》曰:"脾不及,则令人九窍不通。"《素问·藏气法时论》载:"肝病者……虚则耳无所闻……气逆则头痛,耳聋不聪"等。《难经·四十难》云:"肺主声,故令耳闻声。"此后历代医著对于耳与脏腑的关系论述更为详细,如《千金方》所载:"神者,心之脏……心气通于舌,非窍也,其通于窍者,寄见于耳,荣华于耳。"《证治准绳》所载:"肾为耳窍之主,心为耳窍之客。"《厘正按摩要术》中进一步将耳背分为心、肝、脾、肺、肾五部,其云:"耳珠属肾,耳轮属脾,耳上轮属心,耳皮肉属肺,耳背玉楼属肝。"这说明耳与脏腑在生理方面相互联系,在病理方面相互影响,关系密切。

4.2　The relationship between ear and neurohumoral

Anatomically, the auricle is rich in nerve tissue. The main nerves related to the ear are the greater auricular nerve and the lesser occipital nerve from the cervical plexus of the spinal nerve; the branches of the auriculotemporal nerve, facial nerve, glossopharyngeal nerve and vagus nerve from the cerebral nerve; and the sympathetic nerve accompanying the external carotid artery. The four pairs of cranial nerves and two pairs of spinal nerves distributed in the auricle are closely related to the central nervous system, such as the vagus nerve and glossopharyngeal nerve from the medulla oblongata, which have obvious regulatory effects on the respiratory center, cardiac regulatory center, vascular motor center, salivary secretion center(vomiting and cough center), the parasympathetic nerve from the brain and spinal cord, and the thoracic and lumbar nerves from the spinal cord. The splanchnic nerve, which is composed of sympathetic nerves, has dual control over the organs of the whole body. They resist each other and coordinate with each other to maintain the normal operation of the viscera, trunk and limbs of the whole body.

Anatomy also showed that there were various kinds of nerve receptors in auricle epidermis and perichondrium, such as free plexiform sensory nerve endings, hair follicle sensory nerve endings and lamellar corpuscle; simple and complex plexiform sensory nerve endings, Golgi type tendinous organ endings, Ruffini's terminal nerve and muscle spindles were found on ear tendon and ear muscle. These different types of receptors are the premise and basis of stimulating auricular points to produce comprehensive regulation.

In addition, the experimental results show that there is a certain relationship between the ear and the body fluid. Even if all the nerves in the auricle are removed, the resistance points of the auricular points are not completely eliminated. Therefore, the body fluid is also involved in the process of the connection between the auricular points and the viscera.

4.3　The relationship between ear and holographic theory

According to the theory of holography, the parts with life function and relatively independent (also called holographic elements) in each biological individual contain all the information of the whole, and the holographic elements are the epitome of the whole to a certain extent.

Auricle is a relatively independent holographic element, which is the epitome of the whole human body and contains the main

(二) 耳与神经体液的关系

解剖学研究表明,耳郭内富含神经组织。与耳相关的神经主要有来自脊神经颈丛的耳大神经和枕小神经;来自脑神经的耳颞神经、面神经、舌咽神经、迷走神经的分支;以及伴随颈外动脉的交感神经。这些分布在耳郭上的四对脑神经和两对脊神经均与中枢神经系统联系紧密,如延髓发出的迷走神经和舌咽神经对呼吸中枢、心脏调节中枢、血管运动中枢、唾液分泌中枢(呕吐、咳嗽中枢)等都有明显的调节作用;由脑、脊髓部发出的副交感神经和脊髓胸、腰部发出的交感神经所组成的内脏神经,对全身的脏器几乎都有双重支配作用,两者相互抵抗,又相互协调,共同维持全身脏腑和躯干四肢的正常运功。

解剖学研究还表明,耳郭表皮至软骨膜中均含有各种神经感受器,如游离丛状感觉神经末梢、毛囊神经感觉末梢及环层小体;耳肌腱上和耳肌上含有单纯型和复杂型丛状感觉神经末梢、高尔基型腱器官、鲁菲尼末梢及肌梭。这些不同类型的感受器正是刺激耳穴产生综合调节作用的前提和基础。

此外,实验结果表明,耳与体液有一定的关系,即使将耳郭的全部神经切除,耳穴的电阻点也没有完全消除,因此考虑体液也参与了耳穴与内脏联系的作用过程。

(三) 耳与全息理论的关系

全息理论认为每个生物个体中的具有生命功能又相对独立的局部(又称全息元),均包含了整体的全部信息,全息元在一定程度上是整体的缩影。

耳郭就是一个相对独立的全息元,从形式上成为人体整体的缩

information of each part of the human body. According to the law of biological holography, the auricle and the neurons(reflex center) and the body(viscera) which are holographically connected in the brain form a holographic reflex pathway, and act through the holographic connection of neurons in the brain. The holographic connection of neurons in the brain refers to the bidirectional synaptic connection between the projection of each bit area of any relatively independent part of the body in the center and the projection of its corresponding whole part in the center. Therefore, the projection of each auricular point in the central nervous system must have this kind of connection.

In a sense, the bidirectional reflex pathway between "body (viscera)-central system-auricle" is the physiological basis of auricular point stimulation therapy. The abnormalities of all parts of the body will cause corresponding changes in the ear through the holographic reflection path, which provides physiological basis for the diagnosis of ear diseases. All kinds of stimulation to auricular points will also be transmitted to corresponding organs of the body through holographic reflection path, so as to adjust the state of corresponding tissues and organs and make them return to normal state, so as to achieve the purpose of treating diseases.

影,并包含了人体各部分的主要信息。根据生物全息律,耳郭与脑内全息联系的神经元(反射中枢)、躯体(内脏)形成了全息反射路,并通过脑内神经元的全息联系起作用。脑内神经元的全息联系是指机体的任一相对独立部分的每一位区在中枢内的投影,都与其相应的整体部分在中枢内的投射存在着双向突触联系。故每个耳穴在中枢内的投射也必然存在着这种联系。

从某种意义上说,这种"躯体(内脏)—中枢—耳郭"间的双向反射路径是耳穴刺激疗法的生理学基础。全身各部位的异常,通过全息反射路径会在耳部引起相应的改变,从而为耳穴诊断疾病提供了生理学依据。对耳穴实施的各种刺激,也会通过全息反射路径传达给身体相应的器官,从而调节相应组织器官的状态,使其恢复正常状态,从而达到治疗疾病的目的。

Chapter 6　Scalp Acupuncture

Scalp acupuncture refers to the treatment of acupuncture at specific parts of the head. Acupuncture at the head acupoints has a long history in the treatment of diseases. There are clear records on the location, function, main treatment scope and number of the head acupoints in ancient books. However, until the early 1950s to the 1970s scalp acupuncture has become a special treatment method which is different from the traditional acupoint location and stimulation method. From. There are many academic schools of scalp acupuncture, which have great influence in the international acupuncture field.

The clinical application of scalp acupuncture has a history of thousands of years in China. It is pointed out in the book of *Plain Questions—Discourse on the Essentials of Vessels and the Subtleties of the Essence* that "as for the head, it is the palace of essence brilliance" and "the head is the convergence of all yang meridians". The Six Yang Meridians of the hands and feet all go up to the head; the Heart Meridians of the Hand-Shaoyin and the Liver Meridians of the Foot-Jueyin can go up to the head; the divergent of Yin Meridians join their internally-externally related yang regular meridians and reach the head; the Governor Meridians can go up to the Fengfu(GV16) and reach the top of the brain; at the back of the neck, the Yang Link Meridians meet with the Governor Meridians, and the Yang Heel Meridians meet with the Gallbladder Meridians of the Foot-Shaoyang. It indicates that the meridians qi gathers in the head and face through the connection of meridians, branches of the regular meridians and skin, so "the qi street of the head" is the first in the theory of qi street. Zhang jiebin in the Ming Dynasty said, "The essence and qi of the five zang organs and six fu organs are all go up to the face and enter to the empty orifices." It shows that the head and face is an important part of the convergence point of meridian qi, and the head and organs are closely related in physiology and pathology via meridians and collaterals. A large number of experimental results show that the needling scalp region can regulate cortical function, improve cerebral blood flow diagram, relax and contract blood vessels, and improve vascular elasticity. There is a certain refraction relationship between the functions of the cerebral cortex and the corresponding scalp region. When acupuncture and other methods are used to stimulate a certain scalp region, the corresponding function of cerebral cortex can be affected.

So far, more than 100 kinds of diseases have been treated by scalp acupuncture, involving internal medicine, external medicine,

第六章　头　针　法

头针是指在头部特定部位针刺的治疗方法。针刺头部腧穴治疗疾病的方法由来已久,历代典籍对头部腧穴的定位、功能、主治范围以及数目都有较明确的记载,但头针疗法成为一种有别于传统腧穴定位、刺激方法特殊的治疗手段则是在 20 世纪 50 年代初至 70 年代,头针学术流派纷呈,在国际针灸界颇有影响。

头针的临床应用在我国已有数千年历史。《素问·脉要精微论》指出"头者,精明之府""头为诸阳之会"。手足六阳经循行皆上至头面;六阴经中手少阴心经与足厥阴肝经循行可上行至头面部;阴经经别相合于其相表里的阳经经脉而上达头面;督脉可上至风府,入脑上巅;阳维脉至项后与督脉会合;阳跷脉至项后合于足少阳胆经;表明人体经气通过经脉、经别、皮部等联系均汇聚于头面部。明代张介宾曰:"五脏六腑之精气皆上注于面而走空窍。"这说明头面部是经气汇集的重要部位,头与人体其他脏腑组织器官借助经络在生理病理上均有密切联系。大量实验结果表明,针刺头部穴区对皮层功能有调节作用,可改善脑血流图,有舒缩血管、改善血管弹性等作用。大脑皮层的功能在相应的头皮部位存在一定的折射关系,当采用针刺等方法刺激相应的头皮时,可影响相应的大脑皮层功能。

迄今为止,采用头针疗法治疗的疾病种类已达百余种,涉及内、

gynecology, pediatrics and other clinical departments, especially for brain-derived diseases. In order to promote the development and research of scalp acupuncture application, the Western Pacific Region Meeting of the World Health Organization(WHO) approved the "*International Program for the Standardization of Scalp Acupoints Names*" in 1984 formulated by the Chinese Acupuncture Association in accordance with the principle of "dividing the meridians into different regions, selecting the points through the meridians, and combining with the traditional acupoint penetration needing method". In 2008, the General Administration of Quality Supervision, Inspection and Quarantine of the People's Republic of China(AQSIQ) and the Standardization Administration of China (SAC) promulgated and implemented the acupuncture technical operation specifications of scalp acupuncture and international standardization program of scalp acupoint names again.

外、妇、儿等临床各科,其中对脑源性疾病的治疗效果尤为显著。为促进头针应用的发展与研究,1984年世界卫生组织西太区会议通过了中国针灸学会依照"分区定经,经上选穴,结合传统穴位透刺方法"的原则,拟定《头皮针穴名国际标准化方案》。2008年国家质量监督检验检疫总局和国家标准化管理委员会再次颁布和实施了头针针灸技术操作规范以及头针穴名国际标准化方案。

1. Scalp acupuncture stimulation region

There are 14 standardized scalp acupuncture lines, which are respectively located in the scalp of frontal region, parietal region, temporal region and occipital region.

(1) Frontal region(Tab. 6-1, Fig. 6-1).

一、头针刺激部位

标准化头针线共 14 条,分别位于额区、顶区、颞区、枕区 4 个区域的头皮部。

1. 额区(图 6-1,表 6-1)

Tab. 6-1　Frontal region(表 6-1　额区)

Acupoint name (穴名)	Location (定位)	Relationship with meridians (与经脉的关系)	Indication (主治)
Middle line of forehead (额中线)	1 cun long from Shenting(GV24) straight down along the meridian (在额部正中,前发际上下各 0.5 寸,即自神庭穴向下针 1 寸)	Belongs to the Governor Vessel (属督脉)	Headache, forced laughing, crying, insomnia, forgetfulness, dreaminess, epilepsy, nasal disease, etc. (头痛、强笑、哭泣、失眠、健忘、多梦、癫痫、鼻病等)
Lateral line 1 of forehead (额旁 1 线)	1 cun long from Meichong(BL3) straight down along the meridian (在额部,额中线外侧直对目内眦角,发际上下各 0.5 寸,即自眉冲穴起,向下针 1 寸)	Belongs to the Bladder Meridian of Foot-Taiyang (属足太阳膀胱经)	Upper energizer syndrome, such as coronary heart disease, angina, bronchial asthma, bronchitis, insomnia and so on (冠心病、心绞痛、支气管哮喘、支气管炎、失眠等上焦病证)
Lateral line 2 of forehead (额旁 2 线)	1 cun long from Toulinqi(GB15) straight down along the meridian (在额部,额旁 1 线的外侧,直对瞳孔,发际上下各 0.5 寸,即自头临泣穴起,向下针 1 寸)	Belongs to the Gallbladder Meridian of Foot-Shaoyang (属足少阳胆经)	Acute or chronic gastritis, gastroduodenal ulcer, and liver and gallbladder diseases (急慢性胃炎、胃和十二指肠溃疡、肝胆疾病等中焦病证)
Lateral line 3 of forehead (额旁 3 线)	1 cun long from the point 0.75 cun media to Touwei(ST8) straight down (在额部,额旁 2 线的外侧,自头维穴内侧 0.75 寸处,发际上下各 0.5 寸,共 1 寸)	Between the Gallbladder Meridian of Foot-Shaoyang and the Stomach Meridian of Foot-Yangming (属足少阳胆经和足阳明胃经之间)	Functional uterine bleeding, impotence, spermatorrhea, prolapse of uterine, and frequent and urgent urination (功能性子宫出血、阳痿、遗精、子宫脱垂、尿频、尿急等下焦病证)

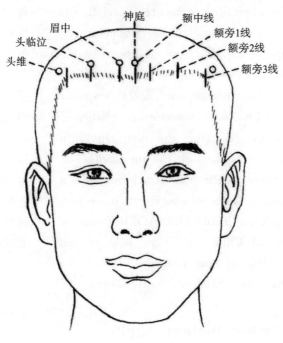

头临泣　眉中　神庭　额中线
头维　　　　　　　额旁1线
　　　　　　　　　额旁2线
　　　　　　　　　额旁3线

图 6-1　额区

（2）Parietal region(Tab. 6-2,Fig. 6-2,Fig. 6-3,Fig. 6-4).　　　　　　　　2. 顶区（表 6-2,图 6-2,图 6-3,图6-4）

Tab. 6-2　Parietal region（表 6-2　顶区）

Acupoint name （穴名）	Location （定位）	Relationship with meridians （与经脉的关系）	Indication （主治）
Middle line of vertex （顶中线）	From Baihui（GV20）to Qianding（GV21）along the midline of head （在头顶正中线上,自百会穴向前 1.5 寸至前顶穴）	Belongs to the Governor Vessel （属督脉）	Syndrome of waist, leg and foot, such as paralysis, numbness, pain, cortical polyuria, prolapse, gastric sagging, uterine prolapse, hypertension, overhead pain and so on （腰腿足病证,如瘫痪、麻木、疼痛,皮质性多尿,脱肛,胃下垂,子宫脱垂,高血压,头顶痛等）
Anterior oblique line of vertex-temporal （顶颞前斜线）	From Qianding（GV21）, 1 cun anterior to Baihui(GV20) obliquely to Xuanli(GB6) （在头部侧面,从前顶穴至悬厘穴的连线）	Oblique wear through the Bladder Meridian of Foot-Taiyang and the Gallbladder Meridian of Foot-Shaoyang （斜穿足太阳膀胱经、足少阳胆经）	Central motor dysfunction of contralateral limb. The whole line was divided into 5 equal parts：upper 1/5 for contralateral lower limb central paralysis, middle 2/5 for contralateral upper limb central paralysis, and lower 2/5 for contralateral central facial paralysis, motor aphasia, salivation, cerebral arteriosclerosis, etc. （对侧肢体中枢性运动功能障碍。将全线分 5 等份,上 1/5 治疗对侧下肢中枢性瘫痪,中 2/5治疗对侧上肢中枢性瘫痪,下 2/5 治疗对侧中枢性面瘫、运动性失语、流涎、脑动脉硬化等）

续表

Acupoint name（穴名）	Location（定位）	Relationship with meridians（与经脉的关系）	Indication（主治）
Posterior oblique line of vertex-temporal（顶颞后斜线）	From Baihui（GV20）obliquely to Qubin(GB7)（在头部侧面，从百会穴至曲鬓穴的连线）	Oblique wear through the Governor Vessel, the Bladder Meridian of Foot-Taiyang and the Gallbladder Meridian of Foot-Shaoyang（斜穿督脉、足太阳膀胱经和足少阳胆经）	Central sensory disturbance of contralateral limb. The whole line was divided into 5 equal parts：upper 1/5 for contralateral lower limb paresthesia，middle 2/5 for contralateral upper limb paresthesia，and lower 2/5 for contralateral head and face paresthesia（对侧肢体中枢性感觉障碍。将全线分为 5 等份，上 1/5 治疗对侧下肢感觉异常，中 2/5 治疗对侧上肢感觉异常，下 2/5 治疗对侧头面部感觉异常）
Lateral line 1 of vertex（顶旁 1 线）	1.5 cun lateral to Middle Line of Vertex，1.5 cun long from Tongtian（BL7）backward along the meridian（在头顶部，顶中线左、右各旁开 1.5 寸的两条平行线，自通天穴起向后针 1.5 寸）	Belong to the Bladder Meridian of Foot-Taiyang（属足太阳膀胱经）	Lower back and limb diseases such as paralysis，numbness，and pain（腰腿足病证，如瘫痪、麻木、疼痛等）
Lateral line 2 of vertex（顶旁 2 线）	2.25 cun lateral to Middle Line of Vertex，1.5 cun long from Zhengying（GB17）backward along the meridian（在头顶部，顶旁 1 线的外侧，两线相距 0.75 寸，距正中线 2.25 寸，自正营穴起沿经线向后针 1.5 寸）	Belong to the Gallbladder Meridian of Foot-Shaoyang（属足少阳胆经）	Shoulders and upper limb diseases such as paralysis，numbness，and pain（肩臂手病证，如瘫痪、麻木、疼痛等）

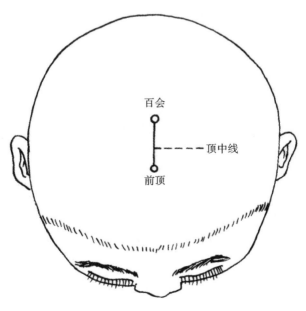

图 6-2 顶区 1

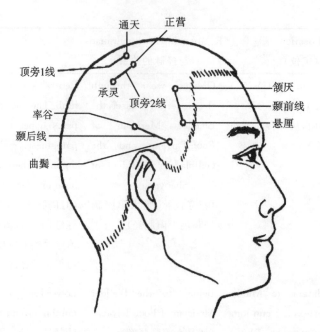

图 6-3　顶区 2

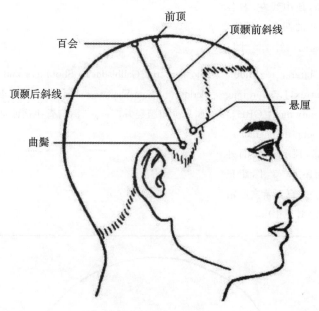

图 6-4　顶区及颞区

（3）Temporal region(Tab. 6-3,Fig. 6-4).　　　　3. 颞区(表 6-3,图 6-4)

Tab. 6-3　Temporal region(表 6-3　颞区)

Acupoint name （穴名）	Location （定位）	Relationship with meridians （与经脉的关系）	Indication （主治）
Anterior temporal line （颞前线）	From Hanyan(GB4) to Xuanli (GB6) （在头部侧面，颞部两鬓内，从额角下部向前发际处，颔厌穴至悬厘穴）	Belong to the Gallbladder Meridian of Foot-Shaoyang （属足少阳胆经）	Migraine, motor aphasia, facial paralysis,and oral diseases （偏头痛、运动性失语、周围性面神经麻痹及口腔疾病等）

续表

Acupoint name （穴名）	Location （定位）	Relationship with meridians （与经脉的关系）	Indication （主治）
Posterior temporal line （颞后线）	From Shuaigu(GB8) to Qubin (GB7) （在头部侧面，颞部耳上方，耳尖直上率谷穴至曲鬓穴）	Belong to the Gallbladder Meridian of Foot-Shaoyang （属足少阳胆经）	Migraines, dizziness, deafness, tinnitus, etc. （偏头痛、眩晕、耳聋、耳鸣等）

（4）Occipital area(Tab. 6-4, Fig. 6-5).　　　　　　　4. 枕区（表 6-4，图 6-5）

Tab. 6-4　Occipital area(表 6-4　枕区)

Acupoint name （穴名）	Location （定位）	Relationship with meridians （与经脉的关系）	Indication （主治）
Upper-middle line of occiput （枕上正中线）	From Qiangjian (GV18) to Naohu(GV17) （在枕部，枕外粗隆上方正中的垂直线，自强间穴至脑户穴）	Belong to the Governor Vessel （属督脉）	Eye diseases （眼病）
Upper-lateral line of occiput （枕上旁线）	0.5 cun lateral and parallel to Naohu(GV17), 1.5 cun long upward （在枕部，枕上正中线平行向外 0.5 寸）	Belong to the Bladder Meridian of Foot-Taiyang （属足太阳膀胱经）	Eye diseases such as cortical visual impairment, cataract, myopia, and red eye swelling and pain （皮质性视力障碍、白内障、近视眼、目赤肿痛等眼病）
Lower-lateral line of occiput （枕下旁线）	2 cun long from Yuzhen(BL9) straight down （在枕部，从膀胱经玉枕穴，向下引一直线，长 2 寸）	Belong to the Bladder Meridian of Foot-Taiyang （属足太阳膀胱经）	Balance disorders caused by cerebellar diseases, as well as posterior headache and lumbodorsal pain （小脑疾病引起的平衡障碍、后头痛、腰背两侧痛）

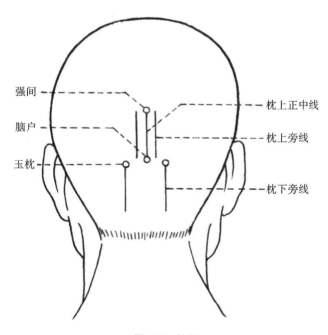

图 6-5　枕区

2. Operation steps and requirements of scalp acupuncture

2.1 Preparation

Different types of filiform needles should be selected according to the illness and the operating position of the disease. Choose a comfortable and convenient treatment position such as seat and recumbent position. According to the disease and the dialectics of TCM, select and disinfect the standardized needling lines.

2.2 Needling method

Generally, the needles should be inserted obliquely with an angle of 15°-30° between the needle body and the skin, and then the needle is inserted horizontally into the skin. Insert the needle into the subgaleal region rapidly and parallel to the skin to reach certain depth. After the needle is inserted into the lower layer of the galea aponeurotica, the resistance is reduced under the finger, and then the needle is parallel to the scalp and should be inserted along the skin; the depth of insertion depends on the patient's condition and the requirements of the prescription.

2.3 Needle manipulation

Generally, there are three methods of needle manipulation: twirling, lifting-thrusting, and handle-flicking.

(1) Twirling method. After the needle body enters the lower layer of the galea aponeurotica, the shoulder, elbow, wrist joint and thumb of the doctor are fixed to keep the needle relatively fixed. The first and second segments of the index finger are semi flexed. The handle of the needle is held by the radial side of the first segment of the index finger and the palmar side of the first segment of the thumb. Then the palmar joint of the index finger is extended and flexed to make the needle rotate rapidly. The twisting frequency is required to be about 200 times per min, lasting for 2-3 minutes.

(2) Lifting-thrusting method. The doctor inserts the needle into the lower layer of the galea aponeurotica along the skin with 3 cm, squeezes the handle tightly with the thumb and index finger, and lifts and thrusts the needle. The finger force should be uniform, and the range should not be too large. Repeat the operation for 3 to 5 minutes. The range and frequency of lifting and thrusting depend on the patient's condition.

(3) Handle-flicking method. During the period of needle retention, the needle handle can be plucked with fingers. The force should be moderate and not be too fast. Generally, it can be used for patients who are not suitable for too strong stimulation.

二、头针操作技术

(一) 针前准备

应根据病情和操作部位选择不同型号的毫针。患者取坐位或卧位。根据辨证与辨病,选定标准线,局部常规消毒。

(二) 进针方法

一般采用快速进针法,针体与头皮成 15°～30°角,将针迅速刺入皮下,当针尖到达帽状腱膜下层时,指下感觉阻力减小,然后使针与头皮平行,根据不同穴线刺入不同深度。进针深度宜根据患者具体情况和处方要求决定。

(三) 行针方法

行针方法一般分为捻转、提插和弹拨针柄三种。

1. 捻转　在针体进入帽状腱膜下层后,医者肩、肘、腕关节和拇指固定不动,以保持毫针相对固定。食指第一、二节呈半屈曲状,用食指第一节的桡侧面与拇指第一节的掌侧面持住针柄,然后食指掌指关节做伸屈运动,使针体快速旋转,要求捻转频率在 200 次/分左右,持续 2～3 分钟。

2. 提插　医者手持毫针沿皮刺入帽状腱膜下层,将针向内推进 3 cm 左右,保持针体平卧,用拇指、食指紧捏针柄,进针提插,指力应均匀一致,幅度不宜过大,如此反复操作,持续 3～5 分钟。提插的幅度与频率视患者的病情而定。

3. 弹拨针柄　在头针留针期间,可用手指弹拨针柄,用力宜适度,速度不应过快,一般可用于不宜过强刺激的患者。

2.4　Needle retention

Generally, it can be divided into static needle retention and dynamic needle retention.

(1) Static needle retention. During the period of needle retention, no acupuncture technique will be used to keep the needle quietly and naturally. In general, the time for retaining the needle should be 15-30 minutes. If the symptoms are serious, the condition is complex and the course of disease is long, the needle can be kept for more than 2 hours.

(2) Dynamic needle retention. It is to repeat the corresponding manipulation intermittently during the period of needle retention, so as to strengthen the stimulation and obtain immediate effect in a short time. Generally, in 15-30 minutes, intermittent needling should be performed 2-3 times, each time for about 2 minutes.

2.5　Withdraw the needle

The needling hand make the needle rotate lightly, if there is no tight feeling under the needle, slowly remove the needle to the subcutaneous area, and then pull out the needle quickly. After pulling out the needle, press the needle hole 1-2 minutes with the sterile dry cotton ball to prevent bleeding.

3.　Clinical application of scalp acupuncture

3.1　Scope of application

(1) Central nervous system disease, including hemiplegia, aphasia and pseudobulbar palsy caused by cerebrovascular disease, infantile nerve hypoplasia and cerebral palsy, sequelae of brain injury and encephalitis, epilepsy, chorea and tremor paralysis, etc.

(2) Mental disorders, including schizophrenia, hysteria, examination room syndrome, depression, etc. It can also be used for Alzheimer's disease and infantile congenital stupidity.

(3) Pain and abnormal sensation, including headache, trigeminal neuralgia, neck pain, shoulder pain, back pain, sciatica, biliary colic, stomachache, dysmenorrhea and other acute and chronic pain; as well as distal limb numbness, skin pruritus and other diseases.

(4) The diseases caused by the dysfunction of cortex and viscera, including hypertension, coronary heart disease, ulcer, sexual dysfunction, irregular menstruation, nervous vomiting and functional diarrhea.

3.2　Principle of acupoint selection by prescription

(1) In the method of cross acupoint selection, the stimulation

（四）留针方法

一般分为静留针与动留针两种。

1. 静留针　在留针期间不再施行任何行针手法，让针体安静而自然地留置在头皮内。一般情况下，头针留针时间宜在 15～30 分钟。如症状严重，病情复杂，病程较长者，可留针 2 小时以上。

2. 动留针　在留针期间间歇重复施行相应行针手法，以加强刺激，在较短时间内获得即时疗效。一般情况下，在 15～30 分钟内，宜间歇行针 2～3 次，每次 2 分钟左右。

（五）出针方法

刺手夹持针柄轻轻捻转松动针身，如针下无紧涩感，即可缓慢退针至皮下，然后迅速出针，出针后必须用消毒干棉球按压针孔，每穴按压 1～2 分钟，以防出血。

三、头针临床应用

（一）适应范围

1. 中枢神经系统疾病　脑血管疾病所致的偏瘫、失语、假性球麻痹，小儿神经发育不全和脑性瘫痪，颅脑外伤后遗症，脑炎后遗症，以及癫痫、舞蹈病和震颤麻痹等。

2. 精神障碍　精神分裂症、癔病（症）、考场综合征、抑郁症等。也可用于阿尔茨海默病和小儿先天愚型者。

3. 疼痛和感觉异常　头痛、三叉神经痛、颈项痛、肩痛、腰背痛、坐骨神经痛、胆绞痛、胃痛、痛经等各种急慢性疼痛病证；以及肢体远端麻木、皮肤瘙痒症等病证。

4. 皮层内脏功能失调所致疾病　高血压、冠心病、溃疡、性功能障碍和月经不调，以及神经性呕吐、功能性腹泻等。

（二）处方选穴原则

1. 交叉选穴法　单侧肢体

area on the opposite side of the disease is generally selected; in the case of bilateral limb disease, the stimulation areas on both sides are also selected; in the case of visceral disease, the stimulation areas on both sides are selected.

(2) According to the location of different diseases in the cerebral cortex, the corresponding stimulation area was selected as the main location, and other stimulation areas were selected according to the syndrome.

3.3　Example from prescription

(1) Migraine: Anterior temporal line, posterior temporal line (the same side).

(2) Trigeminal neuralgia: Lower 2/5 of posterior oblique line of vertex-temporal(the same side).

(3) Lumbago and sciatica: Lateral line 1 of vertex(the opposite side), middle line of vertex.

(4) Apoplexy hemiplegia: Anterior oblique line of vertex-temporal, posterior oblique line of vertex-temporal, middle line of vertex, lateral line 1 of vertex(the opposite side).

(5) Facial paralysis: Middle line of vertex, lower 2/5 of the anterior oblique line of vertex-temporal, lower 2/5 of the posterior oblique line of vertex-temporal, anterior temporal line(the opposite side).

(6) Vertigo and tinnitus: Posterior temporal line (the same side).

(7) Hypertension: Middle line of vertex, anterior oblique line of vertex-temporal, posterior oblique line of vertex-temporal (bilateral).

(8) Coronary heart disease, cough and asthma: Lateral line 1 of forehead(bilateral).

(9) Asynodia, hysteroptosia: Lateral line 3 of forehead (bilateral), middle line of vertex.

(10) Cortical visual impairment: Upper-middle line of occiput and upper-lateral line of occiput(the opposite side).

3.4　Precautions

(1) It is not suitable for infants who do not have ossified fontanelle and bone suture, or patients with skull defect or open brain damage and pregnant women to use scalp needle to treat.

(2) It is not suitable to use in the sites operation, with serious infection, ulcer and trauma of scalp. The treatment line of corresponding scalp needle can be taken on the opposite side.

(3) Patients with severe heart disease, severe diabetes mellitus, severe anemia, acute inflammation, cerebrovascular accident in the

病，一般选用病证对侧刺激区；双侧肢体病，同时选用双侧刺激区；内脏病证，选用双侧刺激区。

2. 对应选穴法　针对不同疾病在大脑皮层的定位，以选用对应的刺激区为主，同时根据兼证选用其他有关刺激区配合治疗。

（三）处方示例

（1）偏头痛：颞前线、颞后线（同侧）。

（2）三叉神经痛：顶颞后斜线下 2/5（同侧）。

（3）腰痛、坐骨神经痛：顶旁 1 线（对侧）、顶中线。

（4）中风偏瘫：顶颞前斜线、顶颞后斜线、顶中线、顶旁 1 线（对侧）。

（5）面瘫：顶中线、顶颞前斜线下 2/5、顶颞后斜线下 2/5、颞前线（对侧）。

（6）眩晕、耳鸣：颞后线（同侧）。

（7）高血压：顶中线、顶颞前斜线、顶颞后斜线（双侧）。

（8）冠心病、咳喘：额旁 1 线（双侧）。

（9）阳痿、阴挺：额旁 3 线（双侧）、顶中线。

（10）皮层性视力障碍：枕上正中线、枕上旁线（对侧）。

（四）注意事项

（1）囟门和骨缝尚未骨化的婴儿、颅骨缺损或开放性脑损伤患者和孕妇不宜用头针治疗。

（2）头颅手术部位，头皮严重感染、溃疡和创伤处不宜使用头针治疗，可在其对侧取相应头针治疗线进行针刺治疗。

（3）严重心脏病、重度糖尿病、重度贫血、急性炎症和脑血管

acute stage or unstable blood pressure should not use scalp acupuncture. It should be used with caution for people who are nervous, full or hungry.

(4) The scalp should be punctured quickly and avoid hair follicle and scars. The depth and direction of acupuncture should be determined according to the treatment requirements, combined with the patient's age, constitution and sensitivity. Do not bump the needle handle to avoid bending and pain.

(5) Scalp acupuncture therapy combined with exercise therapy can improve the clinical effect of some diseases.

意外急性期患者或血压、病情不稳定者不宜使用。对精神紧张、过饱过饥者应慎用。

（4）头针刺入时要迅速，注意避开发囊、瘢痕。针刺深度及方向，应根据治疗需要，并结合患者年龄、体质及敏感性决定。留针时不要随意碰撞针柄，以免发生弯针和疼痛。

（5）头针治疗时配合针对性运动，对部分病证有提高临床疗效的作用。

Chapter 7　Wrist-Ankle Acupuncture

Wrist-ankle acupuncture is a method of treating diseases by needling subcutaneously at the corresponding points of wrist or ankle.

The theory of the twelve cutaneous regions, "standard and origin", and "root and node" are the important theoretical basis for the application of wrist-ankle acupuncture. As the *Plain Questions—Discourse on Skin Sections* describes, "the skin consists of sections [made up] by the vessels" and "the altogether twelve conduit and network vessels constitute the sections of the skin". It shows that the twelve cutaneous regions are not only the parts where the function activities of the twelve meridians are reflected on the body surface, but the distribution area of which is based on the distribution range of the body surface of the twelve meridians. The six divisions of the wrist-ankle acupuncture are similar to the twelve cutaneous regions.

According to the theory of "standard and origin" and "root and node", limbs are the origin of twelve meridians, the position where meridian qi starts. Acupuncture at acupoints below elbow and knee is easier to stimulate meridians to regulate the function of viscera and meridians. The twelve stimulation points of the wrist-ankle acupuncture are all located near the wrist and ankle joints below the elbows and knees of the limbs, which are equivalent to the main part of the 12 meridians. It can not only treat local lesions, but also treat diseases of the viscera and the head, face and five sense organs that are far away from the acupoints. Since the wrist-ankle acupuncture requires that the point reached by the needle is subcutaneous, where the qi of the collaterals spread. Combined with the relationship between the wrist-ankle acupuncture and the twelve cutaneous regions, the acupuncture can adjust the qi of the corresponding meridian and the function of the viscera associated with it, and play a therapeutic effect of removing evil qi and strengthening the healthy qi.

1. Wrist-ankle needle stimulation site

Wrist-ankle acupuncture divides the thoracoabdominal and dorsolateral sides of human body into yin and yang. The thoracoabdominal side belonging to yin is divided into zone 1, zone 2 and zone 3, and the dorsolateral side belonging to yang is divided into zone 4, zone 5 and zone 6. With diaphragm as the boundary, the human body is divided into upper and lower parts according to the distribution of twelve cutaneous regions.

1.1　Division of human body surface

The body surface is divided into six longitudinal regions and

第七章　腕踝针法

腕踝针法是在手腕或足踝部的相应进针点，用毫针进行皮下针刺以治疗疾病的方法。

经络皮部论和标本根结论是腕踝针法运用的重要理论基础。《素问·皮部论》中的"皮者，脉之部也""凡十二经脉者，皮之部也"，说明十二皮部不仅是十二经脉功能活动反映于体表的部位，而且十二皮部的分布区域以十二经脉体表的分布范围为依据。腕踝针的六区划分与十二皮部相似。

标本根结论认为四肢为十二经脉之本，其部位在下，是经气始生始发之地，针刺四肢肘膝以下的腧穴更易激发经气以调节脏腑经络功能。腕踝针的12个刺激点均位于四肢肘膝以下的腕踝关节附近，恰好相当于十二经脉的本部，不仅能治疗局部病变，而且能治疗远离腧穴部位的脏腑病、头面五官病等。由于腕踝针法操作时，要求针尖所达部位为皮下，此处正是络脉之气散布之所在，结合腕踝针与十二皮部的关系，刺之可调整相应经脉之气及与之相联属脏腑的功能，起到祛邪扶正的治疗作用。

一、腕踝针刺激部位

腕踝针法将人体的胸腹侧和背腰侧分为阴阳两个面，属阴的胸腹侧划为1、2、3区，属阳的背腰侧划为4、5、6区。并以横膈为界，将人体分为上下两部分，符合十二经脉及皮部的分布规律。

（一）人体体表分区

人体体表分区将人体体表划

two upper and lower segments(Fig. 7-1,Fig. 7-2,Fig. 7-3).

分为 6 个纵行区和上下两段（图 7-1，图 7-2，图 7-3）。

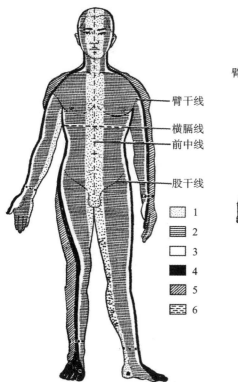

图 7-1　躯干定位分区正面

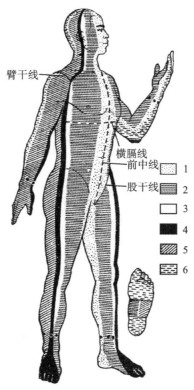

图 7-2　躯干定位分区侧面

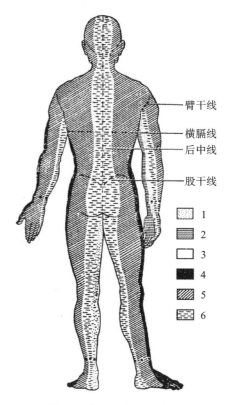

图 7-3　躯干定位分区背面

（1）Longitudinal six areas. The longitudinal six regions include the six regions of head, neck and trunk and the six regions of limbs.

①The anterior posterior midline of six sections of head, neck and trunk is the standard line, and the two sides of the body are divided into six longitudinal areas from the front to back.

Zone 1：The body surface area formed 1. 5 cun by opening each side to the left and right from the front median line. Clinically, the left zone 1 and the right zone 1 are often referred to as zone 1, and the following areas are also the same.

Zone 2：The body surface area formed from the border line of zone 1 to the axillary front, which is symmetrical.

Zone 3：The body surface area formed from axillary front to midaxillary line, which is symmetrical.

Zone 4：The body surface area formed from midaxillary line to posterior axillary line, which is symmetrical.

Zone 5：The body surface area formed from the posterior axillary line to the border line of area 6, which is symmetrical.

Zone 6：The body surface area formed 1. 5 cun to the left and right of the posterior midline, respectively called the left zone 6 and the right zone 6.

②Division of limbs. The brachial trunk line and the femoral

1. 纵行六区　纵行六区包括头、颈、躯干六区和四肢六区两部分。

（1）头、颈、躯干六区。以前后正中线为标线，将身体两侧面由前向后划分为 6 个纵行区。

1 区：从前正中线开始，向左、向右各旁开 1.5 寸所形成的体表区域，分别称为左 1 区、右 1 区。临床常把左 1 区与右 1 区合称为 1 区，以下各区亦同。

2 区：1 区边线到腋前线之间所形成的体表区域，左右对称。

3 区：腋前线至腋中线之间所形成的体表区域，左右对称。

4 区：腋中线至腋后线之间所形成的体表区域，左右对称。

5 区：腋后线至 6 区边线之间所形成的体表区域，左右对称。

6 区：后正中线向左、向右各旁开 1.5 寸所形成的体表区域，分别称之为左 6 区、右 6 区。

（2）四肢六区。以臂干线和

trunk line are the boundary between limbs and trunk. The brachial trunk line(around the attachment margin of the triangulus of the shoulder to the armpit) serves as the boundary between the upper limb and the trunk, while the femoral trunk line(from the groin to the iliac valley) is the boundary between the lower limb and the trunk. When the upper and the lower limbs on both sides are in forward out of position, making the surface between yin and yang of the limbs and trunk of yin and yang in the same direction and close to each other, take the destiny that appears close to each other as the boundary. The front one is equivalent to the anterior midline, and the rear one is equivalent to the posterior midline, so that the division of the limbs can be analogized according to the division of the trunk.

Upper limbs six area: Divide the body surface area of the upper extremity into six equal parts in the longitudinal direction, starting from the inner ulnar edge of the upper extremity, and in turn are zone 1, zone 2, zone 3, zone 4, zone 5 and zone 6, symmetrical.

Lower limbs six area: Divide the body surface area of the lower extremity into six equal parts in the longitudinal direction, starting from the inner Achilles tendon edge of the lower extremity, and in turn are zone 1, zone 2, zone 3, zone 4, zone 5 and zone 6, symmetrical.

(2) The upper and lower two segments. Centered at the junction of the end of the sternum and the costal arch on both sides. Draw a horizontal line around the body called the diaphragm line. The diaphragm line divides the six sides of the body into two upper and lower segments. Above the diaphragm line are upper 1, upper 2, upper 3, upper 4, upper 5 and upper 6. The areas below the diaphragm line are lower 1, lower 2, lower 3, lower 4, lower 5 and lower 6. If you need to indicate whether the symptoms are on the left or right, on the top or on the bottom, you can also write it down as the upper right 2 or the lower left 2.

1.2　Insertion points

(1) Needle insertion points on the wrist and their location and indications.

There are 6 pairs on the left and right sides, about 2 cun (equivalent to PC6 and TE5) on the wrist transverse line, make a horizontal line around the forearm, starting from the medial ulnar margin of the forearm, along the medial center of the forearm, the medial radius margin of the forearm, the lateral radius margin of the forearm, the lateral center of the forearm, and the lateral ulnar margin of the forearm in six equal parts. The midpoint of each equal

股干线为四肢和躯干的分界。臂干线(环绕肩部三角肌附着缘至腋窝)作为上肢与躯干的分界,股干线(腹股沟至髂嵴)为下肢与躯干的分界。当两侧的上下肢处于内侧面向前的外旋位置,也就是使四肢的阴阳面和躯干的阴阳面处在同一方向并互相靠拢时,以靠拢处出现的缘为分界,在前面的相当于前中线,在后面的相当于后中线,这样四肢的分区就可按躯干的分区类推。

上肢六区:将上肢的体表区域纵向六等分,从上肢内侧尺骨缘开始,右侧顺时针,左侧逆时针,依次为1区、2区、3区、4区、5区、6区,左右对称。

下肢六区:将下肢的体表区域纵向六等分,从下肢内侧跟腱缘开始,右侧顺时针,左侧逆时针,依次为1区、2区、3区、4区、5区、6区,左右对称。

2. 上下两段　以胸骨末端和两侧肋弓的交接处为中心,划一条环绕身体的水平线,称为横膈线。横膈线将身体两侧的6个区分成上下两段。横膈线以上各区分别称为上1区、上2区、上3区、上4区、上5区、上6区;横膈线以下的各区称为下1区、下2区、下3区、下4区、下5区、下6区。如需标明症状在左侧还是右侧,在上还是在下,又可记为右上2区或左下2区等。

(二)腕踝针进针点

1. 腕部进针点、定位及主治　左右两侧共6对,约在腕横纹上2寸(相当于内关穴与外关穴)位置上,环前臂作一水平线,从前臂内侧尺骨缘开始,沿前臂内侧中央、前臂内侧桡骨缘、前臂外侧桡骨缘、前臂外侧中央、前臂外侧尺骨缘顺序六等分,每等份的中点为进针点,并分别称为上1、上2、上

part is the needle insertion point, and they are called the upper 1, upper 2, upper 3, upper 4, upper 5, and upper 6, respectively (Tab. 7-1, Fig. 7-4).

3、上 4、上 5、上 6（表 7-1，图 7-4）。

Tab. 7-1　Needle insertion points on the wrist（表 7-1　腕部进针点定位）

Acupoint name（穴名）	Location（定位）	Indications（主治）
Upper 1（上 1）	Between the ulnar margin of the little finger and the flexor carpi ulnaris tendon（在小指侧的尺骨缘与尺侧腕屈肌腱之间）	Syndromes of forehead, eye, nose, mouth, incisors, tongue, throat, sternum, trachea, esophagus, left upper limb area 1 and right upper limb area 1, such as forehead pain, myopia, rhinitis, toothache, wrist joint pain, pain and numbness of little finger, urticaria, hypertension, insomnia, menopause syndrome, diabetes and so on（前额、眼、鼻、口、门齿、舌、咽喉、胸骨、气管、食管及左上肢、右上肢 1 区内的病证。如前额痛，近视，鼻炎，牙痛，腕关节痛，小指疼痛麻木，荨麻疹，高血压，失眠，更年期综合征，糖尿病等）
Upper 2（上 2）	In the middle of the lateral palmar of the wrist, between the long palmar tendon and the flexor tendon of the radial carpal flexor tendon, equivalent to the position where the PC 6 locates（在腕掌侧面中央，掌长肌腱与桡侧腕屈肌腱之间，相当于内关穴处）	Syndromes of frontal angle, eye, posterior teeth, lung, breast, heart (upper left area 2) and left upper limb area 2 and right upper limb area 2, such as ptosis, eye red swelling, infraorbital pain, paranasal sinusitis, toothache, neck pain, chest pain, hypochondriac pain, hyperplasia of mammary gland, breast tenderness, lack of milk, milk withdrawal, palpitations, arrhythmia, adverse wrist joint flexion and extension, wrist joint sprain and contusion, and middle finger and ring finger injury（额角，眼，后齿，肺，乳房，心（左上 2 区）及左上肢、右上肢 2 区内的病证。如眼睑下垂，目赤肿痛，眶下疼痛，副鼻窦炎，牙痛，颈痛，胸痛，胁痛，乳腺增生，乳房胀痛，缺乳，回乳，心悸，心律不齐，腕关节屈伸不利，腕关节扭挫伤，中指和无名指扭挫伤等）
Upper 3（上 3）	Between the edge of the radius and the radial artery（在桡动脉与桡骨缘之间）	Symptomes of cheek, lateral chest, left upper limb area 3 and right upper limb area 3, such as migraine, acute mumps, toothache, tinnitus, otitis media, side chest pain, armpit odor, armpit hyperhidrosis, shoulder joint pain, and thumb and index finger twists and turns（面颊，侧胸及左上肢、右上肢 3 区内的病证。如偏头痛，急性腮腺炎，牙痛，耳鸣，中耳炎，侧胸痛，腋臭，腋窝多汗症，肩关节疼痛，拇指和食指扭挫伤等）
Upper 4（上 4）	Between the inside and outside of the radius on the thumb side（在拇指侧的桡骨内外缘之间）	Symptomes of temporal, ear, lateral thorax, left upper limb area 4 and right upper limb area 4, such as posterior ear pain, sternocleidomastoid myositis, tinnitus, otitis media, side chest pain, armpit hyperhidrosis, shoulder joint pain, wrist joint pain, and bruising of the thumb and index finger（颞，耳，侧胸及左上肢、右上肢 4 区内的病证。如耳后痛，胸锁乳突肌炎，耳鸣，中耳炎，侧胸痛，腋窝多汗症，肩关节疼痛，腕关节疼痛，拇指和食指扭挫伤等）
Upper 5（上 5）	In the middle of the back of the wrist, between the radius and the ulna（在腕背中央，即外关穴处）	Syndromes of posterior head, posterior back, heart, lung, left upper limb area 5, and right upper limb area 5, such as headache, cervical spondylosis, stiff neck, vertigo, shoulder back pain, adverse wrist joint flexion and extension, wrist joint swelling and pain, hand back pain, and middle finger and ring finger pain（后头部，后背部，心，肺及左上肢、右上肢 5 区内的病证。如后头痛，颈椎病，落枕，眩晕，肩背痛，腕关节屈伸不利，腕关节肿痛，手背疼痛，中指和无名指疼痛等）

Acupoint name （穴名）	Location （定位）	Indications （主治）
Upper 6 （上 6）	On the back of the wrist, 1 cm from the edge of the little finger ulna （在距小指侧尺骨缘 1 cm 处）	Syndromes of posterior head, neck and chest segment of spine, left upper limb area 6, and right upper limb area 6, such as headache, neck pain, stiff neck, chest pain, wrist joint swelling and pain, and numbness of little finger （后头部,脊柱颈胸段及左上肢、右上肢 6 区内的病证。如后头痛,颈项强痛,落枕,胸背痛,腕关节肿痛,小指麻木不仁等）

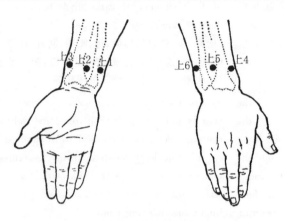

图 7-4　腕部进针点

（2）Needle insertion points, location and indications at the ankle.

There are 6 pairs on the left and right sides, about 3 cun (equivalent to GB39 and SP6) above the high point of the inner ankle and the outer ankle, make a horizontal line around the lower leg, and start from the edge of the achilles tendon on the inside of the lower leg, along the order of the medial center of the lower leg, the tibia edge on the inside of the lower leg, the fibula edge on the outside of the lower leg, the lateral center of the lower leg, and the Achilles tendon edge on the outside of the lower leg. The midpoint of each equal part is the needle insertion point, and they are called lower 1, lower 2, lower 3, lower 4, lower 5 and lower 6, respectively (Tab. 7-2, Fig. 7-5).

2. 踝部进针点,定位及主治

左右两侧共 6 对,约在内踝高点与外踝高点上 3 寸(相当于悬钟穴与三阴交穴)位置上,环小腿作一水平线,并从小腿内侧跟腱缘开始,沿小腿内侧中央、小腿内侧胫骨缘、小腿外侧腓骨缘、小腿外侧中央、小腿外侧跟腱缘的顺序六等分,每等份的中点为进针点,并分别称为下 1、下 2、下 3、下 4、下 5、下 6(表 7-2,图 7-5)。

Tab. 7-2　Needle insertion points on the ankle(表 7-2　踝部进针点定位)

Acupoint name （穴名）	Location （定位）	Indications （主治）
Lower 1 （下 1）	Near the medial edge of the Achilles tendon （靠跟腱内缘）	Syndromes of stomach, bladder, uterus, vulva, left lower limb area 1, and right lower limb area 1, such as stomach pain, nausea, vomiting, periumbilical pain, stranguria, irregular menstruation, dysmenorrhea, pelvic inflammation, vaginitis, impotence, enuresis, spermatorrhea, premature ejaculation, testicular swelling, pain in the knee and Achilles tendon, and heel pain （胃,膀胱,子宫,前阴及左下肢、右下肢 1 区内的病证。如胃痛,恶心呕吐,脐周痛,淋证,月经不调,痛经,盆腔炎,阴道炎,阳痿,遗尿,遗精,早泄,睾丸肿胀,跟腱疼痛,足跟疼痛）

续表

Acupoint name （穴名）	Location （定位）	Indications （主治）
Lower 2 （下 2）	In the center of the medial side of the shin, near the medial humerus （在内侧面中央,靠胫骨后缘）	Syndromes of stomach, spleen, liver, large intestine, small intestine, left lower limb area 2 and right lower limb area 2, such as chest distension, abdominal pain, diarrhea, constipation, knee arthritis, and internal ankle torsion and contusion （胃,脾,肝,大小肠及左下肢、右下肢 2 区内的病证。如胸胁胀满,腹痛,腹泻,便秘,膝关节炎,内踝扭挫伤）
Lower 3 （下 3）	Within 1 cm of the anterior tibia crest and the anterior border of the fibula （在胫骨前嵴向内 1 cm 处）	Syndromes of liver, gallbladder, spleen, flank, left lower limb area 3, and right lower limb area 3, such as flank pain, adverse hip joint flexion and extension, knee arthritis, and ankle joint torsion and contusion （肝,胆,脾,胁部及左下肢、右下肢 3 区内的病证。如胁痛,髋关节屈伸不利,膝关节炎,踝关节扭挫伤）
Lower 4 （下 4）	The midpoint between anterior border of tibia and anterior border of fibula （在胫骨前嵴与腓骨前缘的中点）	Syndromes of flank, liver, spleen, left lower limb area 4 and right lower limb area 4, such as lateral lumbar pain, lateral femoral cutaneous neuritis, knee arthritis, ankle joint torsion and contusion, and sciatica （胁部,肝,脾及左下肢、右下肢 4 区内的病证。如侧腰痛,股外侧皮神经炎,膝关节炎,踝关节扭挫伤,坐骨神经痛）
Lower 5 （下 5）	In the center of the lateral side of the ankle, near the posterior edge of the humerus （在外侧面中央,靠腓骨后缘）	Syndromes of waist, kidney, ureter, buttock, left lower limb area 5, and right lower limb area 5, such as renal colic, lumbar pain, gluteal cutaneous neuritis, sciatica, adverse knee joint flexion and extension or pain, and external ankle torsion and contusion （腰部,肾,输尿管,臀及左下肢、右下肢 5 区内病证。如肾绞痛,腰痛,臀上皮神经炎,股外侧皮神经炎,坐骨神经痛,膝关节屈伸不利或疼痛,外踝扭挫伤）
Lower 6 （下 6）	Near the edge of Achilles tendon （靠跟腱外缘）	Syndromes of spinal lumbosacral, anal, left lower limb area 6, and right lower limb area 6, such as low back pain, acute torsion and contusion, hemorrhoids, eczema around the anus, coccygeal pain, and sciatica （脊柱腰骶部,肛门及左下肢、右下肢 6 区内的病证。如腰痛,急性腰扭伤,痔疮,肛门周围湿疹,尾骨疼痛,坐骨神经痛）

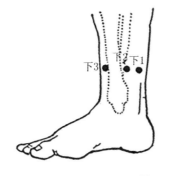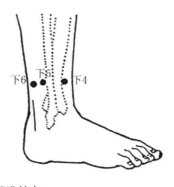

图 7-5　踝部进针点

2. Operation technique of wrist-ankle acupuncture

(1) Preparation. The patient can use sitting position or lying position before needle preparation, or sitting position for wrist needle, and lying position for ankle needle preparation. The position of limbs is very important during puncturing. The muscles should be relaxed as much as possible to avoid the skew of the needle body in the clockwise direction. The acupoint skin should be disinfected regularly. Generally, (0. 32-0. 38) mm×(25-40) mm filiform needle is often used.

(2) Needling method. After selecting the needle point, fix and tighten the skin around the point with pressing hand. Hold the needle with puncturing handle in the ways of the pricking thumb at the bottom and the index finger and middle finger at the top. The needle is at an angle of 15°-30° with the skin, quickly pierce the subcutaneous skin, and then place the needle flat so that the needle body enters 1-1. 2 cun under the dermis in a horizontal position (Fig. 7-6).

二、腕踝针操作技术

1. 针前准备　患者可采用坐位或卧位,或针腕时取坐位,针踝时取卧位。针刺时患者肢体位置非常重要,肌肉尽量放松,以免针刺时针体方向发生偏斜;穴位皮肤常规消毒;一般常选用(0. 32～0. 38)mm×(25～40)mm 毫针。

2. 进针方法　选定进针点后,押手固定在进针点的下部,并拉紧皮肤,刺手拇指在下,食指、中指在上夹持针柄,针与皮肤成 15°～30°角快速刺入皮下,然后将针平放,使针身成水平位沿真皮下进入1～1. 2 寸(图 7-6)。

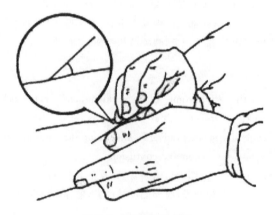

图 7-6　腕踝针进针法

(3) Needle manipulation and manifestation of obtaining qi. It is better to have a soft feeling under the needle without twisting the needle; the patient may have no feeling under the needle, but the main symptoms of the patient can be improved or disappeared. If the patient has the feeling of soreness, numbness, distention and heaviness, it means that the needle is too deep to enter into the lower layer of fascia, so the needle must be withdrawn to the subcutaneous layer, and the needle should be inserted along the dermis again.

(4) Needle retention. The retention time of needle is generally 20-30 minutes. If the patient's condition is serious or the course of disease is long, the retention time of needle can be appropriately extended for 1 to several hours, but the longest time is not more than 24 hours; during the needle retention period, no manual operation.

(5) Withdraw the needle. The method of withdrawing the

3. 行针方法及得气表现　以针下有松软感为宜,不捻针;患者针下无任何感觉,但患者的主要症状可得到改善或消失。如患者有酸、麻、胀、重等感觉,说明针刺入筋膜下层,进针过深,须将针退至皮下,重新沿真皮下刺入。

4. 留针方法　一般情况下留针 20～30 分钟。若病情较重或病程较长者,可适当延长留针时间数小时,但最长不超过 24 小时;留针期间不行针。

5. 出针方法　与毫针出针法

needle is almost the same as that of filiform needling.

3. Clinical application of wrist-ankle acupuncture

3.1 Scope of application

In the treatment of wrist-ankle acupuncture, the diseases treated in each area generally include two aspects: One is various diseases caused by the viscera, tissues, organs, etc. The other is various diseases of which the main symptoms can reflect in the same name area. In general, this method has a wide range of application and quick effect.

3.2 Principle of acupoint selection by prescription

(1) The upper points are taken for the upper disease, and the lower points are taken for the lower disease. The needle for upper and lower diseases should be taken for different zones. If the body surface area of the forehead belongs to the upper part, the treatment of the forehead pain should be based on upper 1.

(2) The left points are taken for the left disease, and the right points are taken for the right disease. For 6 body surface regions symmetrical to the right and left. If the left breast is located at the upper left zone 2, so the left breast carbuncle is mainly treated at the left upper 2.

(3) If the affected areas are not clear, choose upper 1 of both sides. For the diseases which affected areas cannot be determined, such as insomnia, hypertension, systemic pruritus, climacteric syndrome, infantile chorea, and infantile hyperactivity, as well as the diseases with complex etiology and difficult to determine the surface area, both sides can be treated at upper 1.

(4) Take the upper and the lower point at the same time. When the main symptom of the patient is close to the diaphragmatic line, not only the upper needle point, but also the corresponding lower needle point should be taken. For example, according to the division of the body surface area, the epigastric part is generally belonging to double lower zone 1 and the lower right zone 2. Therefore, in the treatment of epigastralgia, we should not only take double lower 1 and the right lower 2, but also take double upper 1 and the right upper 2 according to their symptoms near the diaphragmatic line.

(5) Take the right and the left point at the same time. If the main symptom of the patient is in the zone 1 of the trunk, the double upper 1 or double lower 1 should be taken in clinical treatment. If the main symptom of the patient is in the zone 6 of the trunk, double upper 6 or double lower 6 should be taken in clinical

相同。

三、腕踝针临床应用

（一）适应范围

腕踝针疗法中，每个区所治疗的病证大致包括两个方面：其一是同名区域内所属脏腑、组织、器官等所引起的各种病证；其二，主要症状能反映在同名区域内的各种病证。总的来说，本法适应范围广，见效快。

（二）处方选穴原则

1. 上病取上、下病取下　此原则是针对上下不同分区而言的。如前额的体表区域属上部，故前额部疼痛以选上1治疗为主。

2. 左病取左、右病取右　此原则是针对左右对称的6个体表区域而言的。如左侧乳房位于左上2区，故左侧乳痈以选取左上2治疗为主。

3. 区域不明、选双上1　部分疾病无法确定其所属体表区域，如失眠、高血压、全身瘙痒症、更年期综合征、小儿舞蹈症、小儿多动症等，以及病因复杂难以明确判断其所属体表区域的疾病，均可取双上1进行治疗。

4. 上下同取　患者主要症状的表现位置靠近横膈线时，不仅要取上部的进针点，还要取与之相对应的下部进针点。如按体表区域的划分，胃脘部大致属于双下1区和右下2区，故治疗胃脘痛不仅取双下1、右下2，还应根据其病证表现靠近横膈线而加取双上1和右上2。

5. 左右共针　如患者的主要症状表现在躯干部的1区，临床治疗时应取双上1或双下1。又如患者的主要症状表现在躯干部的6区，临床治疗时应取双上6或双

treatment.

3.3　Prescription example

（1）Headache：Upper 1 and upper 2.

（2）Migraine：Upper 2 and upper 5.

（3）Stomachache：Upper 1 and upper 2.

（4）Pain in liver area：Lower 2.

（5）Dysmenorrhea：Lower 1.

（6）Shoulder pain：Upper 4，upper 5，and upper 6.

（7）Sciatica：Lower 6.

（8）TMJ（temporomandibular arthritis）：Upper 4.

（9）Enteritis：Lower 1 and upper 2.

（10）Pruritus and urticaria：Upper 1.

3.4　Precautions

（1）Wrist-ankle needle insertion generally does not elicit the feeling of pain, distension, or numbness. If the above symptoms appear, it means that the needle insertion depth is too deep, and it should be adjusted to no pain, no distention, no numbness and so on.

（2）Grasp the accurate direction of needle insertion. That is to say, if the disease is manifested in the upper part of the needle point, the needle tip must be inserted centripetally；otherwise，if the disease is manifested in the lower part of the needle point, the needle tip must be inserted centrifug ally.

（3）Sometimes, the position of needling insertion should be adjusted according to the local situation and needling direction. For example，the subcutaneous area to be pierced by the needle has thick veins, scars and wounds, the lower end of the needle handle near bone tuberosity which is inconvenient for puncturing, and the direction of needling should be toward the centrifugal end, the position of the needle insertion point should be shifted towards the heart end properly, but the positioning method of the point should not be changed and should be in the center of the area.

（4）When several symptoms exist at the same time, the primary and secondary symptoms should be analyzed. For example, if there is pain in the symptoms, first select points according to the pain area.

（5）In case of syncope, stagnation, hematoma and other phenomena, they shall be treated according to the treatment method of abnormal situation in filiform needle acupuncture.

（6）Pain, numbness, pruritus and other feelings and some motor symptoms related to pain can be completely disappeared or significantly improved in one acupuncture treatment. If the pain and

下 6。

（三）处方示例

（1）头痛：取上 1，上 2。

（2）偏头痛：取上 2，上 5。

（3）胃痛：取上 1，上 2。

（4）肝区痛：取下 2。

（5）痛经：取下 1。

（6）肩痛：取上 4，上 5，上 6。

（7）坐骨神经痛：取下 6。

（8）颞颌关节炎：取上 4。

（9）肠炎：取下 1，下 2。

（10）皮肤瘙痒，荨麻疹：取上 1。

（四）注意事项

（1）腕踝针法进针一般不痛、不胀、不麻等，如出现上述症状，说明进针过深，须调至以不痛、不胀、不麻为宜。

（2）把握准确的针刺方向。即病证表现在进针点上部者，针尖须向心而刺；病证表现在进针点下部者，针尖须离心而刺。

（3）进针点位置有时要根据针刺局部情况及针刺方向进行调整。如局部皮下有较粗静脉、瘢痕、伤口，或针柄下端有骨粗隆不便针刺，针刺方向要朝向离心端等情况时，进针点位置要朝向心端适当移位，但点的定位方法不变，要处于区的中央。

（4）有几种症状同时存在时，要分析症状的主次，如症状中有痛的感觉，首先按痛所在区选点。

（5）如出现晕针、滞针、血肿等现象者，按毫针刺法中异常情况的处理方法进行处理。

（6）对如疼痛、麻木、瘙痒等感觉及与痛有关联的一些运动症状，在一次针刺治疗中常能立即获

other symptoms cannot be improved or not completely improved after acupuncture, in addition to the causes of the disease itself, it is often related to the factors such as improper body position when acupuncture, the position of the acupuncture point is not in the middle of the area, the subcutaneous needling is not shallow enough, the direction is not straight enough, and the length of the needling is not right, sometimes only slightly worse will affect the curative effect. Therefore, we should pay attention to each step of needling. If it is a problem of needling method, it is necessary to withdraw the needle tip to the subcutaneous area and correct it as appropriate before puncturing the needle.

得疗效,达到疼痛等症状完全消失。若针刺入后疼痛等症状未能改变或改变不全,除疾病本身原因外,往往与针刺时体位不正、针刺点位置在区内不够居中、针刺进皮下不够表浅、方向不够正直、刺入长度不当等因素有关,有时差别甚微都会影响疗效。因此,要注意针刺的各个步骤。如属针刺方法问题,要将针尖退至皮下,酌情纠正后再进针。

Chapter 8　Abdominal Acupuncture

Abdominal acupuncture is a therapy to treat systemic diseases by needle-piercing the specific acupoints of the abdomen to adjust the balance of viscera, meridian, qi and blood, and yin and yang under the guidance of Chinese medicine theory.

Meridians and collaterals are the channels for the whole body to move qi and blood, and the network system for the body to obtain nutrients. Among the 14 meridians, there are 6 meridians running in the abdomen, namely Conception vessel, kidney meridian of Foot-Shaoyin, stomach meridian of Foot-Yangming, spleen meridian of Foot-Taiyin, liver meridian of Foot-Jueyin, and gallbladder meridian of Foot-Shaoyang; 12 divergent meridians are connected with viscera through abdomen; the belt vessel is confined to the waist and abdomen, and connected with the Governor vessel and bladder meridian of the back; the thoroughfare vessel, Yin Link vessel and Yin Heel vessel also move in front of the abdomen. Therefore, the meridians system along the abdomen provides a variety of connections for the transportation of qi and blood to the whole body, it also provides a theoretical basis for abdominal acupuncture therapy in the umbilical cord-centered regulatory system.

Clinical studies have found that shallow needling at abdominal acupoints mainly affects the peripheral system, including the deep and superficial arteries and veins of the abdominal wall, the abdominal segment and cutaneous branches of lymphatic vessels and spinal nerves, as well as some other tissues of the abdominal wall layer; when deep needling at abdominal acupoints, it directly affects the visceral nerve and peripheral nerve tissue in the body cavity, stimulate the visceral nerve and its surrounding tissue in the abdominal cavity, cause the corresponding visceral system and stress response, and thus play a therapeutic effect.

The existence of local parts in organisms is the microcosm of the whole world, and to a certain extent can reproduce the rule of the whole image, which is called the theory of biological holography. The abdominal acupuncture method conforms to the modern theory of biological holographic, that is, any part or specific part of the human body can completely reflect the whole information of the human body, showing the holographic correspondence between parts and parts of the human body and between parts and the whole. The local acupoints reflect the physiological and pathological information of the whole body and organs. Therefore, when a certain organ or part is ill, the

第八章　腹　针　法

腹针法是在中医理论指导下，通过针刺腹部特定穴位以调整脏腑、经络、气血、阴阳的平衡，从而治疗全身性疾病的一种疗法。

经络是全身运行气血的通道，是人体获得营养物质的网络系统。十四经中有6条经脉循行于腹部，即任脉、足少阴肾经、足阳明胃经、足太阴脾经、足厥阴肝经、足少阳胆经；十二经别从腹部经过与脏腑相联系；带脉约束于腰腹部，与背部的督脉、膀胱经相连；冲脉、阴跷脉、阴维脉亦行于小腹或腹前。腹部循行的经络系统为气血向全身输布提供了多种联系，也为以脐为中心的调控系统的腹针疗法提供了理论基础。

有研究认为，浅刺腹部穴位主要影响外围系统，包括腹壁的深浅动静脉、淋巴管和脊神经的腹区段及皮支，以及腹部壁层的一些其他组织；深刺腹部穴位可直接影响体腔的内脏神经及周围神经组织，引起相应内脏系统的应激反应，从而起到治疗作用。

生物体内存在的局部是全局的缩影，并且在一定程度上可再现整体之象的规律，这一规律被称为生物全息律。腹针法符合现代生物全息理论，即人体部分与部分、部分与整体之间的全息对应性。局部穴位反映人体整体和器官的生理以及病理信息，当某一器官或部位出现病变时，相对应的局部穴位会有反应，根据这些反应可进行全息诊断、治疗和预防。由上可

corresponding local acupoints will have reactions, which can be used for holographic diagnosis, treatment and prevention. From above, abdominal acupuncture therapy is closely related to meridian system, nervous system and the theory of biological holography.

1. Stimulating region of abdominal acupuncture

1.1 Abdominal surface division

In order to describe the position of abdominal organs and touch the body surface, the front of abdomen was divided into three parts and nine zones with two horizontal lines and two vertical lines. The upper horizontal line is the line through the lowest point of the rib arches on both sides. The lower horizontal line is the line connecting the highest points of the iliac crest on both sides. The two longitudinal lines are the vertical lines made by the midpoint of the two inguinal ligaments. Two horizontal lines divide the abdomen into three parts: upper abdomen, middle abdomen and lower abdomen. Four lines intersect and divide the abdomen into nine zones. The upper part of the abdomen is divided into the middle upper part of the abdomen and the left and right costal zones on both sides; the middle part of the abdomen is divided into the middle umbilicus zone and the left and right ventrolateral zones on both sides; the lower part of the abdomen is divided into the middle pubic zone(hypogastric zone) and the left and right inguinal zones(iliac zone) on both sides.

In clinical, sometimes with the umbilicus as the "O" point of the horizontal and vertical axis, the anterior abdominal wall is divided into four zones: upper left, upper right, lower left and lower right, which are called the upper left abdomen, upper right abdomen, lower left abdomen and lower right abdomen.

1.2 Take Shenque(CV8) as the core holographic image

The abdominal acupuncture theory holds that the meridian of the abdomen is a multi-layered spatial structure, and that the hologram of the human body in the abdomen resembles a turtle lying on the front abdominal wall. The central part is Shenque (CV8), the head part is Zhongwan(CV12), and the tail is Guanyuan (CV4). The side extending from the center to the left and right are two sides of Daheng(SP15). The neck protrudes from the Shangqu (KI17) of both sides; its head lies up and down near Zhongwan (CV12); the tail extends downward from two Qipang points(5-fen of beside CV6) to the vicinity of Guanyuan(CV4); the forelimbs are led out from the ST24(shoulder), respectively, flexing at the upper rheumatic point(elbow) and ending at the external rheumatic point (upper rheumatic point, located at the upper 5-fen outside the ST24, upper rheumatic external point(wrist), located at the 1 cun

见,腹针疗法与经络系统、神经系统和生物全息论都有着密切关系。

一、刺激部位

(一)腹部体表分区

腹部以 2 条水平线和 2 条垂直线划分成 3 部 9 区。上横线是通过两侧肋弓最低点的连线,下横线是两侧髂嵴最高点的连线,2 条纵线是左、右两侧腹股沟韧带中点所作的垂直线。2 条水平线将腹部分为腹上、腹中和腹下 3 部,4 条线相交将腹部分为 9 区:腹上部分为中间的腹上区和两侧的左、右季肋区;腹中部分为中间的脐区和两侧的左、右腹外侧区;腹下部分为中间的耻区(腹下区)和两侧的左、右腹股沟区(髂区)。

在临床上,有时以脐为坐标横轴与纵轴的交点(原点),将前腹壁分为左上、右上、左下、右下 4 个区,称为左上腹、右上腹、左下腹、右下腹。

(二)以脐为核心的全息影像

腹针理论认为腹部的经络是一个多层次的空间结构,人体在腹部的全息影像酷似一个伏在前腹壁上的神龟。中心部位是神阙穴,头顶部是中脘穴,尾部是关元穴,中心部向左右延伸的边端是大横穴。其颈部从两个商曲穴处伸出,其头部伏于中脘穴上下,尾部从两个气旁穴(位于气海旁开 5 分)处向下延伸至关元穴附近。其前肢分别由滑肉门穴肩部引出,在上风湿点(位于滑肉门穴向外向上 5分)屈曲,止于上风湿外点(位于滑肉门穴外 1 寸),其后肢分别由外

outside the ST24). The hind limbs are divided into lower rheumatic point(knee)from ST26(hip) outwards and downward 5 fen, and the lower rheumatic point is 1-cun outwards to ST27(ankle, extending outwards and ending at the lower rheumatic point (1-cun downwards and 1-cun outwards from ST26). In the thick abdominal wall cover tissue, this image is distributed in the shallow layer of the abdominal wall, forming the main body of the circumference adjustment system of the Shenque control system, and the abdominal positioning acuity method is mainly to regulate the corresponding parts of the human body, therefore, the abdominal positioning method is characterized by the biological hologram of the turtle in the abdomen.

2. The positioning of abdominal acupuncture

According to the holographic distribution characteristics of the abdomen, the positioning of the abdominal acupuncture has the following characteristics. ① The acupoints in the upper abdomen can treat the diseases of head, face, neck, shoulder, upper limb and hand, and the acupoints in the lower abdomen can treat the diseases of lumbosacral portion, knee joint and foot according to the different parts. ② In the treatment of head diseases, the acupoints around Zhongwan(CV12) and Yindu(KI19) are the main points. The neck of abdominal holography extends from Shangqu(KI17), so the treatment of neck diseases is to take Shangqu (KI17), Shiguan(KI18) and nearby acupoints. ③ The abdomen holographic forelegs represent the corresponding upper limbs of the human body, so the treatment of the diseases of the left and right upper limbs is to take the acupoints from Huaroumen(ST24) to the upper rheumatic point, and the same side acupoints between the upper rheumatic external points for treatment; The lower limbs of abdominal holography extend from Wailing (ST26) to the lower part corresponding to the lower limbs of human body, so the corresponding acupoints between Wailing (ST26) to lower rheumatic point, and lower rheumatic lower point are taken for treatment of the diseases of lower limbs. The lumbosacral part of abdominal holography starts from the Qipang points and ends near Guanyuan(CV4), so the disease of lumbar spine is treated by the nearby acupoints(Tab. 8-1.).

陵穴引出,向外伸展于下风湿点(位于外陵穴向外向下 5 分),止于下风湿下点(大巨穴向外 1 寸)。在厚厚的腹壁覆被组织中,这一影像分布于腹壁的浅层,构成了神阙调控系统中外周调节系统的主体,而腹部定位取穴法又主要是调节与人体相对应的部位,因此,腹部定位取穴法以腹部的神龟生物全息影像为特征。

二、定位取穴

根据腹部的全息分布特点,腹针法的定位取穴有以下特点:①腹上部的经穴根据所在部位不同,可分别治疗头、面、颈、肩、上肢及手部的疾病;腹下部的经穴根据所在部位不同,可分别治疗腰骶部、膝关节及足部的疾病。②治疗头部疾病时以中脘、阴都及周围的穴位为主;腹全息图的颈部由商曲穴处伸出,故治疗颈部的疾病以商曲、石关及附近的穴位为主。③腹全息图的前肢代表人体相应的上肢,故治疗左右上肢的疾病选取由滑肉门至上风湿点、上风湿外点之间的同侧穴位进行治疗;腹全息图的后肢由外陵穴向外下方伸展与人体的下肢相应,故治疗下肢疾病选取外陵至下风湿点、下风湿下点之间的相应穴位进行治疗。腹全息图的腰骶部起于气旁终于关元穴附近,故腰椎的疾病选取其附近的穴位进行治疗(表 8-1)。

Tab. 8-1　Abdominal acupuncture acupoints corresponding to body parts(表 8-1　腹针定位取穴表)

Diseased site (患病部位)	Acupoint selection (穴位选择)
Head (头部)	Zhongwan(CV12), Yindu(KI19) and adjacent acupoints (中脘、阴都及邻近穴位)
Neck (颈部)	Shangqu(KI17), Shiguan(KI18) and adjacent acupoints (商曲、石关及邻近穴位)

续表

Diseased site （患病部位）	Acupoint selection （穴位选择）
Upper limbs （上肢）	Huaroumen(ST24) to the upper rheumatic point, and the same side acupoints between the upper rheumatic external points （滑肉门至上风湿点、上风湿外点之间的同侧穴位）
Lower limbs （下肢）	Wailing(ST26) to the lower rheumatic point, and the same side acupoints between the lower rheumatic lower points （外陵至下风湿点、下风湿下点之间的相应穴位）
Lumbosacral part （腰椎）	Points near lumbosacral, Qihai(CV6), Guanyuan(CV4) and adjacent points （腰骶部邻近穴位，气旁、关元及邻近穴位）

Acupoint selection in eight contour profiles is another important feature of the abdominal acupuncture acupoint selection method. Acupoint selection in eight contour profiles are the method of combining Zhouyi gossip with the five elements to dialectically select acupoints in the abdomen. When positioning in the abdomen, taking Shenque(CV8) as the center, divide the abdomen into eight equal parts. For memory convenience, take an acupoint as the core to represent a contour profile. For example, Zhongwan(CV12) is the fire(Li), which is the main part of heart and small intestine; Guanyuan(CV4) is the water (Kan), which is the main part of kidney and bladder; the left upper rheumatic point is the land (Kun), which is the main part of spleen and stomach; the left Daheng(SP15) is the Ze(Dui), which is the main part of lower jiao; the left lower rheumatic point is the sky(Qian), which is the main part of lung and large intestine; the right upper rheumatic point is the wind(Xun), which is the main part of liver and middle jiao; the right Daheng(SP15) is the thunder(Zhen), which is the main part of liver and gallbladder; the right lower rheumatic point is the mountain(Gen), which is the main part of upper jiao. The acupoints in each of the eight contour profiles have a specific therapeutic effect on the main viscera and play an important role in regulating the balance of the viscera.

八廓取穴是腹针定位取穴法的另一个重要特点。八廓取穴是将周易八卦与五行相结合，在腹部进行辨证选穴的方法。在腹部八廓定位时，以神阙为中心将腹部分成大致相等的八个部位。为记忆方便各以一个穴位为核心代表一个部位，如中脘为火，为离，主心与小肠；关元为水，为坎，主肾与膀胱；左上风湿点为地，为坤，主脾胃；左大横为泽，为兑，主下焦；左下风湿点为天，为乾，主肺与大肠；右上风湿点为风，为巽，主肝与中焦；右大横为雷，为震，主肝胆；右下风湿点为山，为艮，主上焦。八廓中每一廓的穴位都对所主脏腑有特定的治疗作用，并对内脏的平衡调节起着重要的作用。

3. Operation technique of abdominal acupuncture

3.1 Preparation before acupuncture

Most patients take supine positions, limbs need to relax, and disinfect acupoint skin routinely.

3.2 Needling instrument selection

(1) Conventional filiform needle.

(2) Professional abdominal needle. Professional abdominal needle can be divided into A, B, and C types. In clinical practice, we should select different types of special abdominal needle according

三、操作技术

（一）针前准备

患者多采取仰卧位，四肢需放松。穴位皮肤常规消毒。

（二）针具选择

（1）常规毫针针具。

（2）腹针专用针具。腹针专用针具一般分 A、B、C 型，临床上可根据疾病的性质选择不同型号。

to the nature of the disease.

• Indications of type A needle: cervical spondylosis, periarthritis of shoulder joint, tennis elbow, carpal tunnel syndrome, lumbar spondylosis, sciatica, osteoarthritis, rheumatic arthritis, rheumatoid arthritis and other painful diseases.

• Indications of type B needle: headache, facial paralysis, upper respiratory tract infection, herpes zoster, allergic asthma, chronic gastritis, chronic pelvic inflammation and other chronic diseases.

• Indications of type C needle: sequelae of cerebrovascular disease, cerebral palsy in children, chronic prostatitis, fundus diseases, senile diseases and other chronic diseases with physical deficiency.

Each type can be divided into three models: Ⅰ, Ⅱ and Ⅲ, which are suitable for obese patients, normal patients and thin patients, respectively.

3.3　Insertion method

Abdominal acupuncture mainly uses skin-spreading needle insertion and finger-press needle insertion, which are basically the same as filiform acupuncture method.

3.4　Needling manipulation

In abdominal acupuncture, the commonly used needling techniques are lifting, inserting and twisting. The abdominal acupuncture is different from the traditional acupuncture, and the operation should be gentle and slow. If the tip reaches the expected depth, the methods of twisting without lifting or inserting and gentle twisting with slow lifting and inserting are generally used. If the effect is not good, the gentle pressing method can be used. This acupuncture method can make the omentum in the abdominal cavity free enough time, avoid the needle body, and avoid stabbing the internal organs.

The indications of abdominal acupuncture are mostly chronic diseases, and chronic diseases can lead to weakness, so most of the abdominal acupuncture operations were reinforcing method. In addition to the manipulation, moxibustion is often used. During moxibustion, warm moxibustion can be performed at each acupuncture acupoint from top to bottom, or moxibustion frame can be placed at Shenque to strengthen vital yang and warm meridians, so as to improve the therapeutic effect of abdominal acupuncture.

3.5　Needle retaining

The retention time of abdominal acupuncture is generally 20-30 minutes. For patients with short course and poor body constitution, the retention time of needle is slightly shorter; for patients with

A型适应证：颈椎病、肩周炎、网球肘、腕管综合征、腰椎病、坐骨神经痛、骨关节病、风湿性关节炎、类风湿性关节炎等疼痛性疾病。

B型适应证：头痛、面神经麻痹、上呼吸道感染、带状疱疹、变应性哮喘、慢性胃炎、慢性盆腔炎等各种慢性疾病。

C型适应证：脑血管病后遗症、小儿脑瘫、慢性前列腺炎、眼底病、老年病等各种体质虚弱的慢性疾病。

每种型号根据针具的不同长度又分为Ⅰ、Ⅱ、Ⅲ三种类型，分别适用于比较肥胖的患者、正常体型的患者和比较消瘦的患者。

（三）进针方法

主要使用舒张进针法和指切进针法，与毫针操作基本相同。

（四）行针方法

一般采用只捻转不提插或轻捻转慢提插的手法，重在轻、缓，如疗效不佳，可采用轻压法。这种手法可使腹腔内网膜有足够的时间游离，避开针体，以避免刺伤内脏。

腹针的适应证以慢性疾病为主，而慢性疾病患者又久病则虚，故腹针操作时补多泻少。并多配灸法，灸时可由上而下地对相应穴位施以温和灸，也可以将艾灸架置于神阙穴，以壮元阳、温经络，进而提高腹针疗效。

（五）留针方法

留针时间一般为20～30分钟。对于病程短和体质较差的患者主张留针时间偏短，对于病程长

long course and better body constitution, the retention time of needle is relatively longer.

3.6 Withdraw the needle

When withdrawing the needle, twist the needle slowly according to the order of inserting the needle. It is not allowed to prick the needle deeply first and then withdraw the needle.

4. Clinical application of abdominal acupuncture

4.1 Scope of application

The indications of abdominal acupuncture are mostly disorder of internal organs diseases or chronic diseases. Clinically, it can be roughly divided into the followings.

（1）Systemic diseases with long course of internal injury, such as sequelae of cerebrovascular disease, dementia, cerebral arteriosclerosis, cardiovascular disease, hypertension, and hysteria.

（2）Diseases caused by imbalance of Zang-Fu organs, such as insomnia, constipation, senile kidney deficiency and frequency urination, headache, and vertigo.

（3）The course of the disease is short, but the diseases related to the deficiency of vital energy in viscera, such as periarthritis of shoulder, sciatica, arthritis, diseases of cervical vertebra and lumbar vertebrae, and tennis elbow.

（4）Other indications of acupuncture and moxibustion, with poor efficacy after treatment, can be abdominal acupuncture indications.

4.2 Principle of acupoint selection by prescription

The commonly used basic prescription combinations of abdominal acupuncture are heaven and earth needle, drawing qi to its origin, abdominal Siguan, regulate spleen and rheumatic points.

（1）Heaven and earth needle.

Composition: Zhongwan(CV12) and Guanyuan(CV4).

Function: Tonifying the spleen and kidney.

（2）Drawing qi to its origin.

Composition: Zhongwan(CV12), Xiawan(CV10), Qihai(CV6) and Guanyuan(CV4).

Function: To treat heart and lung, regulate spleen and stomach, tonify liver and kidney.

（3）Abdominal Siguan.

Composition: Huaroumen(ST24) and Wailing(ST26).

Function: Regulate qi and blood, dredge meridians, guide the qi of the viscera to the whole body.

（4）Regulate spleen.

Composition: Daheng(SP15).

和体质较好的患者主张留针时间偏久。

（六）出针方法

出针时按照进针的顺序缓慢捻转出针,不允许先向内深刺然后出针的操作。

四、临床应用

（一）适应范围

腹针的适应证以内伤性疾病或慢性疾病为主。包括:①病程较久的内伤脏腑的全身性疾病,如脑血管病后遗症、痴呆,脑动脉硬化、心血管疾病、高血压、癔症等;②脏腑失衡后引起的疾病,如失眠、便秘、老年肾虚尿频、头痛、眩晕等;③虽病程较短,但与脏腑正气不足相关的疾病,如肩周炎、坐骨神经痛、关节炎、颈椎腰椎疾病、网球肘等;④其他的针灸适应证,经治疗疗效不佳者,均可为腹针适应证。

（二）基本处方

常用的腹针基本处方主要有天地针、引气归元、腹四关、调脾气、风湿点等组合。

1. 天地针

组成:中脘、关元。

功能:补脾肾。

2. 引气归元

组成:中脘、下脘、气海、关元。

功能:治心肺、调脾胃、补肝肾。

3. 腹四关

组成:滑肉门、外陵。

功能:通调气血,疏理经气,引脏腑之气向全身布散。

4. 调脾气

组成:大横。

Function: Regulate spleen function, remove dampness, strengthen spleen and smooth joints. It is often used to treat waist diseases and sciatica with abdominal Siguan, and to treat systemic arthritis or periarthritis of shoulder with rheumatic points.

(5) Rheumatic points.

Composition: Upper rheumatic point and lower rheumatic point.

Function: Combined with Daheng(SP15), it can dispel wind, smooth joints, reduce swelling and pain, and disperse blood stasis. Upper rheumatic points can be used in the treatment of shoulder and elbow diseases; lower rheumatic points can be used in the treatment of lower extremity diseases.

4.3　Prescription example

(1) Neck stiffness.

Acupoint selection: Zhongwan (CV12), KI17 (affected side, shallow), ST24(affected side).

Addition and subtraction: Bilateral neck pain, Shangqu(KI17) (bilateral, shallow), Huaroumen (ST24) (bilateral); posterior middle neck pain, Xiawan (CV10) (shallow), Shangqu (KI17) (bilateral, shallow).

(2) Scapulohumeral periarthritis of shoulder joint.

Main acupoint: Zhongwan(CV12).

Auxiliary acupoints: Shangqu (KI17) (healthy side), Huaroumen(ST24) triangle(affected side, shallow).

Addition and subtraction: When the range of shoulder pain is large, the triangle distance with Huaroumen(ST24) as the vertex is slightly longer(affected side); the range of shoulder pain is shorter, the triangle distance with Huaroumen (ST24) as the vertex is slightly shorter.

(3) Lumbar disc herniation.

Main acupoints: Qihai(CV6), Guanyuan(CV4).

Auxiliary acupoint: Shuifen(CV9).

Addition and subtraction: For acute lumbar disc herniation, Renzhong(GV26) and Yintang(GV29). Antiquated lumbar disc herniation, choose Qixue(KI13)(bilateral). Mainly low back pain, choose Wailing(ST26)(bilateral), Qixue(KI13)(bilateral), Siman (KI14) (bilateral), when low back pain with sciatica, combined Qipang points(contralateral), Wailing(ST26)(affected side), lower rheumatic point(affected side)and lower point of lower rheumatism (affected side).

(4) Headache.

Acupoint selection: Zhongwan(CV12), Yindu(KI19).

Addition and subtraction: Headache due to external pathogenic factors, Quchi(LI11) or bleeding at twelve jing-well points. Blood

功能:调脾健脾、祛风湿、利关节。常与腹四关合用治疗腰部疾病和坐骨神经痛;与风湿点合用治疗全身关节炎或肩周炎等症。

5. 风湿点

组成:上风湿点、下风湿点。

功能:与大横合用可加强祛风湿、利关节、消肿痛、散瘀血之效。治疗肩、肘疾病时可仅用上风湿点,治疗下肢疾病时可仅配下风湿点。

(三) 处方示例

1. 落枕

取穴:中脘、商曲(患,浅)、滑肉门(患)。

加减:颈项双侧疼痛,商曲(双、浅)、滑肉门(双);颈项后正中疼痛,下脘(浅)、商曲(双、浅)。

2. 肩周炎

主穴:中脘。

辅穴:商曲(健)、滑肉门三角(患、浅)。

加减:肩部疼痛的范围较大时以滑肉门为顶点的三角取穴距离略长(患);肩部疼痛的范围较局限时以滑肉门为顶点的三角取穴距离缩短。

3. 腰椎间盘突出症

主穴:气海、关元。

辅穴:水分。

加减:急性腰椎间盘突出症加人中、印堂;陈旧性腰椎间盘突出症加气穴(双);腰痛甚者加外陵(双)、气穴(双)、四满(双);合并坐骨神经痛加气旁(对侧)、外陵(患侧)、下风湿点(患侧)、下风湿下点(患侧)。

4. 头痛

取穴:中脘、阴都。

加减:外感头痛加曲池或十二井放血;血虚头痛加气海、天枢

deficiency headache,Qihai(CV6),Tianshu(ST25)(bilateral);blood stasis headache,Qihai(CV6),Guanyuan(CV4),Huaroumen(ST24)(double).

（5）Pain of elbow and wrist.

Acupoint selection：Zhongwan（CV12），Huaroumen（ST24）（affected side），upper rheumatic point（affected side），Shangqu（KI17）（healthy side）.

Addition and subtraction：Severe elbow pain plus upper rheumatic point triangle(affected side). Pain on the thumb side of wrist plus Lieque(LU7)(affected side). Pain in the middle of the wrist plus Waiguan(TE5).

4.4　Precautions

The stimulating part of abdominal acupuncture is abdomen,so some abdominal diseases should not use abdominal acupuncture.

（1）All acute abdomen with unknown causes is contraindications to avoid misdiagnosis due to acupuncture.

（2）Abdominal acupuncture cannot be used in patients with acute peritonitis,umbilical varices caused by hepatosplenomegaly,intra-abdominal tumor and extensive metastasis.

（3）Pregnant women should not use abdominal acupuncture,especially in pregnancy more than 28 weeks.

（4）Abdominal acupuncture should not be used in the site of broken skin and ulcers.

（5）For the patients who are weak due to long-term chronic diseases,acupuncturist should also be cautious during operation.

（6）Treatment should be carried out half an hour after meals,and patients should drain the stool before treatment.

（双）；瘀血头痛加气海、关元、滑肉门（双）。

5. 肘、腕痛

取穴：中脘、滑肉门（患侧）、上风湿点（患侧）、商曲（健侧）。

加减：肘痛较剧加上风湿点三角（患侧）；腕部拇指侧疼痛加列缺（患侧）；腕部正中疼痛加外关。

（四）注意事项

腹部是腹针法的主要刺激部位，某些腹部疾病应该禁用腹针。包括以下几点。

（1）一切原因不明的急腹症均为禁忌证，以免因针刺而引起误诊。

（2）急性腹膜炎、肝脾肿大引起的脐静脉曲张，腹腔内部肿瘤并广泛转移者禁用。

（3）孕妇不宜采用腹针法，尤其孕期28周以上者禁用。

（4）针刺部位有皮肤破损及溃疡者不宜用腹针疗法。

（5）对长期慢性疾病而致体质虚弱的患者，在施术时亦须谨慎处理。

（6）饭后半小时方可进行治疗，治疗应排空大小便。

Chapter 9　Three-Edged Needle Therapy

The three-edged needle, known as the "sharp needle" in ancient times. The three-edged needle therapy is a method of puncturing the selected site to bleed with a three-edged needle to treat diseases, known as puncturing collateral therapy in the ancient time and bleeding therapy in the recent time.

The ancients attached great importance to the three-edged needle therapy. For example, *Miraculous Pivot—Theory of Nine Classical Needles* referred that the lance needle is mainly used for "removing pathogenic heat by bleeding". *Plain Questions—Blood and Qi*, *Physical Appearance and Mind* illustrated, "Whenever one treats the disease, one must first remove their blood." *Miraculous Pivot—Nine Needles and Twelve Source* put forward the therapeutic principle of "what has accumulated over an extended period of time, that is to be discarded". There are many methods in *Miraculous Pivot—Official Acupuncture*, such as "collateral needling" "repeated shallow needling" and "leopard-spot needling". Although there are different needle tools and methods, they all belong to the category of three-edged needle therapy. *Miraculous Pivot—The Theory of Pivot Blood Collateral* further clarified the application scope of three-edged needle therapy by the discription that "when the blood vessels are filled to abundance, when they run hard across and are of red color... with the small ones being thin like a needle, and the big ones resembling a sinew" and pointed that only when there was obvious blood stasis could the use of a drainage result in a cure in myriad cases. It can be seen that the ancients have rich experience in three-edged needle therapy.

1.　Needle instrument

The three-edged needle presently made of stainless steel. It can be divided into three types: large, medium and small. Large size is 2.6 mm × 65 mm, medium size is 2 mm × 65 mm, and small size is 1.6 mm × 65 mm. The handle of the needle is thick and cylindrical, the shaft of the needle is triangular, and the tip of the needle with three edges is sharp(Fig. 9-1).

2.　Operation method

2.1　Preparation before operation

The needle should be sterilized by high pressure steam before use or soaked in 75% ethanol for 30 minutes. The local skin should

第九章　三棱针法

三棱针法也称刺络泻血法,是用三棱针刺破血络或腧穴,放出适量血液或挤出少量液体,或挑断皮下纤维组织,以治疗疾病的方法。其中放出适量血液以治疗疾病的方法属刺络法或刺血法,又称放血疗法。此法来源于古代九针之一的"锋针"。

古人对三棱针法非常重视。如《灵枢·九针论》谈到九针中的锋针主要用于"泻热出血"。《素问·血气形志》曰:"凡治病必先去其血。"《灵枢·九针十二原》提出了"宛陈则除之"的治疗原则。《灵枢·官针》中有"络刺""赞刺""豹文刺"等方法,虽针具和方法不尽相同,但都属于三棱针法的范畴。《灵枢·血络论》进一步阐明了三棱针法的应用范畴,如"血脉者,盛坚横以赤……小者如针""大者如筋"等,并指出有明显瘀血现象的才能"泻之万全",可见古人对三棱针法是有丰富经验的。

一、针具

三棱针一般用不锈钢制成,分为大、中、小3种型号,大号规格2.6 mm×65 mm,中号规格2 mm×65 mm,小号规格1.6 mm×65 mm,针柄较粗呈圆柱形,针身呈三棱形,尖端三面有刃,针尖锋利(图9-1)。

二、操作方法

(一)操作前准备

针具使用前应进行高压消毒,或放入75%酒精内浸泡30分钟。

be disinfected with 2％ tincture of iodine and then deiodinated with 75％ alcohol cotton before insertion.

2.2 Needle-holding posture

Generally, hold the middle part of the handle with the thumb and index finger of the right hand, and the belly of the middle finger is close to the side of the needle body, exposing the tip of the needle for 2-3 mm(Fig. 9-2).

施针前在局部皮肤用 2％碘伏进行消毒,再用 75％酒精脱碘。

（二）持针姿势

一般以右手持针,用拇指、食指捏住针柄中段,中指指腹紧靠针身侧面,露出针尖 2～3 mm（图 9-2）。

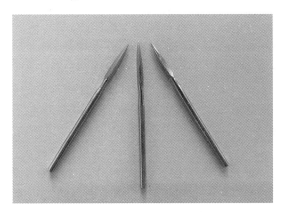

图 9-1 三棱针针具

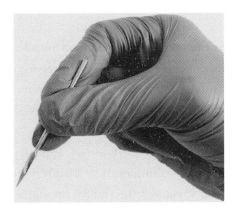

图 9-2 持针法

2.3 Manipulation

The operation methods of the three-edged needle are generally divided into four kinds: spot needling, collateral needling, scattered needling and piercing method.

（1）Spot needling method. Pinch and press the area to be treated to cause localized congestion. Sterilize the area with 2％ tincture of iodine and then with 75％ alcohol-soaked cotton balls. Prick the area with the three-edged needle swiftly to a depth of 2-3 mm with the needling hand and withdraw the needle immediately. Squeeze and press around the pinprick to discharge a few drops of blood and then compress the pinhole with a dry sterilized cotton ball to stop the bleeding. This method is mainly used on points at the end of four extremities, face and ear, such as Shixuan（EX-UE11）, the twelve Jing-Well Points(Fig. 9-3).

（三）操作方法

三棱针的操作方法一般分为点刺法、刺络法、散刺法、挑治法 4 种。

1. 点刺法 即点刺腧穴出血或挤出少量液体的方法。此法是用三棱针点刺腧穴或血络以治疗疾病的方法。

针刺前,医者在预定针刺部位上下用左手拇指、食指向针刺处推按,使血液积聚于点刺部位。常规消毒后,医者左手拇指、食指、中指夹紧被刺部位,右手持针,直刺 2～3 mm,快进快出,轻轻挤压针孔周围,使出血数滴,或挤出少量液体。然后用消毒干棉球按压针孔。为了刺出一定量的血液或液体,点刺穴位的深度不宜太浅。此法多用于指趾末端、面部、耳部的穴位,如十宣、十二井穴等处（图 9-3）。

（2）Collateral needling. Including superficial needling and deep needling.

①Superficial needling. The method is used in superficial venules that appear with the diseases to cause bleeding by puncturing. After routine disinfection, the needling hand holds the

2. 刺络法 有浅刺和深刺两种。

（1）浅刺:点刺随病显现的浅表小静脉使其出血的方法。常规消毒后,医者持针垂直点刺,快进

needle to prick vertically, fast in and fast out, and the movement is required to be stable, accurate and quick. One bleeding was 5-10 mL. This method is often used in the areas with venules, such as the back of lower limbs, forehead, temporal area, and dorsum of feet.

②Deep needling. The method is used in deep and large veins to release a certain amount of blood. It's called bloodletting as well. First, ligate the upper end(near the heart) of the acupuncture site with a belt or rubber tube, and then sterilize it quickly. When puncturing, press with thumb of pressing hand on the lower end of the acupuncture site, hold the three-edged needle with the needling hand to aim at the vein of the acupuncture site, stab the vein 1-2 mm deep, and the needle exits quickly. After the bleeding stops, press the pinhole with a sterile cotton ball. This method has a large amount of bleeding. A single treatment can bleed tens or even hundreds of milliliters. It is mainly used in the vein of elbow and popliteal fossa and the small vein stasis(Fig. 9-4).

快出,动作要求稳、准、快。一次出血5～10 mL。此法多用于有小静脉显现的部位,如下肢背面、额部、颞部、足背等部位。

(2)深刺:点刺较深、较大静脉放出一定量血液的方法,称为泻血法。先用带子或橡皮管结扎在针刺部位上端(近心端),然后迅速消毒针刺部位皮肤,针刺时医者左手拇指压在被针刺部位下端,右手持三棱针对准被针刺部位的静脉,刺入静脉1～2 mm深即将针迅速退出,出血停止后,再用消毒棉球按压针孔。本法出血量较大,一次治疗可出血几十甚至上百毫升,多用于肘窝、腘窝的静脉及小静脉瘀滞处(图9-4)。

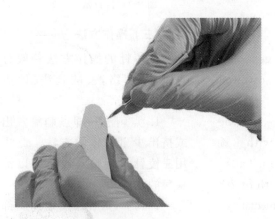

图9-3 点刺法

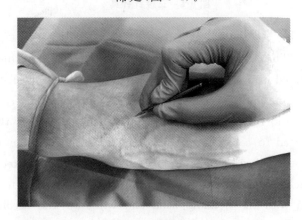

图9-4 刺络法

(3) Scattered needling method. This method is used to prick around the affected area(Fig. 9-5). In clinical practice, one area may be pricked in more than 10 spots. The pricking is conducted from the outside to the center in a circular manner. It is mainly used to treat local blood stasis, hematomas, edema and stubborn tinea.

3. 散刺法 医者用一手固定被刺部位,另一手持针在施术部位点刺多处(图9-5)。根据病变部位大小不同,可刺数针,甚至十余针,由病变外缘环形向中心点刺,以促使瘀血或水肿的排泄,达到"宛陈则除之"、通经活络的目的。针刺深度根据局部肌肉厚薄、血管深浅而定。此法多用于局部瘀血、水肿、顽癣等。

(4) Piercing method. This method uses a three-edged needle to break the subcutaneous fibrous tissue of acupoints to treat diseases. After local disinfection, the doctor pinches the skin of the operation parts with the left hand, pricks the skin with the needle in the right hand at an angle of 15°-30°, and then picks up the

4. 挑治法 此法是以三棱针挑断穴位皮下纤维组织以治疗疾病的方法。局部消毒后,医者左手捏起施术部位皮肤,右手持针先以15°～30°角进入皮肤,然后上挑针

needle tip to break the skin or subcutaneous tissue, squeezes out a certain amount of liquid or blood, and then protects the wound with a sterile dressing(Fig. 9-6). For those who are afraid of pain, local anesthesia with 2% lidocaine can be used before pricking. Pricking parts can choose meridians and acupoints, extra-points and Ashi acupoints. When selecting the positive reaction point, we should pay attention to distinguish it from nevus, folliculitis, pigmented spot and Back-Shu point.

尖,挑破皮肤或皮下组织,并可挤出一定量的血液或少量液体,然后用无菌敷料保护创口,以胶布固定(图 9-6)。对于一些畏惧疼痛者,可先用 2% 利多卡因局麻后再挑刺。挑刺的部位可以选用经穴,也可选用奇穴,多选用阿是穴。在选用阳性反应点时,应注意与痣、毛囊炎、色素斑及背俞穴相鉴别。

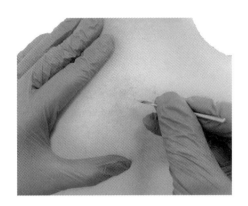

图 9-5 散刺法

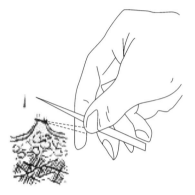

图 9-6 挑治法

3. Clinical application

3.1 Scope of application

Three-edged needle therapy may unblock the meridian and free the collateral vessels, open the orifices to clear heat, disperse swelling and relieve pain.

It is widely applied in clinical practice especially for excesses, heat conditions, blood stasis, and pain. At present, it is commonly used for many acute diseases, such as fainting, high fever, apoplexy with blocking syndrome, acute pharyngitis, heatstroke, etc. And it is also suitable for several chronic diseases, such as stubborn tinea, sprains, headache, scapulohumeral periarthritis, erysipelas, numbness in the extremities, etc.

3.2 Precautions

(1) The three-edged needle therapy may induce a strong reaction, thus an adequate explanation to the recipient is necessary before starting the technique in order to disperse any worries on behalf of the patient.

(2) Strict disinfection should be carried out to prevent infection.

(3) The pricking should be done superficially, quickly and accurately. Be sure not to injure the arteries and other tissues.

三、临床应用

(一) 适应范围

三棱针刺络放血具有通经活络、开窍泻热、消肿止痛等作用,适应范围较为广泛,凡各种实证、热证、瘀血、疼痛等均可应用。

目前较常用于急症,如昏厥、高热、中风闭证、急性咽喉肿痛、中暑等;某些慢性疾病,如顽癣、扭挫伤、头痛、肩周炎、丹毒、指(趾)麻木等。

(二) 注意事项

(1) 对患者要做必要的解释工作,以消除其思想顾虑,尤其是对放血量较大者。

(2) 严格消毒,防止感染。

(3) 操作时手法宜轻、稳、准、快,不可用力过猛,防止刺入过深、创伤过大,损害其他组织,更不可伤及动脉。

(4) This method should not be used in patients with a weak constitution, anemia, hypotension, pregnant or postpartum women, or patients with hemorrhagic diseases.

(5) This therapy is usually performed once every 2-3 days, and the patients with more bleeding can be treated once every 1-2 weeks.

（4）对体弱、贫血、低血压,妇女怀孕和产后等,均要慎重使用。凡有出血倾向和血管瘤的患者,不宜使用本法。

（5）刺血治疗一般隔2~3天1次,出血量较多者可间隔1~2周1次。

Chapter 10　Dermal Needle Therapy

Dermal needle therapy is used to prick some parts(acupoints) of human body superficially with a specialized dermal needle that with several short needles. It originates from the ancient needling techniques of "half needling""skin needling" and "shallow surround needling". As *Miraculous Pivot—The Official Acupuncture* said, half needling meant that the insertion was superficial, and the needle was withdrawn quickly, as if one were to pluck a hair without doing harm to the flesh. Skin needling is to be pierced at the surface in the skin. As for shallow surround needling, there are five needles, one〔needle〕is to be inserted straight〔into the location of the disease〕, and four〔needles〕are to be inserted sideways, and superficially. This serves to cure massively pounding cold qi. By tapping and pricking the skin, this therapy can unblock the meridians, free the collaterals, balance qi and blood and promote the functions of body to recover, so as to prevent or treat diseases.

1. Needle instrument

Dermal needle is a kind of needle with small hammer shape. Generally, the handle of the needle is 15-19 cm long, with a lotus shaped needle disk at one end and a stainless-steel short needle embedded at the bottom. There are two types of needle handle: soft handle and hard handle. Soft handle is generally made of plexiglass or hard plastic. According to the number of inserted needles, they are also called plum-blossom needles (five needles), seven-star needles (seven needles) (Fig. 10-1), Luohan needles (eighteen needles), etc. The needle tip should not be too sharp, but instead in the shape of a loose needle. The handle of the needle should be firm and elastic, and the whole needle tip should be flush to prevent deflection, hook bending, corrosion and defect. For the inspection of the needle, dry absorbent cotton can be used to lightly touch the needle tip. If the needle tip has a hook or a defect, the cotton wool is easy to be driven.

2. Operation method

2.1　Preparation before operation

Sterilize the needle before puncturing. The local skin was disinfected with 2% tincture of iodine and deiodinated with 75% alcohol cotton before insertion.

2.2　Needle-holding posture

The needle-holding posture of soft handle and hard handle skin needles are different, which are described as follows.

第十章　皮肤针法

皮肤针法是以多支短针浅刺人体一定部位(穴位)的一种针刺方法,它是我国古代"半刺""毛刺""扬刺"等针法的发展。《灵枢·官针》曰:"半刺者,浅内而疾发针,无针伤肉,如拔毛状""毛刺者,刺浮痹皮肤也""扬刺者,正内一,旁内四而浮之,以治寒气之博大者也"。皮肤针法通过叩刺皮部,以疏通经络、调和气血,促使机体恢复正常,从而达到防治疾病的目的。

一、针具

皮肤针是针头呈小锤形的一种针具,一般针柄长15～19 cm,一端附有莲蓬状的针盘,下边散嵌着不锈钢短针。针柄有软柄和硬柄两种类型,软柄一般用有机玻璃或硬塑料制作。根据所嵌针数的不同,又分别称为梅花针(五支针)、七星针(七支针)(图10-1)、罗汉针(十八支针)等。针尖不宜太锐,应呈松针形。针柄要坚固具有弹性,全束针尖应平齐,防止偏斜、钩曲、锈蚀和缺损。针具的检查,可用干脱脂棉轻触针尖,如果针尖有钩或有缺损则棉絮易被带动。

二、操作方法

(一) 操作前准备

针刺前将针具灭菌。施针前在局部皮肤用2%碘酊进行消毒,再用75%酒精棉脱碘。

(二) 持针姿势

软柄和硬柄皮肤针的持针姿势不同,分述如下。

(1) Place the end of the handle of the soft handle skin needle in the palm, with the thumb on the top, the index finger on the bottom, and the remaining fingers clenching to fix the end of the handle(Fig. 10-2).

1. 软柄皮肤针　将针柄末端置于掌心，拇指居上，食指在下，余指呈握拳状固定针柄末端（图10-2）。

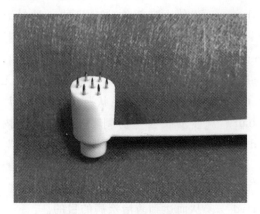

图 10-1　皮肤针针具（七星针）

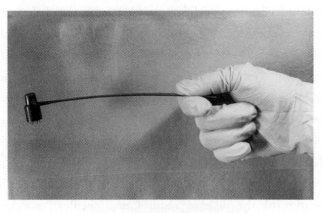

图 10-2　软柄皮肤针持针姿势

(2) Hold the handle of the hard handle skin needle with the right hand, and fix the end of the handle at the small thenar with the ring finger and the little finger. Generally, the end of the handle is exposed 2-5 cm behind the palm of the hand, and the handle is clamped with the thumb and the middle two fingers, and the index finger is placed above the middle part of the handle(Fig. 10-3).

2. 硬柄皮肤针　用右手握针柄，以无名指、小指将针柄末端固定于小鱼际处，一般针柄末端露出手掌后 2～5 cm，以拇指、中指夹持针柄，食指置于针柄中段上面（图10-3）。

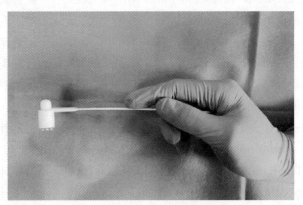

图 10-3　硬柄皮肤针持针姿势

2. 3　Manipulation

After routine skin disinfection, the tip of the needle is aimed at the percussion site, and the flexible wrist force is used to percussion vertically, that is, the tip of the needle is percussed vertically on the skin, and immediately bounced up. When tapping, we should use flexible wrist force to stab directly, elastically and rapidly. The speed of percussion and stabbing should be uniform. The rise and fall of the needle tip should be in a vertical direction, that is, the needle should be stabbed vertically and lifted vertically, and the operation should be repeated. Prevent the needle from entering obliquely and pulling backward to lift the needle, which will

（三）叩刺方法

皮肤常规消毒后，针尖对准叩刺部位，运用灵活的腕力垂直叩刺，将针尖垂直叩击在皮肤上，并立刻弹起，如此反复进行。叩刺时要运用灵活的腕力直刺、弹刺、速刺。叩刺速度要均匀，防止快慢不一、用力不匀地乱刺。针尖起落要成垂直方向，即将针垂直地刺下、垂直地提起，如此反复操作。防止针尖斜着刺入和向后拖拉着起针，

increase the patient's pain. The position of acupuncture should be accurate. The distance between each needle should be 1. 0-1. 5 cm.

2. 4　Stimulus intensity

According to the patient's condition, constitution, age and location of percussion, mild stimulation, moderate stimulation and strong stimulation can be used respectively.

（1）Mild stimulation. Tap the skin gently with the needle using wrist action until the area becomes red and slightly congested, and make sure the patient has no pain. The less time the needle tip contacts the skin, the better. It is suitable for the elderly, the frail, children, newly diagnosed patients, and areas with thin muscles like head, face and facial features.

（2）Moderate stimulation. Tap the skin with a moderate force using wrist action until the area is congested but not bleeding, and the patient may feel a little pain. The intensity of the tapping should be between mild and strong stimulations. This is used mainly for common illnesses or patients with normal constitutions. It is applicable to most patients and most parts of body except for the areas with thin muscles such as head, face and facial features.

（3）Strong stimulation. Tap the skin heavily with the needle using wrist action until the area bleeds slightly. This is applied to young patients with strong constitutions, and areas with strong muscles such as shoulder, back, waist, hip and limbs.

2. 5　Tapping areas

It can be divided into three types: tapping along meridians, around acupoints and around affected areas.

（1）Tapping along the meridian route related to the disease. It is mainly used in the Governor Vessel and Bladder meridian of the neck, back, waist and sacrum, followed by the three yin and three yang channels under the elbow and knee of the limbs. It can be used to treat the pathological changes of viscera and meridians.

（2）Select the disease-related acupoints for percussion. It is mainly used in Back-Shu point, Jiaji（EX-B2）and positive reaction point.

（3）Tapping around the affected area. Such as the treatment for the facial features, joints and local sprains, ringworm and other diseases can be locally tapped and punctured.

这样会增加患者的疼痛。针刺部位须准确，按预定应刺部位下针，每一针之间的距离，一般在 1.0～1.5 cm。

（四）刺激强度

根据患者病情、体质、年龄和叩刺部位的不同，可分别采用弱刺激、中等刺激和强刺激。

1. 弱刺激　用较轻的腕力叩刺，冲力小，针尖接触皮肤的时间越短越好，局部皮肤略见潮红，患者无疼痛感觉。适用于年老体弱、小儿、初诊患者，以及头面五官肌肉浅薄处。

2. 中等刺激　叩刺的腕力介于强、弱刺激之间，冲力中等，局部皮肤潮红，但无出血，患者稍觉疼痛。适用于多数患者，除头面五官等肌肉浅薄处，其他部位均可选用。

3. 强刺激　用较重的腕力叩刺，冲力大，针尖接触皮肤的时间可稍长，局部皮肤可见出血，患者有明显疼痛的感觉。适用于年壮体强，以及肩、背、腰、臀、四肢等肌肉丰厚处。

（五）叩刺部位

可分为循经叩刺、穴位叩刺和局部叩刺 3 种。

1. 循经叩刺　沿着与疾病有关的经脉循行路线叩刺。主要用于项、背、腰、骶部的督脉和膀胱经，其次是四肢肘、膝以下的三阴经、三阳经。可治疗相应脏腑经络病变。

2. 穴位叩刺　选取与疾病相关的穴位叩刺。主要用于背俞穴、夹脊穴和阳性反应点。

3. 局部叩刺　在病变局部叩刺。如治疗头面五官、关节及局部扭伤、顽癣等疾病可叩刺病变局部。

Specific tapping sequences of each part are as follows.

①Head. According to the circulation of Governor Vessel, Bladder meridian and Gallbladder meridian, the head is punctured from the front to the back of Naohu(GV17), Yuzhen(BL9) and Fengchi(GB20). Both sides of the temporal part are tapped from the top to the bottom.

②Posterior neck. Puncture acupoints from Naohu(GV17) to Dazhui(GV14), or from Fengchi(GB20) and Tianzhu(BL10)to both sides of the 6th cervical spine.

③Neck. The first line of the neck should puncture the posterior margin of sternocleidomastoid muscle; the second line of the neck should puncture downward from the anterior margin of sternocleidomastoid muscle; and the third line of the neck should puncture forward from the back of the lower frontal angle.

④Scapula. Firstly, tap the internal edge of the scapula from the top to the bottom, and then the upper edge of the scapula from the inside to the outside, and finally the lower edge of the scapula from the inside to the outside. If it is difficult to lift the arm, you can heavily tap around the shoulder joint at the upper back and the upper front of the armpit.

⑤Dorsal part of spine. In the first row, tap the first lateral line of the Bladder Meridian on both sides of the spine; in the second row, tap the second lateral line of the Bladder Meridian on both sides of the spine.

⑥Sacral region. From the tip of the tailbone to the top of the external percussion, tap each side for 3 lines.

⑦Upper limb. According to the three yin and three yang meridians of the hand, percussion can be conducted around the joint.

⑧Face. Tap locality.

⑨Eyes. The first line is from the inside tip to the outside tip along the eyebrow; the second line is from the inner canthus of the eye to Tongziliao(GB1) through the upper eyelid; the third line is from the inner canthus of the eye to the Tongziliao(GB1) through the infraorbital edge.

⑩Nose. Focus on the cartilaginous part above the bilateral alar.

⑪Ear. Focus on the back and front of the earlobe.

3. Clinical application

3.1 Scope of application

(1) Pain, such as headache, post herpetic pain, shoulder and back pain, lumbago, dysmenorrhea, and arthralgia.

各部位的具体叩刺顺序如下。

(1) 头部：按督脉、膀胱经、胆经各经的循行，由前发际叩刺至后发际之脑户穴、玉枕穴、风池穴。两侧颞部由上向下叩刺。

(2) 项部：由脑户叩刺至大椎穴；由风池穴、天柱穴叩刺至第6颈椎棘突两旁。

(3) 颈部：第1线叩刺胸锁乳突肌后缘；第2线由胸锁乳突肌前缘向下叩刺；第3线从下颌角后向前叩刺。

(4) 肩胛部：先由肩胛骨内缘从上向下叩刺，其次在肩胛冈上缘由内向外叩刺，最后由肩胛冈下缘从内向外叩刺。如举臂困难可着重刺腋窝后上方和前上方的肩关节周围处。

(5) 脊背部：第1行叩刺脊柱两侧膀胱经第1侧线；第2行叩刺脊柱两侧膀胱经第2侧线。

(6) 骶部：由尾骨尖向外上方叩刺，每侧叩刺3行。

(7) 上肢：按手三阴经、手三阳经循经叩刺，在关节周围可进行环形叩刺。

(8) 面部：按局部叩刺。

(9) 眼部：第1行从眉头沿眉毛向眉梢部叩刺；第2行由目内眦经上眼睑叩刺至瞳子髎；第3行由目内眦经眶下缘叩刺至瞳子髎。

(10) 鼻部：以两侧鼻翼上方软骨部为重点。

(11) 耳部：以耳垂后和耳前为重点。

三、临床应用

(一) 适应范围

(1) 疼痛类疾病，如头痛、疱疹后遗痛、肩背痛、腰痛、痛经、痹证等。

（2）Digestive system diseases，such as hiccup，epigastralgia，and abdominal pain.

（3）Respiratory diseases，such as nasal obstruction and asthma.

（4）Diseases of urogenital system，such as enuresis and spermatorrhea.

（5）Others，such as insomnia，facial paralysis，alopecia areata，urticaria，impotence syndrome，skin numbness，infantile convulsion，and cerebral palsy.

3.2　Precautions

（1）The needle should be checked regularly，keeping the tips of the needles even and free from hooking.

（2）The needles and the local skin should be disinfected. After stabbing repeatedly，the local skin should be disinfected with alcohol cotton ball and the location should be kept clean to prevent infection.

（3）Use the wrist force to tap and puncture vertically and lift it immediately. Do not stab sideways，press，slow or drag. Do not use arm strength.

（4）This method should not be used for local skin with trauma，ulcer or scar.

（2）消化系统疾病，如呃逆、胃脘痛、腹痛等。

（3）呼吸系统疾病，如鼻塞、哮喘等。

（4）泌尿生殖系统疾病，如遗尿、遗精等。

（5）其他，如失眠、面瘫、斑秃、荨麻疹、痿证、皮肤麻木、小儿惊风、脑瘫等。

（二）注意事项

（1）注意检查针具，当发现针尖有钩毛或缺损、针锋参差不齐时，须及时修理。

（2）针具及针刺局部皮肤均应消毒。重刺后，局部皮肤需用酒精棉球消毒并应注意保持针刺局部清洁，以防感染。

（3）操作时运用腕力垂直叩刺，并立即抬起。不可斜刺、压刺、慢刺、拖刺，避免使用臂力。

（4）局部皮肤有创伤、溃疡及瘢痕者，不宜使用本法。

Chapter 11 Intradermal Needle Therapy

Intradermal needle therapy is a kind of method to treat the disease by inserting intradermal needle into the skin or subcutaneously fixed at the acupoint site and stimulating for a long time. This method is originated from the opinion on "staying in peace for a long time" in the theory of *Huangdi Neijing—Plain Questions*. It is applicable to chronic diseases requiring continuous needle retention and painful diseases occurring frequently.

1. Needle instrument

There are two types of intradermal needles: thumbtack type and grain-like type.

(1) Thumbtack type needle. The length of the needle is 2-3 mm, 0.28-0.32 mm diameter. The needle handle is round with a diameter of 4 mm, and the needle body is vertical to the needle handle(Fig. 11-1). In clinic, the needle of the 2 mm length and 0.28 mm diameter is the most commonly used. Thumbtack type needle is also called push pin needle.

(2) Grain-like type needle. The length of the needle is 5-10 mm, the diameter of the needle body is 0.28 mm, and the needle handle is round with a diameter of 3 mm. The needle body and the needle handle are in the same plane(Fig. 11-2). Grain type needle is also called pellet type needle.

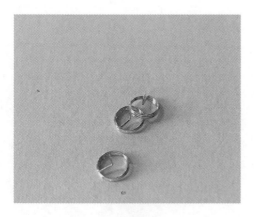

图 11-1　撖钉型皮内针

2. Operation method

2.1 Preparation before operation

Before puncturing, the needles should be sterilized by high pressure steam or soaked in 75% alcohol for 30 minutes. The local skin should be disinfected with 2% tincture of iodine and deiodinated with 75% alcohol cotton before insertion.

第十一章　皮内针法

皮内针法是以皮内针刺入并固定于腧穴部位的皮内或皮下,进行较长时间刺激以治疗疾病的方法。本法源于《黄帝内经·素问》中"静以久留"的方法,适用于需要持续留针的慢性疾病以及经常发作的疼痛性疾病。

一、针具

皮内针是用不锈钢制成的小针,有撖钉型和麦粒型两种。

1. 撖钉型　针身长 2～3 mm,针身直径 0.28～0.32 mm,针柄呈圆形,其直径 4 mm,针身与针柄垂直(图 11-1)。临床以针身长度为 2 mm 和针身直径 0.28 mm 者最常用。撖钉型也称图钉型。

2. 麦粒型　针身长 5～10 mm,针身直径 0.28 mm,针柄呈圆形,其直径为 3 mm,针身与针柄在同一平面(图 11-2)。麦粒型也称颗粒型。

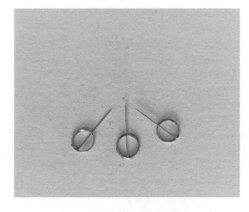

图 11-2　麦粒型皮内针

二、操作方法

(一) 操作前准备

针刺前针具高压蒸汽灭菌,或以 75%酒精浸泡 30 分钟消毒。施针前在局部皮肤用 2%碘酊进行消毒,再用 75%酒精棉脱碘。

2. 2　Manipulation

（1）Inserting the needle.

①Thumbtack type needle. Fix the skin of the acupoint with one hand, and hold the needle tail with tweezer and stab into the skin of the acupoint vertically with the other hand.

②Grain-like type needle. Extend the skin of the both sides of acupoint with one hand, and hold the needle tail with tweezer and stab into the skin of the acupoint horizontally with the other hand.

（2）Fixing the needle.

①Thumbtack type needle. Cover the end of the needle with desensitized adhesive tape, paste and fix it.

②Grain-like type needle. First, put a rubber paste under the end of the needle, and then use desensitized adhesive tape to cover, paste and fix the needle from the end along the needle body to the direction of penetration.

（3）Stimulation. Press the adhesive tape 3-4 times a day for about 1 minute each time, with the patient tolerance as the degree, and the interval between the two times is about 4 hours. During the embedding period, the patient can press several times a day to enhance the stimulation.

（4）Withdraw the needle. Fix the skin on both sides of the needle part with one hand, take off the adhesive tape with the other hand, and then hold the end of the needle with tweezer and take out the needle.

The duration of intradermal needle retention can be determined according to the condition of the patient, generally 3-5 days, up to 1 week. If the weather is hot, the needle retention time should not exceed 2 days to avoid infection.

3. Clinical application

3. 1　Scope of application

（1）Chronic refractory diseases, such as hypertension, neurasthenia, bronchial asthma, soft tissue injury, irregular menstruation, and infantile enuresis.

（2）Recurrent pain diseases, such as migraine, trigeminal neuralgia, facial spasm, dysmenorrhea, epigastralgia, biliary colic, and arthralgia.

（3）Others, such as drug treatment and weight loss.

3. 2　Precautions

（1）The acupoints that are easy to fix and do not hinder the movement of limbs should be selected for embedding needles.

（2）After embedding the needle, if the patient feels local tingling, take out the needle and bury it again or use other acupoints instead.

（二）针刺方法

1. 进针

（1）撳钉型皮内针：一手固定腧穴部皮肤，另一手持镊子夹持针尾直刺入腧穴皮内。

（2）麦粒型皮内针：一手将腧穴部皮肤向两侧舒张，另一手持镊子夹持针尾平刺入腧穴皮内。

2. 固定

（1）撳钉型皮内针：用脱敏胶布覆盖针尾、粘贴固定。

（2）麦粒型皮内针：先在针尾下垫一橡皮膏，然后用脱敏胶布从针尾沿针身向刺入的方向覆盖、粘贴固定。

3. 固定后刺激　每日按压胶布 3～4 次，每次约 1 分钟，以患者耐受为度，两次间隔约 4 小时。埋针期间，患者可自行每日按压数次，以增强刺激量。

4. 出针　一手固定埋针部位两侧皮肤，另一手取下胶布，然后持镊子夹持针尾，将针取出。

皮内针可根据病情决定其留针时间，一般为 3～5 日，最长可达 1 周。若天气炎热，留针时间不宜超过 2 日，以防感染。

三、临床应用

（一）适应范围

（1）慢性难治性疾病，如高血压、神经衰弱、支气管哮喘、软组织损伤、月经不调、小儿遗尿等。

（2）反复发作的疼痛类疾病，如偏头痛、三叉神经痛、面肌痉挛、痛经、胃脘痛、胆绞痛、关节痛等。

（3）其他，如戒毒、减肥等。

（二）注意事项

（1）埋针宜选用较易固定和不妨碍肢体运动的穴位。

（2）埋针后，若患者感觉局部刺痛，应将针取出重埋或改用其他穴位。

(3) Do not touch water during embedding to avoid infection.

(4) The needle embedding time should not be too long in hot days with more sweating.

(5) If local infection is found, the needle should be removed and local symptomatic treatment should be given.

(6) It is forbidden to embed needle in ulcer, inflammation and swelling area of unknown cause.

(3) 埋针期间,埋针处不要碰水,以免感染。

(4) 炎热天气出汗较多,埋针时间不宜过长。

(5) 若发现埋针局部感染,应将针取出,并对症处理。

(6) 溃疡、炎症、不明原因的肿胀部位,禁忌埋针。

Chapter 12   Fire Needle Therapy

Fire needle therapy is a method to treat diseases by burning a needle specially made of metal to red and rapidly piercing it into a certain part or acupoint of human body and then withdraw it quickly. The fire needle is called "Fanzhen", and the fire needle method is called "red-hot needling" in ancient time. As *Miraculous Pivot—The Official Acupuncture* said, "Red-hot needling means piercing with a heated needle to remove cold blockages." Gao Wu in Ming Dynasty said in his book *Collection of Gems of Acupuncture and Moxibustion*, "Fire needle therapy has a very satisfactory effect of removing the toxin turbidity. It can be used at the initial stage of boils or carbuncle with pus inside, and the skin without ulceration, with touch of swelling, softness but not firmness." Wu hegao in Ming Dynasty also said, "Red-hot needling, burning the needle body first to become a red-hot needle, then inserting it into the skin, is used to treat cold blockages located at bones."

This method is commonly used in patients with persistent pain, cold and chronic diseases in various clinical departments. The selected acupoints are mainly focused on localized lesions and the treatment had advantages of fewer points, quicker effect and fewer treatment time.

1. Needle instrument

Fire needle is made of tungsten alloy or stainless-steel wire which can withstand high temperature, is not easy to degrade heat, not easy to deform, not easy to break, and has high hardness under high temperature. They are shaped like filiform needles, the diameter of the needle is thicker, and the handle of the needle is twisted with copper wire. Clinically, according to the difference in the depth and size of the site of the acupuncture, the single-headed fire needle, the three-headed fire needle, the flat-headed fire needle, and the three-edged fire needle can be selected to use. Single-headed fire needles have different thickness and can be divided into fine fire needle(about 0.5 mm in diameter) and thick fire needle(about 1.2 mm in diameter)(Fig. 12-1).

2. Operation method

2.1 Acupoint selection and disinfection

(1) Acupoint selection. The principle of selecting acupuncture acupoints is basically the same as that of the filiform needle acupuncture, but the choice of acupoints should be less, and the acupoints should be mostly local acupoints.

第十二章 火 针 法

火针法是将特制的金属针具烧红,迅速刺入人体的一定部位或腧穴,并快速退出以治疗疾病的一种方法。火针古称"燔针",火针刺法称为"焠刺"。《灵枢·官针》曰:"焠刺者,刺燔针则取痹也。"明代高武的《针灸聚英》云:"火针者,宜破痈毒发背,溃脓在内,外皮无头者,但按肿软不坚者以溃脓。"明代吴鹤皋说:"焠针者,用火先赤其针而后刺,此治寒痹之在骨也。"

本法临床上常用于持续性疼痛、寒性、慢性疾病,涉及临床各科。多以病灶局部选穴为主,具有选穴少、奏效快、治疗次数少的优势。

一、针具

火针针具多选用能耐高温、不退热、变形少、不易折、高温下硬度强的钨合金或不锈钢丝制作,形似毫针,针型较粗,针柄多用铜丝缠绕而成。临床上根据火针所刺部位深浅、大小等情形的不同,可选用单头火针、三头火针、平头火针、三棱火针等。单头火针又有粗细不同,可分为细火针(针头直径约0.5 mm)和粗火针(针头直径约1.2 mm)(图 12-1)。

二、操作方法

(一) 选穴与消毒

1. 选穴   与毫针刺法选穴原则基本相同,但选穴宜少,多以局部腧穴为主。

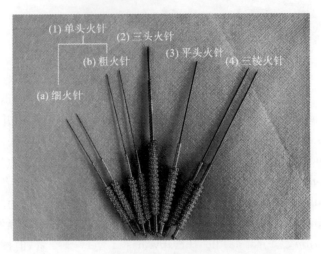

图 12-1　火针针具

(2) Disinfection. Before puncturing, sterilize the local area strictly, disinfect with 2% iodine first, then deiodinated with 75% alcohol, or disinfect with 0.5%-1% iodine.

2.2　Commonly used method of fire needle

(1) Spot puncture. A method of acupuncture with a single needle pricking on the acupoint.

(2) Multiple needle puncture. Multi-needle intensive stimulation is performed on the lesion of the body surface, with no more than 1 cm apart.

(3) Clumpy puncture. A method of applying multi-needle intensive stimulation on the lesion of the body surface, about 2 cm interval of each needle.

(4) Surrounding puncture. A method of applying multi-needle stimulation around the lesion of the body surface, and the acupuncture points are at the junction of the lesion and normal tissue.

(5) Collateral needling. A method of using a fire needle to penetrate into the superficial venules in state of blood stasis on body surface and release a proper amount of blood.

2.3　Burning needles and acupuncture

(1) Burning needles. It is a key step in the use of a fire needle. Burning red or not can directly affect its effect. The *Compendium of Acupuncture and Moxibustion* clearly pointed out, "If the needle is burned on the lamp until it is red, it will be effective when used. If it is not red, it will not cure diseases, but damage people." Therefore, the needle must be redden before using the fire needle. Burn the needle body first, then burn the tip. The degree of burning of the needle can be burnt to white, red or reddish, depending on the treatment needs(Fig 12-2). If the acupuncture is deeper, it

2. 消毒　针刺前对局部皮肤进行严格消毒,先用2%碘酒消毒,再以75%酒精脱碘,或用0.5%~1%碘酒消毒。

(二)火针常用刺法

1. 点刺法　在腧穴上施以单针点刺的方法。

2. 密刺法　在体表病灶上施以多针密集刺激的方法,每针间隔不超过1 cm。

3. 散刺法　在体表病灶上施以多针密集刺激的方法,每针间隔2 cm左右。

4. 围刺法　围绕体表病灶施以多针刺激的方法,针刺点在病灶与正常组织的交接处。

5. 刺络法　用火针刺入体表血液瘀滞的血络,放出适量血液的方法。

(三)烧针与针刺

1. 烧针　使用火针的关键步骤,针烧的红与不红可直接影响疗效。《针灸大成》明确指出:"灯上烧,令通红,用方有功。若不红,不能去病,反损于人。"因此,在使用火针前必须将针烧红,多先烧针身,后烧针尖。对于火针烧灼的程度,根据治疗需要,可将针烧至白亮、通红或微红(图12-2)。若针刺

needs to be burned to the white light, fast forward and out, otherwise not easy to penetrate, also not easy to pull out, with sharp pain. If the acupuncture is relatively shallow, it can be burned to the red, fast forward and out, shallow puncture; if the acupuncture is shallow, burned to a reddish color, and burn the skin lightly and slightly.

较深，需烧至白亮，速进疾出，否则不易刺入，也不易拔出，而且剧痛；若针刺较浅，可烧至通红，速入疾出，轻浅点刺；若针刺表浅，烧至微红，在表皮部位轻而稍慢地烙熨。

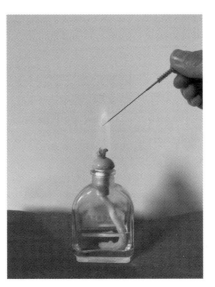

图 12-2　烧针

（2）Acupuncture. The doctor uses the left hand to hold the lit alcohol lamp, the right hand to hold the needle, as close as possible to the place of the treatment, acupuncture vertical point after burning needle, fast forward and out. To relieve pain and prevent bleeding, apply a sterile dry cotton ball to the pinhole after the acupuncture. The operator is required to concentrate and be dexterous.

2. 刺针　医者左手拿点燃的酒精灯，右手持针，尽量靠近施治部位，烧针后对准穴位垂直点刺，速入疾出。出针后用无菌干棉球按压针孔，以减少疼痛并防止出血。医者要全神贯注，动作熟练敏捷。

2.4　Depth of acupuncture

The depth of acupuncture should be determined according to the patient's condition, constitution, age and muscle thickness of the acupoint, the depth of blood vessels, and the distribution of nerves. Generally speaking, the limbs, lumbar and abdominal acupuncture is slightly deep, around 2-5 mm; the chest and back acupuncture should be shallow, almost 1-2 mm; as for the needle depth of the mole wart, it is appropriate to stab the depth of the base.

（四）针刺的深度

针刺的深度应根据患者病情、体质、年龄和针刺部位的肌肉厚薄、血管深浅、神经分布等而定。一般而言，四肢、腰腹部针刺稍深，可刺 2～5 mm 深；胸背部针刺宜浅，可刺 1～2 mm 深；至于痣疣的针刺深度以刺至基底的深度为宜。

3. Clinical application

3.1　Scope of application

This method has the function of warming meridians to dispel dampness and cold, freeing the channels, softening hardness and dispersing mass, and removing slough and promoting growth of tissue regeneration, etc. It is commonly used in such syndromes as

三、临床应用

（一）适应范围

本法具有温经散寒、通经活络、软坚散结、祛腐生肌等作用。常用病证如下。

follows.

(1) Pain as the main symptoms and touching refractory disease, such as various kinds of poliomyelitis(rheumatic arthritis and rheumatoid arthritis), tennis elbow, periarthritis of shoulder, osteoarthritis, synovitis, tenosynovitis, lumbar disease, strain of lumbar muscles, dysmenorrhea, stomachache, and trigeminal neuralgia.

(2) Skin diseases, such as neurodermatitis, snake string sores, elephantiasis, eczema, moles, and warts.

(3) Surgical infectious diseases, such as gangrene, erysipelas, and scrofula.

(4) Chronic diseases, such as chronic colitis, epilepsy, impotence, varicose veins, and infantile chancre.

3.2 Precautions

(1) Safety precautions should be taken to prevent abnormal conditions such as burns.

(2) It is forbidden to use on the face in addition to treating moles and warts, and the parts with large vessels and nerve trunk.

(3) It is a normal phenomenon that the pinhole after acupuncture has a slight red, hot, mild pain, itching and so on, so there is no need to deal with it, but should not scratch it, in case of infection.

(4) If the depth is 1-3 mm, no special treatment is needed after withdrawing the needle; but 4-5 mm deep, cover the pinhole with sterile gauze and fix it with adhesive for 1-2 days in case of infection.

(5) This treatment should be used with caution in pregnant women, puerpera and infants; and it is forbidden to use in patients with diabetes, hemophilia or impairment of coagulation mechanism.

(6) For patients who are treated with fire needle therapy for the first time, explanations should be given to eliminate fear, so as to prevent fainting during treatment.

（1）以疼痛为主要症状且缠绵难愈的病证，如各种痹证（风湿性关节炎与类风湿性关节炎）、网球肘、肩周炎、骨性关节炎、滑膜炎、腱鞘炎、腰椎病、腰肌劳损、痛经、胃脘痛、三叉神经痛等。

（2）皮肤病，如神经性皮炎、蛇串疮、象皮腿、湿疹、痣、疣等。

（3）外科感染性疾病，如痈疽、丹毒、瘰疬等。

（4）慢性疾病，如慢性结肠炎、癫痫、阳痿、下肢静脉曲张、小儿疳积等。

（二）注意事项

（1）施术时应注意安全，防止烧伤等异常情况。

（2）除治疗痣、疣外，面部禁用火针；有大血管、神经干的部位禁用火针。

（3）针刺后针孔局部若出现微红、灼热、轻度疼痛、瘙痒等表现，属正常现象，可不做处理，且不宜搔抓，以防感染。

（4）针刺1～3 mm深，出针后可不做特殊处理，若针刺4～5 mm深，出针后用消毒纱布敷盖针孔，用胶布固定1～2日，以防感染。

（5）孕妇、产妇及婴幼儿慎用；糖尿病、血友病、凝血机制障碍患者禁用火针。

（6）对初次接受火针治疗的患者，应对其做好解释工作，消除恐惧心理，以防晕针。

Chapter 13　Elongated Needle Therapy

Elongated needle therapy is a method to treat the disease by using elongated needles to prick a certain meridian or an acupoint. The elongated needle developed from the "long needle" of "nine classical needles" in the ancient times. Made of fine and flexible stainless-steel wire, its shape is slender as wheat tips, so it is called the elongated needle. *Miraculous Pivot—Treatise of Nine Needle* said, "The eighth is called long needle. It is modeled after the sewing needle. Its length is 7 inches. It controls the removal of deep lying evil [qi] and distant blockage-illnesses."

This method is generally applicable to the disease which has few responds to ordinary filiform needles, and needs to use longer needle to deep puncture.

1.　Needle instrument

The elongated needle structure is the same as the filiform needle, divided into five parts, namely needle tip, needle shaft, needle root, needle handle and needle tail. The elongated needles are mostly made of silver, copper or stainless steel. The needles made of fine stainless steel with better elasticity and toughness are more commonly used. The length, thickness, and size of the elongated needles are mainly determined by the shaft of needle. Clinically, needle lengths of 5 to 8 cun and diameter 26-28 are commonly used.

2.　Operation method

2. 1　Needle selection

According to the needs of the disease treatment and the operating site, different models of needles are selected. The selected needles should be smooth and non-corrosive. The needle tip should be straight, unbiased, clean and with a little round.

2. 2　Needle insertion

The needle should be inserted by both hands coordination. To avoid or reduce patient's pain during needle inserting, on one hand, it is necessary to distract the patient's attention to eliminate fear; On the other hand, doctor's operation techniques must be skillful.

Before needling, routinely sterilize the skin of acupoints. The needling hand handles the lower end of the needle handle. The fingers of the pressing hand to pinch the lower part of the needle with a sterile dry cotton ball to fix the needle, exposed the elongated needle tip and point to the acupoint. When the needle tip approaches the skin of the acupoint, use finger force and wrist force

第十三章　芒　针　法

芒针法是用芒针针刺一定的经络或腧穴以治疗疾病的方法。芒针由古代"九针"中的"长针"发展而来,用较细而富有弹性的不锈钢丝制成,因形状细长如麦芒,故称为芒针。《灵枢·九针论》曰:"八曰长针,取法于綦针,长七寸,主取深邪远痹者也。"

本法一般适用于普通毫针难以取得显著疗效,必须用长针深刺的疾病。

一、针具

芒针的结构与毫针一样,分为五个部分,即针尖、针体、针根、针柄和针尾。芒针多用银质、铜质材料或不锈钢制成,临床上以弹性、韧性较好的细不锈钢丝制成的芒针较为常用。芒针的长短、粗细规格主要是指针体,临床上针长以5~8寸、粗细以26~28号的较为常用。

二、操作方法

(一)针具选择

根据病情需要和操作部位选择不同型号的芒针,所选择的芒针针体应光滑、无锈蚀,针尖宜端正不偏,光洁度高,尖中带圆。

(二)进针法

进针采用双手夹持进针法。应避免或减少疼痛,施术时,医者一方面要分散患者的注意力,消除其恐惧心理,另一方面操作技术必须熟练。

针刺前,将穴位局部皮肤进行常规消毒,医者刺手持针柄下端,押手的拇指、食指用消毒干棉球捏住针体下段以固定针体,露出针尖,并将针尖对准穴位,当针尖接近穴位皮肤时,利用指力和腕力,

to complete the action of pressing and twisting, then forcefully insert the needle with both hands(Fig 13-1). According to different acupoints, slowly insert the needle to the desired depth, and use needle manipulation to achieve supplement or draining such as twirling, lifting-thrusting method after arrival of qi.

压捻结合,双手同时用力迅速将针刺入(图13-1)。根据不同穴位,缓慢运针,将针刺至所需深度。得气后可施以捻转、提插或捻转提插相结合的补泻手法,也可结合使用其他补泻手法。

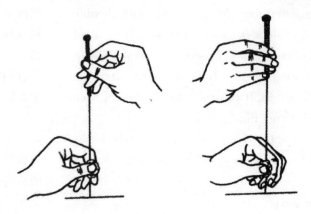

图 13-1　芒针进针法

2.3　Angle of needle insertion

(1) Perpendicular acupuncture. The elongated needle penetrates the skin vertically reaching the deep part of the body. Generally, it's suitable for acupoints on the abdomen, buttocks and other sites with fat muscles.

(2) Oblique acupuncture. The needle is inserted into the skin with an angle of about 45°. Generally, it's applicable to acupoints on the limbs, trunk, head and face.

(3) Horizontal acupuncture (also known as transverse insertion). The needle is inserted about 15° from the skin. Generally, it's suitable for shallow acupoints on the head and back.

2.4　Withdrawing the needle

After the treatment, the needle should be slowly and gently withdrawn to reduce the pain. If there is bleeding, pressed the site with a dry cotton ball until the bleeding stopped.

（三）针刺角度

1. 直刺法　芒针垂直刺入皮肤,直达人体深部。一般适用于腹部、臀部及肌肉丰厚处的穴位。

2. 斜刺法　进针时,针体与皮肤约成45°角倾斜刺入。一般适用于四肢、躯干、头项部、面部的穴位。

3. 平刺法　进针时,针体与皮肤约成15°角刺入。一般适用于头及背部等皮肤浅薄处的穴位。

（四）出针法

施针完毕后,应缓慢将针退至皮肤表层,再轻轻抽出,边退针边揉按针刺部位,以减轻疼痛。如出针后有血液溢出,应迅速以干棉球按压针孔,直至停止出血为止。

3.　Clinical application

3.1　Scope of application

The range of adaptation of the elongated needle is the same as that of ordinary filiform needle. It is mainly used for the treatment of the diseases of nervous system, motor system, digestive system, respiratory system, urogenital system, immune system, etc.

(1) Nervous system diseases, such as paralysis, sequela of

三、临床应用

（一）适应范围

芒针的适应范围与普通毫针一样,范围较广。主要用于治疗神经系统、运动系统、消化系统、呼吸系统、泌尿生殖系统、免疫系统等的疾病。

1. 神经系统疾病　如瘫痪、

cerebrovascular disease, neuralgia, and nerve root inflammation. Neuralgia includes sciatica, trigeminal neuralgia, migraine, neuropathic headache, facial paralysis, facial muscle spasm, etc.

（2）Motor system diseases, such as joint pain, soft tissue injury, periarthritis of shoulder joint, acute lumbar sprain, piriformis syndrome, lumbar disc herniation, costal cartilage, and knee osteoarthritis.

（3）Digestive system diseases, such as gastritis, gastroptosis, and various spasmodic pain in the internal organs including ulcer of the digestive tract, stomach convulsion, gastric neurosis, cholecystitis, cholelithiasis and so on.

（4）Respiratory system diseases, such as asthma, emphysema, and bronchitis.

（5）Diseases of the urogenital system, such as prostatic hypertrophy and prostatitis, urinary retention caused by spinal cord injury, urinary incontinence and urinary tract stones, uterine prolapse, menstrual disorders, infertility, pruritus vulvae, and functional impotence.

（6）Immune system diseases, such as rheumatism and rheumatoid arthritis.

（7）Other diseases, such as varicose veins of the lower limbs, pharyngeal heterosis, epilepsy, and schizophrenia.

3.2　Precautions

（1）For those patients receiving the elongated needle treatment first time, explanations should be given to eliminate his/her fear. At the same time, it is appropriate to choose fewer points, with gentle and skilled needle manipulation.

（2）Due to its needle shaft is very long and thin, and the puncture is deeper than other needles, the patient must be admonished not to move the position at random during needle retention, so as to avoid the needle becoming bent, stuck or even broken.

（3）When puncturing, it must be slow and avoid rapid insertion, so as not to cause damage to blood vessels, nerves or internal organs.

（4）It is forbidden in such conditions as too hungry, stuffed, exhausted and drunk, as well as old patient with weak constitution, pregnant woman, children and some of those who do not cooperate with the treatment.

（5）The doctor should be serious and never careless in case of any accidents.

脑血管病后遗症、神经痛、神经根炎。神经痛包括坐骨神经痛、三叉神经痛、偏头痛、神经性头痛、面神经麻痹、面肌痉挛等。

2. 运动系统疾病　如关节痛、软组织损伤、肩关节周围炎、急性腰扭伤、梨状肌综合征、腰椎间盘突出症、肋软骨炎、膝骨关节炎等。

3. 消化系统疾病　　如胃炎、胃下垂、内脏的各种痉挛性疼痛包括消化道溃疡、胃痉挛、胃神经官能症、胆囊炎、胆石症等。

4. 呼吸系统疾病　如哮喘、肺气肿、支气管炎等。

5. 泌尿生殖系统疾病　如前列腺肥大和前列腺炎，脊髓损伤导致的尿潴留、尿失禁以及泌尿系结石、子宫脱垂、月经紊乱、不孕不育症、阴痒、功能性阳痿等。

6. 免疫系统疾病　　如风湿、类风湿性关节炎等。

7. 其他疾病　如下肢静脉曲张、喉异感症、癫痫、精神分裂症等。

（二）注意事项

（1）对初次接受芒针治疗的患者，应对其耐心做好解释工作，消除其恐惧心理。同时选穴宜少，手法宜轻而且必须熟练，减少患者疼痛。

（2）由于芒针的针身长而细，针刺穴位较深，应告诫患者进针以后不可移动体位，以免造成弯针、滞针或断针。

（3）针刺时必须缓慢，切忌快速提插，以免损伤血管、神经或内脏。

（4）过饥、过饱、过劳、醉酒、年老体弱、孕妇儿童，以及某些不配合治疗者忌针。

（5）医者态度要严肃认真，不可马虎轻率，避免针刺事故的发生。

Chapter 14　Spoon Needle Therapy

Spoon needle therapy is a method of treating diseases by pressing a meridian or acupoint with spoon needle. The spoon needle is used to press acupoint as one of the nine classical needles in the ancient. Because the operation is based on pushing the acupoints, not by the caved, people also call it as push needle. *Miraculous Pivot—Nine Needles and Twelve Source* said, "The third is called spoon needle. It is 3.5 cun long. Its end is sharp like the tip of a millet grain. It serves to exert pressure on the vessels without having them cave in, so that their qi can be reached." *Miraculous Pivot—Official Acupuncture* said, "If a disease is located in the vessels, and if the qi are diminished to a degree that they are to be supplemented, the [evil qi] are to be removed with the arrowhead needle." It can be seen that pressing on the surface of the meridians or acupoints with spoon needles has the effect of dredging the meridians, reconciling qi and blood, and reinforcing deficiency.

In clinic, this method can be used both for treatment and auxiliary diagnosis.

1. Needle instrument

Spoon needle length is 3.5 cun, the needle body is a cylinder, the needle tip is dull and smooth as millet, and diameter of 2-3 mm (Fig. 14-1). It is made of stainless steel, brass, silver and other metal materials. Currently combining with modern electromagnetic technology, the variety of spoon needle becomes more diverse, such as electricity spoon needle, acoustoelectric spoon needle, electric heating spoon needle, magnetic spoon needle, and wood or bone spoon needle.

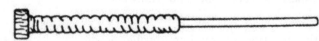

图 14-1　鍉针针具

2. Operation method

Clamping the needle handle with the thumb, middle finger and ring finger, fixing the tail of the needle with the index finger or using the style of writing to hold the needle(Fig. 14-2). The needle body is perpendicular to the pressed meridians or acupoints, each press lasts for 1-10 minutes, and it can be combined with twisting or trembling to strengthen the intensity of stimulation. According to the patient's constitution and condition, the intensity of stimulation can be divided into two kinds: mild stimulation and strong stimulation.

第十四章　鍉　针　法

鍉针法是以鍉针按压经脉或腧穴以治疗疾病的一种方法。鍉针为古代九针之一,为按压腧穴用具。因操作时以推按腧穴(按脉勿陷)为主,故又称为推针。《灵枢·九针十二原》曰:"三曰鍉针,长三寸半……锋如黍粟之锐,主按脉勿陷,以致其气。"《灵枢·官针》曰:"病在脉,气少当补之者,取以鍉针于井荥分输。"可见用鍉针在经络或腧穴表面进行按压,具有疏通经络、调和气血、补虚泻实的作用。

在临床上本法既具有治疗作用,又有辅助诊断的作用。

一、针具

鍉针针体长 3.5 寸,针身呈圆柱体,针头圆钝光滑如黍粟形,针头直径 2～3 mm(图 14-1)。多选用不锈钢、黄铜、银等金属材料制成。目前结合现代电磁技术,鍉针的种类更为多样化,有电鍉针、声电鍉针、电热鍉针、磁鍉针、木或骨鍉针等。

二、操作方法

医者以刺手的拇指、中指及无名指夹持针柄,食指抵押针尾或采用执笔式持针(图 14-2),针体与所按压的经脉或腧穴皮肤垂直,每次按压持续 1～10 分钟,按压时可结合捻转或震颤法以加强刺激。根据患者的体质与病情,刺激的强度可分为弱刺激和强刺激两种。

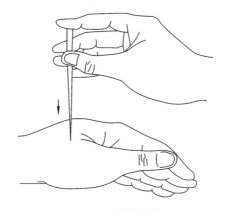

图 14-2　鍉针持针法

（1）Mild stimulation. That is, the pressure is small and light, and the sag is shallow, with local acid distention. When there is a red halo or symptom relief around the area of pressure, slowly raise the needle and slightly knead it.

（2）Strong stimulation. That is, the pressure is large and heavy, forming deep sag. When the patient has a feeling of pain in the local area, or if the needle is up and down, the needle should be shot quickly without rubbing.

The treatment can be performed 1-2 times daily, the severe can be treated 3-4 times, 10 times 1 course of treatment. As it is easy to operate, and does not need to be inserted into the skin, this method is safe and convenient and can be taught to patients to use it themselves.

3. Clinical application

3.1 Scope of application

This method has the function of dredging the meridians and collaterals, harmonizing qi and blood, reinforcing for the deficiency syndrome and reducing for the excess syndrome, and it can also be used for auxiliary diagnosis.

（1）For the treatment of coronary heart disease, hypertension, migraine, stomachache, abdominal pain, vomiting, indigestion, biliary colic, intercostal neuralgia, scapulohumeral periarthritis, tennis elbow, regular menstruation, dysmenorrhea, insomnia, neurasthenia and other diseases.

（2）It can be used to probe the meridians and acupoints of the lesion to assist the diagnosis in meridian differentiation and can also be used in the opening of the eight methods of intelligent turtle and day-prescription of acupoints and hour-prescription of acupoints of the midnight-noon ebb-flow acupuncture therapy.

3.2 Precautions

（1）The needle tip must be smooth round and spoon, not be

1. 弱刺激　即按压力度小而轻,形成的凹陷浅,局部有酸胀感,当按压部位周围发生红晕或症状缓解时,慢慢起针,并在局部稍加揉按。

2. 强刺激　即按压力度大而重,形成的凹陷深,待患者感觉局部有胀痛感,或循经向上下传导时,迅速起针,不加揉按。

每日治疗 1～2 次,重症患者每日可治疗 3～4 次,10 次为 1 个疗程。该法的操作简便,无须刺入皮肤,安全简便,可指导患者自行使用。

三、临床应用

（一）适应范围

鍉针按压具有疏通经络、调和气血、补虚泻实的作用,也可用于辅助诊断。

（1）治疗冠心病、高血压、偏头痛、胃脘痛、腹痛、呕吐、消化不良、胆绞痛、肋间神经痛、肩周炎、网球肘、月经不调、痛经、失眠、神经衰弱等病证。

（2）经络辨证时探查病变的经络、穴位,以辅助诊断;在灵龟八法和子午流注针法的开穴时亦可选用本法。

（二）注意事项

（1）所选用的鍉针,针头要光

too sharp, otherwise, there will be pain and discomfort.

(2) Press vertically, do not puncture obliquely in order to prevent the injury of skin.

(3) It shouldn't be used for local infection or ulcer area.

滑圆钝，不宜过尖，否则会产生疼痛等不适感。

（2）垂直按压，不宜斜刺，防止损伤皮肤。

（3）局部感染或有溃疡的部位，不宜使用。

Chapter 15 Superficial Needle Therapy

Superficial needle therapy, is a kind of double structure soft trocar needle therapy based on ancient filiform needle therapy. Superficial needle therapy is mainly used for the treatment of localized pain, with the characteristics of simple operation, safety, quick response, and wide indications. It is a combination of traditional acupuncture and modern medicine.

1. Needle instrument

Superficial needle mainly consist of three parts (Fig. 15-1): ①needle core: Being made of stainless steel, the needle tip is in a slope shape. ②Soft sleeve and needle base: the soft sleeve wraps the needle core, which is the main structure of the Superficial needle, so that the needle has enough flexibility to facilitate the retention of the needle for a long time. The needle base is an accessory structure of the floating needle, by which the soft sleeve retained in the body can be fixed. ③Protective sleeve: to protect the needle core and soft sleeve from collision and wear with other objects, and also to help maintain the sterile state.

第十五章 浮 针 法

浮针是在古代针具毫针的基础上,改革创新的复式结构软套管针。浮针法是传统针灸学与现代医学相结合的产物,主要用于局限性疼痛的治疗,具有操作简单、安全速效、适应证广的特点。

一、针具

浮针为复合套管针,其结构为复式结构,分为三部分(图 15-1)。①针芯:由不锈钢制成,针尖呈斜坡形。②软套管及针座:软套管包裹针芯,是浮针的主要结构,具有足够的柔软度以利于长时间留针;针座是浮针的附属结构,借此可以固定留置于体内的软套管。③保护套管:为保护针芯和软套管不与他物碰撞产生磨损,同时也为了有利于保持无菌状态。

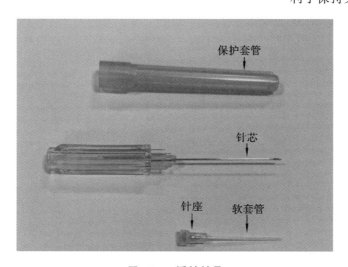

图 15-1 浮针针具

2. Operation method

2.1 Inserting needle

The local skin should be properly tightened and disinfected before injection. Clinically, the needle handle is usually held by the thumb, index finger and middle finger of the right hand, and the auxiliary needle body is held by the thumb and index finger of the left hand. The needle is punctured at an angle of 15°-25°, with moderate force and fast penetration. Do not pierce too deep, just slightly reach the muscle layer. Then release the left hand and

二、操作方法

(一)进针

进针时局部皮肤要松紧适度。进针前严格消毒,临床上一般用右手拇指、食指、中指三指夹持针柄,左手拇指、食指夹持辅助针身。针体与皮肤成15°～25°角刺入,用力适中,快速透皮,不要刺入太深,略达肌层即可,然后松开左手,右手

gently pull the right hand to make the needle body leave the muscle layer, fall back under the skin, and then lay down the needle body to prepare for the delivery of the needle.

2.2　Manipulating needle

When manipulating the needle, use only the right hand to advance along the subcutaneous. Lift slightly when pushing, so that the tip of the needle does not penetrate. When the needle is dripped, the skin is linear. In the whole process of needle delivery, the right hand feels soft and easy to enter, and the patient does not have the feeling of acid swelling or numbness. Or else the needle is too deep or too shallow. The depth of the needle is generally controlled between 25-35 mm. For the pain with large scope and long course, the depth of needle delivery can be long, otherwise, it will be short.

Then, take the needle feeding point as the fulcrum, hold the needle seat, and make the needle tip take fan-shaped movement. During the operation, hold the patient's skin with the middle finger of the right hand to separate the needle base from the skin slightly. The doctor lifts the superficial needle to uplift the skin and buries the needle body under the skin. The operation should be gentle and rhythmic, the operation time is generally 2 minutes, and the frequency is about 200 times. The operation time and frequency depend on the patient's condition. If the pain has disappeared or no longer relieved, stop the operation. If the pain still exists after sweeping, reselect the injection point closer to the pain point and reinject the needle. After inserting needle, take out the needle core and discard it at the safe place to prevent stabbing. Then, the adhesive tape is attached to the needle base to fix the soft casing left under the skin. At the injection point, cover the pinhole with a small dry cotton ball, and then apply with adhesive tape to prevent infection.

2.3　Direction of needling

The direction of acupuncture is strictly required by superficial needle therapy. The needle tip must be straight to the painful part from far to near, otherwise the effect is not satisfactory.

2.4　Retaining and withdrawing the needle

During needle retention, the needle seat of the soft sleeve can be fixed on the skin surface, and the needle entry point can be covered with a thin layer of sterilized dry cotton ball and then applied with adhesive tape. The needle retention time should be determined by the weather, and the patient's reaction and condition.

轻轻提拉，使针身离开肌层，退至皮下，再放倒针身，做好运针准备。

（二）运针

运针是指针入皮下后到针刺完毕之间的一段操作过程。运针时，医者单用右手沿皮下向前推进。推进时稍稍提起，使针尖勿深入。运针时可见皮肤呈线状隆起。在整个运针过程中，医者右手感觉松软易进，患者没有酸胀麻等感觉，否则就是针刺太深或太浅。运针深度一般掌握在 25～35 mm 之间。对范围大、病程长的病痛，运针深度可长，反之则短。

以进针点为支点，医者手握针座，使针尖做扇形运动。操作时医者以右手中指抵住患者皮肤，使针座微微脱离皮肤，医者稍稍平抬浮针，使埋藏于皮下的针体微微隆起。操作时要柔和、有节律，操作时间和次数视病痛的情况而定。如果疼痛已经消失或不再减轻，则停止此动作。扫散时间一般为 2 分钟，次数为 200 次左右。如果扫散后，疼痛依旧存在，可再选更靠近病痛点的进针点重新进针。进针完毕，抽出针芯弃置安全处，防止刺伤。然后将胶布贴敷于针座，以固定留于皮下的软套管。在进针点处，用一个小干棉球盖住针孔，再用胶布贴敷，以防感染。

（三）针刺的方向

浮针法对针刺的方向要求较为严格。针尖必须由远而近地直对病痛部位，偏差后效果不理想。

（四）留针和出针

在留针时多用胶布贴敷，把软套管的针座固定于皮肤表面即可，进针点处可用消毒干棉球覆盖一薄层后用胶布贴敷。留针时间的长短还要根据天气情况、患者的反应和病情的性质决定。

3. Clinical application

3.1 Scope of application

This method is applied to chronic headache, cervical spondylosis, scapulohumeral periarthritis, tennis elbow, tenosynovitis, carpal tunnel syndrome, lumbar disc herniation, lumbar muscle strain, knee arthritis, old ankle injury and other soft tissue pain.

In addition, the superficial needle therapy often has a good effect on the miscellaneous diseases in traditional Chinese medicine, such as cholecystitis, cholelithiasis, chronic stomachache (chronic gastritis, gastric ulcer), urinary calculi, chronic appendicitis, cervicitis, stubborn facial paralysis, and asthma attack.

3.2 Precautions

(1) If the patient is too hungry, tired or nervous, acupuncture should not be done immediately.

(2) Patients with spontaneous bleeding or bleeding after injury are not suitable for acupuncture.

(3) Patients with skin infection, ulcer, scar or tumor parts are not suitable for acupuncture.

(4) Compared with the traditional acupuncture therapy, the superficial needle therapy has a long needle retention time and is more susceptible to infection. Superficial needle apparatus can only be used for one time and should be disinfected at the same time. Especially for the patients who are easy to be infected, such as diabetic patients, we should be more careful to prevent infection.

(5) During the retention of the needle, it is necessary to pay attention to the sealing of the needle mouth and fixation of the needle body and instruct the patient to avoid strenuous activities and bathing, so as to avoid infection caused by sweat and water.

(6) When the body is swollen, use other treatment. For example, in the treatment of systemic lupus erythematosus and rheumatoid arthritis, edema caused by a lot of hormones, in this case, the effect of superficial needle therapy on analgesia is poor.

(7) For soft tissue pain, if the superficial needle therapy has only a short-term effect after treatment, and the disease is recurrent, the immune system disease should be considered.

(8) For positional pain without a clear pain point (pain only appears when the joint is in a certain position), the treatment effect is not good.

三、临床应用

（一）适应范围

慢性头痛、颈椎病、肩周炎、网球肘、腱鞘炎、腕管综合征、腰椎间盘突出症、腰肌劳损、膝关节炎、踝关节陈旧性损伤等软组织伤痛。

另外，针对中医内科的杂病，浮针法常有很好的疗效，如胆囊炎、胆石症、慢性胃痛（慢性胃炎、胃溃疡）、泌尿系结石、慢性附件炎、宫颈炎、顽固性面瘫、哮喘发作等。

（二）注意事项

（1）患者在过于饥饿、疲劳、精神紧张时，不宜立即针刺。

（2）常有自发性出血或损伤后出血不止者，不宜针刺。

（3）皮肤有感染、溃疡、瘢痕或肿瘤的部位，不宜针刺。

（4）浮针法留针时间长，相对传统针刺疗法而言，较易感染。浮针器具只能一次性使用，同时要注意消毒。特别是对容易感染的患者，如糖尿病患者，当加倍小心，慎防感染。

（5）留针期间，应注意针口密封和针体固定，嘱患者避免剧烈活动和洗澡，以免汗液和水进入机体引起感染。

（6）当肢体水肿时，效果不佳，改用其他方法治疗。例如，系统性红斑狼疮、类风湿性关节炎的治疗，大量的激素导致水肿，在这种情况下，浮针法镇痛效果差。

（7）对软组织伤痛，如果浮针法治疗后只有短期效果，病情反复发作，要考虑免疫系统疾病所致。

（8）对于没有明确痛点的位置性疼痛（只有关节处于某一位置时，疼痛才显现出来），治疗效果往往不佳。

Chapter 16　Other Kind of Therapy

Section 1　Electronic Acupuncture Therapy

The electronic acupuncture therapy is a method based on the puncture of the needle and arrival of qi, which use the pulse current output by the electronic acupuncture instrument, and conduct electricity to the needle and the acupoint, to prevent and cure the disease. The electronic acupuncture is a combination of filiform needle and electrophysiological effect, not only can improve the therapeutic effect of acupuncture, reduce the operator's continuous needling, but also enlarge the scope of acupuncture treatment. It has become a commonly used clinical acupuncture treatment.

Since the 1930s, there has been a trial of electronic acupuncture instrument in China. By the late 1950s, electronic acupuncture has been developed rapidly and has been flourished ever since. At present, there are various types of electronic acupuncture instruments, such as G6805 electro-acupuncture treatment instrument, Han's acupoint nerve stimulator, electronic needle apparatus, music electronic acupuncture instrument, etc.

1. Electronic acupuncture instrument

At present, the widespread electronic acupuncture apparatus belongs to the type of pulse generator. Take G6805 type for example, the basic structure of which is made of the power supply circuit, square wave generator circuit, control circuit, pulse main resonance circuit and output circuit(Fig. 16-1).

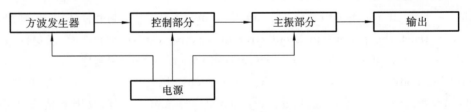

图 16-1　G6805 型电针仪原理方框图

There are many kinds of electronic acupuncture instruments. This section introduces two kinds of common electronic acupuncture therapy apparatus.

1.1　G6805-Ⅱ Electronic acupuncture treatment instrument

G6805-Ⅱ therapeutic apparatus is developed on the basis of G6805-type Ⅰ. It has been improved according to clinical demands, adopting the electronic integrated circuits. It has advantages of small volume, simple operation, easy to carry and so on. Its performance is relatively stable, equipped with alternating current

---

第十六章　其他疗法

第一节　电针法

电针法是在毫针针刺得气的基础上,应用电针仪输出脉冲电流,通过毫针作用于人体一定部位以防治疾病的一种针刺方法。电针法将毫针作用与电生理效应相结合,不仅可以提高毫针的治疗效果,减少操作者的持续行针操作,还扩大了针灸的治疗范围,已经成为临床普遍使用的针灸治疗方法。

自20 世纪30 年代以来我国有人试制电针仪,至 50 年代后期,电针法得到迅速发展,一直兴旺至今。目前,电针仪的类型多种多样,如 G6805 型电针仪、韩氏穴位神经刺激仪、电子针疗仪、音乐电针仪等。

一、电针仪

目前我国普遍使用的电针仪均属于脉冲发生器的类型,以 G6805 型电针仪为例,其基本结构由电源电路、方波发生器电路、控制电路、脉冲主振电路和输出电路5 部分组成(图 16-1)。

电针仪种类很多,本节介绍两种比较通用的电针仪。

(一) G6805-Ⅱ 型电针仪

G6805-Ⅱ型电针仪是在 G6805-Ⅰ型的基础上,根据临床需要而改进的电针仪,该仪器采用电子集成电路,具有体积小、操作简单、便于携带等优点。其性能比较稳定,可使

and DC power supply. Continuous wave, dense wave, intermittent wave can be output. Continuous wave frequency is 1-100 Hz adjustable. The dense wave is made up of sparse wave of 4 Hz and condensation wave of 20 Hz. The intermittent wave is 1-100 Hz adjustable. The positive pulse amplitude(peak) is 50 V and the negative pulse amplitude (peak) is 35 V. The positive pulse width is 500 μs and the negative pulse width is 250 μs.

1.2 Han's acupoint nerve stimulator(HANS-200)

The product has various functions. It is not only simple to operate and easy to carry. The performance and characteristics of the machine mainly include: the microcomputer controls the stimulus parameters; the stimulus intensity can be accurate to 0.1 mA and the LCD display is used; constant current output symmetrical bidirectional pulse wave to ensure the same amount of stimulation between two electrodes; 2-100 Hz with a specific time interval was selected to optimize the density wave, and the treatment effect was good. The wave width changes with frequency and has the advantage of both transcranial nerve stimulation (TENS)and acupuncture therapy. Besides, there are functions such as timing, remaining power display, automatic locking of keys, and automatic reset on startup. The power supply is 9 V DC stack battery, the output current is 0-50 mA(through skin mode)or 0-9.9 mA(through needle mode), the waveform frequency is 2-100 Hz, there are 15 modes, such as density, equal amplitude, amplitude modulation, pulse width from 0.2 to 0.6 ms, and the mode can be widened by 1.5 times. It can be used for both electro-acupuncture and transcutaneous electrical acupoint stimulation.

2. Operation method

2.1 Manipulation

Taking G6805-Ⅱ electronic acupuncture apparatus as an example, the use of the instrument is introduced.

Before using the instrument, we should first check the output knob or button of the electronic acupuncture instrument and adjust it to the "zero" position, and then insert the power plug into the 220 V AC socket.

There are 5 parallel knobs on the front of the instrument. The adjustment intensity of each knob is coordinated with the corresponding mainframe output jack. Each output intensity can be adjusted according to the clinical needs and patient tolerance.

用交、直流两用电源，能够输出连续波、疏密波、断续波。连续波频率为1～100 Hz可调；疏密波其疏波为4 Hz，密波为20 Hz；断续波为1～100 Hz可调。正脉冲幅度（峰值）为50 V，负脉冲幅度（峰值）为35 V。正脉冲波宽为500 μs，负脉冲波宽为250 μs。

（二）韩氏穴位神经刺激仪（HANS-200）

该产品功能多样，操作简便，携带方便。本机性能与特点主要有：微电脑控制刺激参数，刺激强度可精确到0.1 mA，并用液晶屏显示；恒流输出对称双向脉冲波，保证两电极间刺激量相同；具有特定时间间隔的2～100 Hz优选疏密波，治疗效果好；波宽随频率变化，兼具有经皮电神经刺激疗法（TENS）与针刺疗法两者的优势；而且还有定时、剩余电量显示、按键自动锁定和开机自动复位等功能。该机电源为9 V直流层叠电池，输出电流0～50 mA（经皮模式）或者0～9.9 mA（经针模式），波形频率2～100 Hz，有疏密、等幅、调幅等15种模式，脉冲宽度0.2～0.6 ms，可选择加宽1.5倍模式。该机既可作电针使用，又可作经皮穴位电刺激使用。

二、操作方法

（一）使用方法

以G6805-Ⅱ型电针仪为例，介绍仪器的使用方法。

在使用该仪器之前，首先应该逐一检查电针仪各输出旋钮或按键并调整到"零"位，然后将电源插头插入220 V交流电插座内。

该仪器正面有5个并排旋钮，每只旋钮调节强度与相应输出插孔相对应，使用时，将电极线插头端插入相应的主机输出插孔，每路输出强度的大小可以根据临床需要和患者耐受性任意调节。

During the treatment, the wire clips of the two poles of the output end of the electrode line are connected to the needle handle or the needle body respectively, forming a current loop, which requires that the connection is reliable, and the electrical conductivity is good. As usual acupoints in pairs are selected in the course of electroacupuncture treatment, with 1-3 pairs(2-6 points) appropriate. When a single acupoint is selected for treatment, unrelated electrodes should be used. Acupoints through which the main nerve trunk passes, such as the Huantiao(GB30)of the lower extremities, can be selected. After needle insertion, one electrode is connected to the electronic acupuncture instrument; the other is wrapped in a saline soaked gauze as an independent electrode and fixed on the skin of the same side of the meridian. Special attention should be paid to the same pair of output electrodes connected to the same side of the body. When electronic acupuncture is used on acupoints on the chest and back, two electrodes cannot be connected to the two sides of the body to avoid the current circuit passing through the heart.

Usually, the main point is connected to the negative pole, and the compatible point is connected to the positive pole. Open the power switch of the electronic acupuncture instrument, select the wave and frequency required for the treatment, adjust the corresponding output knob, increase the current intensity gradually and slowly from zero position, adjust to the appropriate stimulation intensity, avoid the sudden increase of current intensity and sudden stimulation to the patient.

With a long-time electronic acupuncture treatment, the patient will produce adaptability, that is to feel the stimulation gradually weakened, at this time the intensity of stimulation can be appropriately increased or the method of intermittent power can be used. If it is necessary to adjust the waveform and frequency in the process of electronic acupuncture treatment, we should first adjust the current intensity to the minimum, and then change the waveform and frequency. After the electroacupuncture treatment is completed, the knobs should be slowly transferred to zero position, the power switch of the electronic acupuncture instrument should be closed, and the electrode line should be removed from handle or shaft of the needle.

The course of treatment of all kinds of diseases is different. Generally, 5-10 days is one course of treatment, every day or on alternate days a treatment is necessary. The emergency patient can be treated with electroacupuncture twice a day. The interval between two courses can be 3-5 days.

治疗时，电极线输出端两极的导线夹分别连接于毫针针柄或针体，形成电流回路，应确保连接牢靠、导电良好。通常电针治疗选穴宜成对，以1～3对（2～6个穴位）为宜。当选择单个腧穴进行治疗时，应使用无关电极，可选取有主要神经干通过的穴位（如下肢的环跳穴），将针刺入后连接电针仪的一个电极；另一个电极则用盐水浸湿的纱布裹上，作为无关电极，固定在同侧经脉的皮肤上。应该特别注意，一般将同一对输出电极连接在身体的同侧，在胸、背部的穴位上使用电针时，更不可将两个电极跨接在身体两侧，避免电流回路经过心脏。

通常主穴接负极，配穴接正极。打开电针仪电源开关，选择治疗所需的波形、频率，调节对应输出旋钮，从零位开始逐级、缓慢加大电流强度，调节至合适的刺激强度，避免突然加大电流强度而给患者造成突然的刺激。

如进行较长时间的电针治疗，患者会产生适应性，即感到刺激逐渐变弱，此时可适当增加刺激强度，或采用间歇通电的方法。如有必要在电针治疗过程中对波型、频率进行调整，应首先调节电流强度至最小，然后再变换波型和频率。电针治疗完成后，应首先缓慢将各个旋钮调至零位，关闭电针仪电源开关，然后从针柄或针体取下电极线。

各种不同疾病的疗程不尽相同，一般5～10日为1个疗程，每日或隔日治疗1次，急症患者每日可电针2次。2个疗程中间可以间隔3～5日。

2.2　Acupoints selection of electronic acupuncture

In addition to the syndrome differentiation, the acupoints around the nerve trunk and the muscle nerve are usually used. Examples are as follows:

Head and face region: Facial nerve, select the Tinghui(GB2), Yifeng(TE17); Trigeminal nerve, Xiaguan(ST7), Yangbai(GB14), Sibai(ST2), Jiachengjiang.

Upper extremity: select the 6-7th Jiaji(EX-B2); Brachial plexus nerve, Tian ding (LI17); Ulnar nerve, Qingling (HT2), Xiaohai (SI8); Radial nerve, Shouwuli(LI13), Quchi(LI11); Median nerve, Quze(PC3), Ximen(PC4), Neiguan(PC6).

Lower extremity: Around sciatic nerve, select Huantiao(GB30) and Yinmen(BL37). Around tibial nerve, select Weizhong(BL40). Around common peroneal nerve, select Yanglingquan (GB34). Around femoral nerve, select Chongmen(SP12).

Lumbosacral part: Around lumbar nerve, select Qihaishu (BL24); Around sacral nerve, select Shangliao (BL31), Ciliao (BL32), Zhongliao(BL33) and Xialiao(BL34).

If the nerve function is damaged, acupoints can be chosen in accordance with the characteristics of nerve distribution. If facial nerve palsy exists, Xiaguan(ST7), Yifeng(TE17) can be selected as main acupoints. With wrinkling obstacle, add Yangbai (GB14), Yuyao(EX-HN4). If the nasolabial groove becomes shallow, add Shuigou(GV26) and Yingxiang(LI20). With the mouth askew, add Dicang (ST4) and Jiache (ST6). For patients with Sciatica, in addition to the Huantiao(GB30) and Dachangshu(BL25), Yinmen (BL37), Weizhong(BL40), Yanglingquan(GB34) can be selected.

The selection of the above acupoints is only for reference and should be matched and adjusted according to the location of the disease, the physical conditions and the distance between the acupoints.

2.3　Stimulus parameters

The output of an electronic acupuncture is a pulse currency, which is about a sudden change in the voltage or current that occurs in a very short period of time. That is to say, the sudden change in the quantity of electricity constitutes the pulse of the electricity. The basic waveform output by a electronic acupuncture is generally the alternating current pulse, which is usually bi-directional or bidirectional rectangular pulse(Fig. 16-2).

The parameters include waveform, amplitude, wave width, frequency and duration, etc., which are embodied in the stimulus quantity. Amplitude generally refers to the difference between the

（二）电针选穴

电针的选穴方法除了按经络辨证、脏腑辨证取穴外，通常还可选用神经干通过和肌肉神经运动点取穴。举例如下。

头面部：选取听会、翳风（面神经）；下关、阳白、四白、夹承浆（三叉神经）。

上肢部：选取 C6～C7 颈夹脊、天鼎（臂丛神经）；青灵、小海（尺神经）；手五里、曲池（桡神经）；曲泽、郄门、内关（正中神经）。

下肢部：选取环跳、殷门（坐骨神经）；委中（胫神经）；阳陵泉（腓总神经）；冲门（股神经）。

腰骶部：选取气海俞（腰神经）；八髎（骶神经）。

穴位的配对，若属神经功能受损，可按照神经分布特点取穴。如面神经麻痹，可取下关、翳风；皱额障碍配阳白、鱼腰；鼻唇沟变浅配水沟、迎香；口角歪斜配地仓、颊车。坐骨神经痛除取环跳、大肠俞外，配殷门、委中、阳陵泉等穴。

以上电针腧穴的选用仅供参考，还应根据患病部位、病情需要、腧穴间的距离等进行配对和调整。

（三）刺激参数

电针仪输出的是脉冲电，所谓脉冲电是指在极短时间内出现的电压或电流的突然变化，即电量的突然变化构成了电的脉冲。一般电针仪输出的基本波型是交流电脉冲，常为双向尖脉冲或双向矩形脉冲（图 16-2）。

电针刺激参数包括波型、波幅、波宽、频率和持续时间等，集中体现为刺激量。波幅一般指脉冲

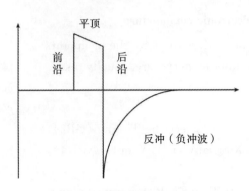

图 16-2　交流电脉冲波型

maximum and minimum value of a pulse voltage or current, or the jump amplitude of a change from one state to another. In clinical practice, the general adjustable stimulus parameters are waveform, frequency, intensity and time.

(1) Waveform. The pulse waveforms set by the common electronic acupuncture stimulator include square wave, spike wave, triangle wave and sawtooth wave (Fig. 16-3). There is also waveform square in the positive direction and sharp in the negative direction. But the single pulse wave form the continuous wave, the dilatational wave, the intermittent wave and so on according to the frequency and the different output mode(Fig. 16-4).

电压或电流的最大值与最小值之差, 也指它们从一种状态变化到另一种状态的跳变幅度值。临床操作时, 一般选择和可调节的刺激参数是波型、频率、强度和时间。

1. 波型　常见电针刺激仪所设置的脉冲波型有方形波、尖峰波、三角波和锯齿波(图 16-3), 也有正向是方形波, 负向是尖峰波的。但单个脉冲波根据频率和不同输出方式组合形成了连续波、疏密波、断续波等(图 16-4)。

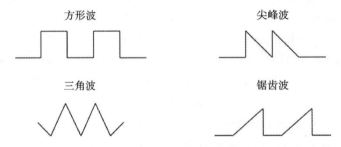

图 16-3　直流电脉冲波型

①Continuous wave. It is a continuous pulse with the same time interval. According to the change in frequency, it can be divided into two kinds of waveforms, as follows.

Sparse wave: The continuous wave with frequency lower than 30 Hz is generally called sparse wave. The continuous wave below 10 Hz are often applied in clinical practice. The stimulation of sparse waves can cause muscle contraction, produce strong tremor, improve the tension of muscle ligament and promote the recovery of neuromuscular function. It's often used in the treatment of impotence, chronic pain, all kinds of muscle, joint and ligament injury and so on.

Dense wave: the continuous wave with frequency higher than 30 Hz is generally called dense wave. The continuous waves above

(1) 连续波: 连续波是一种时间间隔相同的连续脉冲, 有频率可调性。根据频率变化, 又可分为疏波和密波。

疏波: 频率低于 30 Hz 的连续波一般称为疏波。临床运用疏波时多采用 10 Hz 以下的连续波。疏波刺激作用较强, 能引起肌肉收缩, 产生较强的震颤感, 提高肌肉韧带张力, 促进神经肌肉功能的恢复。常用于治疗痿证、慢性疼痛、各种肌肉、关节及韧带的损伤等。

密波: 频率高于 30 Hz 的连续波一般称为密波。临床运用密波

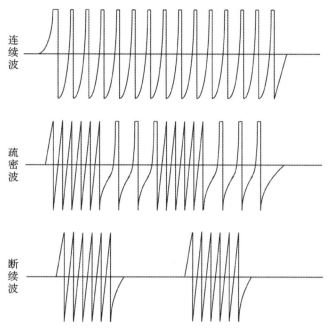

连续波

疏密波

断续波

图 16-4　连续波、疏密波、断续波

50 Hz are often used in clinical practice. Dense wave can reduce nerve stress function and inhibit spinal cord excitability. It is often used to relieve pain, tension or anxiety, muscle spasm and vasospasm, and regain composure, etc., especially in acute pain.

②Dilatational wave. It is a combination wave with a fixed frequency which occurs alternately with the sparse wave and the dense wave, and the duration of the sparse wave and dense wave alternating is about 1.5 seconds each. This wave has the characteristics of overcoming the electric adaptation of a single waveform, causing rhythmic muscle contraction, stimulating the release of various analgesic mediators, strengthening blood circulation and lymphatic circulation, regulating the nutritional metabolism of tissues, eliminating inflammation, edema and so on. It's often used in all kinds of pain, soft tissue injury, arthritis, facial paralysis, muscle weakness, etc.

③Intermittent wave. It is the rhythmic intermittent automatic combination wave, the frequency is adjustable. No pulse outputs when off, dense wave outputs continuously when on, generally in about 1.5 seconds. This waveform has a strong sense of tremor to human body, the body is not easy to produce electrical adaptability. It can improve the excitability of muscle tissue and has good stimulation and contraction to striated muscle which is often used in the treatment of impotence syndrome and paralysis.

(2) Frequency. Frequency is the number of pulses per second, the unit of which is Hertz(HZ). The commonly used frequency of

时多采用 50 Hz 以上的连续波。密波能降低神经应激功能，抑制脊髓兴奋性。常用于止痛、镇静、缓解肌肉和血管痉挛等，尤用于急性疼痛。

（2）疏密波：疏波和密波交替出现的频率固定的组合波，疏密交替持续的时间各 1.5 秒左右。该波具有能够克服单一波型产生电适应的特点，能引起肌肉有节奏的舒缩，刺激各类镇痛介质的释放，加强血液循环和淋巴循环，调节组织的营养代谢，消除炎症水肿等。常用于各种痛证、软组织损伤、关节炎、面瘫、肌肉无力等。

（3）断续波：有节律的时断时续自动出现的组合波，频率可调。断时无脉冲电输出，续时密波连续输出，一般均在 1.5 秒左右。这种波型对人体有强烈的震颤感，机体不易产生电适应性，能提高肌肉组织的兴奋性，对横纹肌有良好的刺激收缩作用。常用于治疗痿证、瘫痪。

2. 频率　频率是指每秒钟内出现的脉冲个数，其单位为赫兹

the electronic acupuncture instrument currently in use is 1-100 Hz. Continuous waves can be combined into different stimulus waveforms by adjusting the frequency, electronic acupuncture with different frequencies can induce central nervous system to release different types of neurotransmitters. As far as pain relief is concerned, low frequency(2 Hz)stimulates the release of enkephalin and endorphin in the high central nervous system, whereas high frequency(100 Hz)stimulates the release of dynorphin from spinal cord, because of the difference in their biological effects, appropriate selection should be made according to different conditions in clinical use.

(3) Intensity. The intensity of electronic acupuncture stimulation mainly depends on the amplitude. The unit of measure for amplitude is volt(V), a sudden and repeated jump from 0 V to 30 V, as in the case of a voltage, the amplitude of the pulse is 30 V, the treatment is usually not more than 20 V. The intensity can also be expressed by current or as a product of voltage and current. Wave width refers to the duration of the pulse. The pulse width is also related to the intensity of the stimulus. The larger the width is, the greater is the amount of stimulus to the patient. The output pulse width of the electronic acupuncture instrument is about 0.4 milliseconds.

The stimulation intensity of electronic acupuncture is generally implemented by the intensity adjustment key at the output end of the electrode. When the current reaches a certain strength, the patient has a sense of tingling. The current stimulation intensity at this time is called "sensory threshold". When the current intensity increases, the patient has a tingling sensation, the current intensity at this point is called the "pain threshold". The generally appropriate current stimulation intensity is between "sensory threshold" and "pain threshold". Generally speaking, when stimulated by electronic acupuncture, local muscle should be rhythmically contracted. The intensity of electroacupuncture stimulation should not be too large, but should be acceptable and tolerable for patients. It is easy to adapt to current stimulation when electronic acupuncture stimulation is performed for a long time. Thus, generally, strength adjustment should be made.

(4) Time. The single time of electroacupuncture stimulation is 15～60 minutes. The length of stimulation time depends on illness and varies from person to person. For analgesia generally 30 minutes and more of the electronic acupuncture stimulation time are needed. It may not be effective when electroacupuncture stimulation

（Hz），目前使用的电针仪设置的常用频率为 1～100 Hz。连续波可通过频率的调整而组合成不同的刺激波型，不同频率的电针可引起中枢释放不同类型的神经递质。就镇痛而言，低频(2 Hz)主要刺激高位中枢释放脑啡肽和内啡肽等，而高频(100 Hz)刺激脊髓释放强啡肽，因其生物效应不同，临床使用时应根据不同病情适当选择。

3. 强度　电针的刺激强度主要取决于波幅的高低，波幅的计量单位是伏特(V)，如电压在 0～30 V 间进行反复的突然跳变，则脉冲的幅度为 30 V，治疗时通常不超过 20 V。也有以电流表示或以电压和电流乘积表示的。波宽即指脉冲的持续时间。脉冲宽度也与刺激强度有关，宽度越大则意味着给患者的刺激量越大。电针仪一般采用适合人体的输出脉冲宽度约为 0.4 毫秒。

电针刺激强度一般通过电极输出端强度调节键实施，当电流开到一定强度时，患者有麻刺感，这时的电流刺激强度称"感觉阈"；当电流强度增加，患者产生刺痛感时，这时的电流刺激强度称为"痛阈"。一般适宜的电流刺激强度介于"感觉阈"和"痛阈"之间。但总体来说，电针刺激时，局部肌肉应呈节律性收缩，但也无需过强刺激，应以患者能接受和耐受的强度为宜。因机体对电流刺激极易适应，做较长时间电针刺激时，一般应做强度调整。

4. 时间　电针单次刺激的时间一般为 15～60 分钟，刺激时间的长短需因病、因人而异，用于镇痛一般需有 30 分钟及以上的电针刺激时间。电针刺激时间过短可

time is too short, whereas excessive stimulation time might induce adaptability for patients.

3. Clinical application

3.1 Indications

The indications of electronic acupuncture are basically the same as that of filiform needling. It can also be used for acupuncture anesthesia, especially for headache, trigeminal neuralgia, sciatica, toothache, dysmenorrhea, facial paralysis, polyneuritis, schizophrenia, epilepsy, neurasthenia, optic atrophy, periarthritis of shoulder, rheumatic arthritis, rheumatoid arthritis, lumbar muscle strain, hyperosteogeny, joint contusion, sequelae of cerebrovascular disease, tinnitus, deafness, uterine prolapse, enuresis, urinary retention, etc.

3.2 Precautions

(1) The performance and output of the electronic acupuncture instrument must be checked before use.

(2) It is supposed to adjust the output intensity slowly. Output intensity should be gradually adjusted from small to large when powering on. Forbid increasing the intensity suddenly to avoid accidents.

(3) When using electronic acupuncture near the medulla oblongata, spinal cord and other parts, the current should be small. The circuit of the current should not cross the central nervous system and the intensity should not be too strong.

(4) Forbid the current flow directly through the heart, and do not allow the two points of the left and right upper limbs to receive one output at the same time.

(5) In the process of electroacupuncture treatment, when the patient feels dizzy, the electroacupuncture treatment should be stopped immediately, the power supply should be turned off, and the treatment of acupuncture syncope reaction should be followed.

(6) As the needle used in warm needles, the surface of the needle handle is often oxidized but not conductive. The thread should be clamped on the needle body of the filiform needle or the new filiform needle shall be used.

(7) Patients with following conditions: old, weak, drunk, hungry, overfed, overworked, etc, should not be treated with electronic acupuncture.

(8) Electroacupuncture is contraindicated in special parts, such as site of skin lesions, near tumors, pregnant women's abdomen, near the heart, chest of those who has pacemaker installation, and

能尚未起效,过长则容易产生耐受。

三、临床应用

(一) 适应范围

电针的适应范围和毫针刺法基本相同,还可用于针刺麻醉,尤适用于头痛、三叉神经痛、坐骨神经痛、牙痛、痛经、面神经麻痹、多发性神经炎、精神分裂症、癫痫、神经衰弱、视神经萎缩、肩周炎、风湿性关节炎、类风湿关节炎、腰肌劳损、骨质增生、关节扭挫伤、脑血管病后遗症、耳鸣、耳聋、子宫脱垂、遗尿、尿潴留等。

(二) 注意事项

(1) 电针仪使用前必须检查其性能是否良好,输出是否正常。

(2) 调节输出量时应缓慢,开机时输出强度应逐渐从小到大,切勿突然增大,以免发生意外。

(3) 靠近延髓、脊髓等部位使用电针时,电流量宜小,并注意电流的回路不要横跨中枢神经系统,不可过强刺激。

(4) 禁止电流直接流过心脏,不允许左右上肢的两个穴位同时接受一路输出治疗。

(5) 电针治疗过程中患者出现晕针现象时,应立即停止电针治疗,关闭电源,按毫针晕针的处理方法处理。

(6) 作为温针使用过的毫针,针柄表面往往氧化而不导电,应用时须将输出线夹在毫针的针体上或使用新的毫针。

(7) 年老、体弱、醉酒、饥饿、过饱、过劳等情况,不宜使用电针。

(8) 皮肤破损处、肿瘤局部、孕妇腹部、心脏附近、安装心脏起搏器、颈动脉窦附近禁忌电针。

carotid sinus area.

Section 2　Acupoint Application Therapy

Acupoint application therapy is a method of applying drugs to certain acupoints to treat diseases through the joint action of drugs and acupoints. Among them, some of the stimulant drugs such as ranunculus, cantharides, white mustard, euphorbia kansu, castor and so on are smashed or grounded and pasted on the acupoint. If the local foaming is caused by "moxibustion", it is called "natural moxibustion" or "self-moxibustion", which is also known as vesiculation therapy. If the drug is applied to the Shenque(CV8) to obtain the goal of treating diseases through the umbilical region absorbing the drug, the therapy above is also called "umbilical compress therapy" or "umbilical therapy". If the drug is applied to the Yongquan(KI1) to treat diseases through the foot absorbing the drugs, then the therapy is known as "foot therapy" or "surge therapy".

Acupoint pasting, which is characterized by dual therapeutic effect—both acupoint stimulation and the absorption of active ingredients by skin tissue can exert obvious pharmacological effects. On one hand, drugs are absorbed through the skin, rarely through the liver or through the digestive tract, which can prevent the liver, various digestive enzymes and digestive juices from decomposing and destroying the drug components. Thus, the drug can be more effective and can play a better therapeutic role. On the other hand, it also avoids some adverse reactions caused by the drug's stimulation to the gastrointestinal tract. Therefore, this method can make up for the shortages of medicine. Except for using a few toxic drugs, this method is generally not dangerous and poisonous, relatively safe and simple, especially for the old, the young, the weak and who are prone to vomiting when taking medicine.

There is a similarity between acupoint application therapy and the "transdermal drug delivery system" of modern medicine. With the in-depth study of "transdermal drug delivery system" in modern medicine, the combination of endothelial therapy and meridional acupoints will open up a wide application prospect for external treatment methods of TCM.

1. Medicine for pasting

1.1　Medicine selection

Any clinically effective decoction or pill can be used as an

第二节　穴位贴敷法

穴位贴敷法是指在某些穴位上贴敷药物，通过药物和腧穴的共同作用以治疗疾病的一种方法。其中将一些带有刺激性的药物如毛茛、斑蝥、白芥子、甘遂、蓖麻子等捣烂或研末，贴敷穴位，如果引起局部发疱化脓如"灸疮"，则称为"天灸"或"自灸"，现代也称为发疱疗法。若将药物贴敷于神阙穴，通过脐部吸收或刺激脐部以治疗疾病时，又称为"敷脐疗法"或"脐疗"。若将药物贴敷于涌泉穴，通过足部吸收或刺激足部以治疗疾病时，又称为"足心疗法"或"涌泉疗法"。

穴位贴敷的特点在于具有双重治疗作用，既有穴位刺激作用，又可通过皮肤组织对药物有效成分的吸收，发挥明显的药理效应。一方面药物经皮肤吸收，极少通过肝脏，也不经过消化道，可避免肝脏及各种消化酶、消化液对药物成分的分解破坏，从而使药物保持更多的有效成分，能更好地发挥治疗作用；另一方面也避免了因药物对胃肠的刺激而产生的一些不良反应。因此，本法可以弥补内服药物的不足。除使用极少数有毒药物作为贴敷药物的情况外，本法一般无危险性和毒副作用，较为安全简便，对于老幼体弱者、药入即吐者尤宜。

穴位贴敷与现代医学的"透皮给药系统"有相似之处，随着现代医学对"透皮给药系统"的深入研究，中药透皮治疗与经络腧穴相结合将为中医外治法开拓广阔的应用前景。

一、贴敷药物

（一）药物的选择

凡是临床上有效的汤剂、丸

ointment for acupoint application therapy. As Wu Shiji said in *Li Yue Pian Wen*, "the principle of external treatment is the same as that of internal treatment. The medicine of external treatment is also the same as that of internal treatment. It is the method that varies." It shows that external treatment and internal treatment are different methods, but the principles of treatment are the same. Whereas compared with the internal medicine, the selection of medicine in acupoint application therapy has the following characteristics.

（1）Many selected herbs have the functions of channeling through the meridians and resuscitating the collaterals. *The Li Yue Pian Wen* contained, "The ointment must be guided by drugs with the effect of channeling through the meridians and resuscitating the collaterals, opening orifice and penetrating bone, and pulling poison out", so as to lead the group of drugs to disperse blood stasis and stagnation of qi and reach the lesion site and remove the evil qi from the body. Commonly used drugs are borneol, musk, cloves, pepper, mustard seed, frankincense, myrrh, cinnamon, asarum, angelica, ginger, onion, garlic and so on. These drugs have strong irritation and can not only treat the corresponding diseases themselves, but also promote the permeation of other drugs to the body and achieve the best efficacy.

（2）Many selected herbs are heavily tasty and poisonous, such as raw Tiannanxing(rhizoma arisaematis), the raw Banxia(pinellia tuber), the raw Chuanwu(Kunwu), the raw Caowu(Kwu), Badou (croton fruit), Banmao (blister beetle), Gansui (gansui root), Maqianzi(nux vomica), Bimazi(castor seed), Daji(Japanese thistle root), etc. The smell of these drugs is thick and strong, and they are toxic to the liver and kidney. However, through point pasting or transdermal administration herb properties can directly arrive to the location of diseases through meridians and acupoints, avoiding damage to organs such as liver and kidney and taking curative effect quickly.

（3）Choose the right solvent to mix the medicine or the ointment so as to achieve the purpose of specific drug strength, fast absorption, and quick effect. Patch drug mixed with vinegar can play the role of detoxification, removing blood stasis, collecting sores and so on. Although the drug is fierce, it can be slowed down. Pasting medications mixed with wine has the effect of activating qi and blood circulation, dredging the collaterals, eliminating swelling and relieving pain. Although the drug is slow, it can be irritable. Pasting medications mixed with oil can emolliate the muscle. Commonly used solvents are water, liquor or rice wine, vinegar, ginger juice, honey, egg white, vaseline, etc. In addition, the infusion

剂,一般都可以熬膏或研末用作穴位贴敷。正如吴师机在《理瀹骈文》中所说:"外治之理即内治之理,外治之药亦即内治之药,所异者,法耳。"说明外治与内治只是方法不同,治疗原则是一样的。但与内服药物相比,贴敷用药的选用具有以下特点。

1. 多用通经走窜、开窍活络之品 《理瀹骈文》载"膏中用药味,必得通经走络、开窍透骨、拔毒外出之品为引",以领群药开结行滞,直达病所,祛邪外出。常用的药物有冰片、麝香、丁香、花椒、白芥子、乳香、没药、肉桂、细辛、白芷、姜、葱、蒜等。这些药物刺激性较强,不仅本身能治疗相应的病变,而且通经活络、走而不守,能促进其他药物向体内渗透,以发挥最佳效应。

2. 多选气味俱厚、生猛有毒之品 如生天南星、生半夏、生川乌、生草乌、巴豆、斑蝥、甘遂、马钱子、蓖麻子、大戟等。这些药物气味俱厚,药性猛烈,口服有毒,对肝肾等脏器有损害。但通过穴位贴敷,透皮给药,能通过经络腧穴直达病所,避免了对肝肾等脏器的损害,又能起到速捷的效果。

3. 选择适当的溶剂调和 选择适当的溶剂调和贴敷药物或熬膏,以达到药力专、吸收快、收效速的目的。醋调贴敷药,能起到解毒、化瘀、敛疮等作用,虽用药猛,可缓其性;酒调贴敷药,则有行气、活血、通络、消肿、止痛作用,虽用药缓,可激其性;油调贴敷药,又可润肤生肌。常用溶剂有水、白酒或黄酒、醋、姜汁、蜂蜜、蛋清、凡士林等。此外,还可针对病情应用药物

of drugs can also be used as a solvent according to the disease.

1.2　Common forms and production

(1) Powder. A powdery agent is made by crushing or mixing one or more kinds of drugs.

(2) Ointment. The medicine is added into the suitable matrix to make the semi solid external preparation which is easy to be applied to the skin, mucosa or wound.

(3) Pills. Pills should be made into thin ends and mixed with suitable adhesives, such as water or honey or medicine juice, to make round pills of various sizes.

(4) Paste. The medicine is crushed into fine powder, or the extract is made by percolation or other methods, and then crushed into fine powder, and a proper mixture of adhesive or wetting agent (such as water, vinegar, wine, egg white or ginger juice) is mixed and blended into a paste.

(5) Iron patch. Put the traditional Chinese medicine into a cloth bag to paste on the acupoint, or apply the powder or the wet medicine cake to the acupoint directly, and then use Moxa fire or other heat source to do the hot ironing on the applied medicine.

(6) Fresh potion. Use fresh herbs to crush or rub into clumps, or cut them into sheets, then apply them to acupoints.

(7) Other dosage form. Other dosage forms commonly used in acupoint application therapy are mud, membrane, lozenge, extract, water(liquor), etc.

2.　Manipulation

2.1　The prescriptions of acupoints

The acupoint application therapy is based on the theory of viscera and meridians, and the acupoints are selected and applied according to syndrome differentiation. In addition, it should combine the following characteristics to choose acupoints.

(1) Use the local acupoints of the lesion to apply the drug, such as sticking to the Dubi(ST35)to treat knee osteoarthritis.

(2) Use the Ashi points to apply the drug, such as the local tenderness point of the lesion.

(3) Use empiric acupoints to apply the medicine, such as Yongquan(KI1) applied with Wuzhuyu(medicinal evodia fruit) to treat children's saliva, and Shenzhu(GV12) applied with Weilingxian(Chinese clematis root)to treat pertussis.

的浸剂作溶剂。

(二) 常用剂型及制作

1. 散剂　将一种或数种药物经粉碎、混匀而制成的粉状药剂。

2. 膏剂　将所选药物加入适宜基质中,制成容易涂布于皮肤、黏膜或创面的半固体外用制剂。

3. 丸剂　将药物研成细末,用适宜的黏合剂(如水或蜜或药汁等)拌和均匀,制成大小不一的药丸。

4. 糊剂　将药物粉碎成细粉,或将药物按所含有效成分以渗漉法或其他方法制得浸膏,再粉碎成细粉,加入适量黏合剂或湿润剂(如水、醋、酒、鸡蛋清或姜汁等),搅拌均匀,调成糊状。

5. 熨贴剂　将中药研成细末装于布袋中贴敷穴位,或直接将药粉或湿药饼贴敷于穴位上,再用艾火或其他热源在所敷药物上进行温熨。

6. 鲜药剂　采用新鲜中草药捣碎或揉搓成团块状,或将药物切成片状,然后将其贴敷于穴位上。

7. 其他剂型　穴位贴敷常用的其他剂型还有泥剂、膜剂、锭剂、浸膏剂、水(酒)渍剂等。

二、操作方法

(一) 选穴处方

穴位贴敷法以脏腑经络学说为基础,通过辨证选取贴敷的腧穴,腧穴力求少而精。此外,还应结合以下特点选取腧穴。

(1) 选用病变局部的腧穴贴敷药物,如贴敷犊鼻穴治疗膝关节炎。

(2) 选用阿是穴贴敷药物,如取病变局部压痛点贴敷药物。

(3) 选用经验穴贴敷药物,如吴茱萸贴敷涌泉穴治疗小儿流涎,威灵仙贴敷身柱穴治疗百日咳等。

(4) Choose commonly used acupoints to apply the medicine, such as Shenque(CV8), Yongquan(KI1), Gaohuang(BL43) and so on.

2.2　Pasting method

According to the selected acupoints, take the appropriate position, so that the drug can be applied safely. Before applying the medicine, locate the acupoints precisely, clean the area with warm water, or wipe it with ethanol cotton ball, and then apply the medicine. The infiltration aid can also be used before dressing. Apply the infiltration aid to acupoints or mix the infiltrating agent with the drug before applying the medicine. As for the medicine applied to acupoints, whatever the form is, all should be fixed well, in order to avoid falling off. It can not only be directly fixed with tape, but also be covered with the gauze or oiled paper firstly and then reoccupied with tape. At present, there are specially designed dressings for acupoints, which are convenient to use.

When it is necessary to change a dressing, we can use disinfectant dry cotton ball to dip in warm water or all sorts of vegetable oil, or paraffin oil to gently wipe the medicine that adheres to the skin, wipe dry and then apply the drug. Generally, for the mild medicine, change the medicine one time every 1-3 days; for medicine that do not need solvents time period of changing a dressing can be extended to 5-7 days; as for irritant drugs, we should see the reaction of the patients and foaming degree to determine the pasting time, varying from a few minutes to several hours. If you need to attach again, acupoint application should be used after the local skin has healed or switched to other effective acupoint alternately. The application of umbilical therapy should be applied for 3-24 hours each time, and one time every other day. The selected drugs should not be stimulant and foaming. The acupoint application therapy applied to specific acupuncture points during the sanfu(the three summer days of the most intense heat) in order to treat diseases of a chronic and cold nature, often occuring in the winter should be used once every 7-10 days, 3-6 hours each time, and 1 course of treatment for 3 years.

For the blisters, small ones usually do not need special treatment to make natural absorption; large ones should be disinfected with sterilized needles to break the bottom, drain and disinfect to prevent infection; the blisters should be covered with sterile application after sterilized to prevent infection.

3.　Clinical application

3.1　Indications

This method has a wide range of indications. It can not only

（4）选用常用腧穴贴敷药物，如神阙穴、涌泉穴、膏肓俞等。

（二）贴敷方法

根据所选腧穴，让患者采取适当体位，使药物能贴敷稳妥。贴敷药物之前，定准穴位，用温水将局部洗净，或用酒精棉球擦净，然后敷药。也可使用助渗剂，在敷药前先在穴位上涂以助渗剂或将助渗剂与药物调和后再贴敷。对于所敷之药，无论是何种剂型，均应将其固定好，以免移位或脱落，可直接用胶布固定，也可先将纱布或油纸覆盖其上，再用胶布固定。目前有专供贴敷穴位的特制敷料，使用固定都很方便。

如需换药，可用消毒干棉球蘸温水或各种植物油，或石蜡油轻轻擦去粘在皮肤上的药物，擦干后再敷药。一般情况下，刺激性小的药物，每隔1～3日换药1次；无需溶剂调和的药物，还可适当延长到5～7日换药1次；刺激性大的药物，应视患者的反应和发疱程度确定贴敷时间，数分钟至数小时不等，如需再贴敷，应待局部皮肤愈后再贴敷，或改用其他有效穴位交替贴敷。敷脐疗法每次贴敷3～24小时，隔日1次，所选药物不应为刺激性大及发疱之品；冬病夏治穴位贴敷从每年入伏到末伏，每7～10日贴1次，每次贴3～6小时，连续3年为1疗程。

对于贴敷部位起水疱者，小的水疱一般不需特殊处理，让其自然吸收；大的水疱应以消毒针具挑破其底部，排尽液体，消毒以防感染；破溃的水疱应在消毒之后外用无菌纱布覆盖，以防感染。

三、临床应用

（一）适应范围

本法适应范围较为广泛，既可

treat certain chronic diseases but also some acute diseases. Such as cold, acute and chronic bronchitis, bronchial asthma, rheumatoid arthritis, trigeminal neuralgia, facial nerve paralysis, neurasthenia, gastroptosis, gastrointestinal neurosis, diarrhea, coronary heart disease, angina, diabetes, empathy, impotence, irregular menstruation, dysmenorrhea, uterine prolapse, toothache, aphthosis, pediatric night cry, anorexia, enuresis, saliva and so on. In addition, it can also be used for disease prevention and health care.

3.2　Application examples

（1）Bronchial asthma. Take mustard seed, dahurica angelica root, gansui root, and pinellia tuber in the same amount. The ginger juice is evenly mixed and distributed, paste on Feishu(BL13), Gaohuangshu(BL43), Dingchuan(EX-B1), Danzhong(CV17) and Zhongfu(LU1). Paste 2-3 h for each time, one time every 10 days;3 times as a cource. It can prevent asthma attacks.

（2）Spontaneous sweating and night sweating. ①Take Yuliren 6 g and Wubeizi 6 g and grind them into fine powder, then the powder is made into paste with pear juice and applied to Neiguan (PC6) on both sides. ② Take the fine powder made of Yujin (turmeric root tuber)6 g and Muli(oyster)12 g, and mix it with vinegar, paste on the umbilicus, covered with gauze, fixed with adhesive tape, and dressing once every day.

3.3　Precautions

（1）When using the solvent to compress the drug, it should be applied as it is compounded to prevent volatilization.

（2）If paste is applied, the temperature of the ointment should be well controlled（the temperature of the ointment should not exceed 45 degrees Celsius）, so as to prevent scalding or sticking.

（3）For those allergic to adhesive tape, apply non-woven products or bandage to apply drugs.

（4）Pigmentation, flushing, itching, burning sensation, pain, slight redness, and slight blister are the normal skin reactions of acupoint application. However, if the skin red spots, blisters and itching of the skin are larger and more serious after the application, the drug should be stopped immediately, and the symptomatic treatment should be carried out. If there is a systemic skin allergy, patients should go to the hospital in time.

（5）For strong and toxic drugs, such as Banmao(blister beetle), Maqianzi(nux vomica), and Badou(croton fruit), the dosage and acupoint should be less, the area should be small and the time should be short, so as to prevent the excessive vesiculation or drug

治疗某些慢性疾病,又可治疗一些急性病证。如感冒、急慢性支气管炎、支气管哮喘、风湿性关节炎、三叉神经痛、面神经麻痹、神经衰弱、胃下垂、胃肠神经官能症、腹泻、冠心病、心绞痛、糖尿病、遗精、阳痿、月经不调、痛经、子宫脱垂、牙痛、口疮、小儿夜啼、厌食、遗尿、流涎等。此外,还可用于防病保健。

(二)应用举例

1. 支气管哮喘　白芥子、白芷、甘遂、半夏各等份。共为细末,鲜姜汁调匀,贴肺俞、膏肓俞、定喘、膻中、中府。1 次敷 2～3 小时,隔 10 天敷 1 次,3 次为 1 疗程。可预防哮喘发作。

2. 自汗、盗汗　①取郁李仁 6 g、五倍子 6 g。研末,用生梨汁调成糊状,敷两侧内关穴。②取郁金 6 g、牡蛎 12 g。共为细末,用醋调敷于脐部,覆以纱布,胶布固定,每日换药 1 次。

(三)注意事项

（1）凡用溶剂调敷药物时,需随调制随贴敷,以防挥发。

（2）若用膏剂贴敷,应掌握好温化膏剂的温度(膏剂温度不应超过 45 ℃),以防烫伤或贴不住。

（3）对胶布过敏者,可改用无纺布制品或用绷带固定贴敷药物。

（4）色素沉着、潮红、微痒、烧灼感、疼痛、轻微红肿、轻度出水疱属于穴位贴敷的正常皮肤反应。但贴敷后若出现范围较大、程度较重的皮肤红斑、水疱、瘙痒现象,应立即停药,进行对症处理;若出现全身性皮肤过敏症状者,应及时到医院就诊。

（5）对刺激性强、毒性大的药物,如斑蝥、马钱子、巴豆等,贴敷药量与穴位宜少、面积宜小、时间宜短,防止发疱过大或发生药物

poisoning.

（6）Be cautious about long illness, weakness, emaciation, pregnant women, young children and those with severe heart, liver and kidney dysfunction.

（7）Pasting is forbidden to regarding wounds and ulcers.

（8）Drugs that cause skin foaming should not be applied to face and joints.

（9）For the ointment remaining on the skin, it cannot be scrubbed with irritating articles such as gasoline or soap.

（10）After applying the medicine, pay attention to the local waterproof.

Section 3　Acupoint Thread-Embedding Therapy

Acupoint thread-embedding therapy is to embed the medical catgut into the acupoint, stimulating the meridians continuously, so as to prevent and treat diseases by regulating qi and blood. In clinical practice, the acupoints selected for acupoint thread-embedding therapy are based on the principle of syndrome differentiation according to the characteristics of the disease. The combination of needling, acupoint and "catgut" has stimulating and curative effects. It can be widely used in various diseases treatment.

1.　Thread-Embedding appliance

Skin disinfectant products, hole towel, syringes, hemostatic forceps, tweezers, and modified No. 12 lumbar puncture needles(the front end of the needle is polished), triangular stitch, embedded wire needle, disposable No. 7 injection needle, surgical blade, surgical tool shank, disposable No. 30 2-cun acupuncture needles, 0-1 chromium sheep gut, 2% lidocaine, scissors, sterile gauze and dressing, etc.

Different equipment should be selected according to different embedding methods. Embedded catgut needle is a tough and special metal crochet. The length is 12-15 cm, the tip of the needle is triangular, and there is a gap at the bottom(Fig. 16-5). If the needle is embedded, we can use No. 12 puncture needle of lumbar vertebra and smooth the front end of the needle. If use simple method of acupoint burying line, use disposable No. 30, 2-inch acupuncture needle, cut off the tip of the needle, from a disposable No. 7 injection needle at the end of the needle. If it is cut and embedded, the catgut should be equipped with a sharp blade, a knife handle, a triangular stitch, etc.

中毒。

（6）对久病、体弱、消瘦、孕妇、幼儿以及有严重心肝肾功能障碍者慎用。

（7）贴敷部位有创伤、溃疡者禁用。

（8）能引起皮肤发疱的药物不宜贴敷面部和关节部位。

（9）对于残留在皮肤的药膏等，不可用汽油或肥皂等有刺激性物品擦洗。

（10）贴敷药物后注意局部防水。

第三节　穴位埋线法

穴位埋线法是将医用羊肠线埋入穴位内，利用线对穴位的持续刺激作用，激发经气、调和气血，以防治疾病的方法。在临床上，穴位埋线根据病证特点，辨证取穴，发挥针刺、经穴和"线"的综合作用，具有刺激性强、疗效持久的特点，可广泛应用于临床各科病证。

一、埋线用具

皮肤消毒用品、洞巾、注射器、止血钳、镊子、经改制的12号腰椎穿刺针（将针芯前端磨平）、三角缝针、埋线针、一次性7号注射针头、手术刀片、手术刀柄、一次性30号2寸针灸针，0～1号铬制羊肠线，2%利多卡因、剪刀、消毒纱布及敷料等。

临床应根据不同的埋线方法选用不同的器材。埋线针是坚韧特制的金属钩针，长12～15 cm，针尖呈三角形，底部有一缺口（图16-5）；如采用穿刺针埋线法，可用12号腰椎穿刺针，并将针芯前端磨平；如采用简易穴位埋线，可用一次性30号2寸针灸针，剪去针尖，从一次性7号注射针头尾部穿入；如采用切开埋线法则需备尖头手术刀片、手术刀柄、三角缝针等。

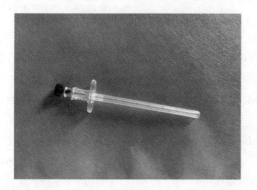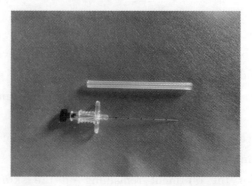

图 16-5　埋线针

2. Manipulation

2.1　The prescriptions of acupoints

Generally, acupoints can be selected according to the prescription principle of acupuncture and moxibustion treatment. The points at the muscular parts are often selected for acupoint catgut embedding, and the most commonly used is the back waist and abdominal points. If asthma takes Feishu(BL13), stomach disease takes Pishu(BL20), Weishu(BL21), Zhongwan(CV12) and so on. The principle of acupoint selection is the same as that of acupuncture therapy, but the acupoints should be simplified, and 1-3 points should be buried at intervals of 2-4 weeks for 1 time.

2.2　Catgut embedding method

(1) Traditional catgut embedding method. Traditional catgut embedding method is represented by puncture needle embedding method, catgut embedding method, triangular needle embedding method and incision and embedding method. They are respectively described as follows.

①Puncture needle embedding method. Routinely disinfect the local skin, take a medical catgut 1-2 cm long, place it at the front end of the lumbar puncture needle, and then connect the needle core. The thumb and index finger of one hand are used to fix the acupuncture point to be inserted, and the other hand is used to puncture acupoint to reach the required depth, and appropriate lifting-thrusting and twirling method are applied. When the needle sensation appears, the needle core is pushed and the needle tube is retreated. The medical catgut is buried in the subcutaneous tissue or the muscle layer of the acupoint. After drawing the needle, the needle hole is pressed with the sterile dry cotton ball to stop bleeding, and then covered with a sterile dressing.

②The catgut embedding method. Routinely disinfect the local skin and 2% lidocaine is used as the infiltration anaesthesia, and a length of 1 cm medical catgut was taken. It was placed on the double notch of the needle tip of the catgut embedding, and the two ends were

二、操作方法

(一) 选穴处方

一般可根据针灸治疗时的处方原则辨证取穴。穴位埋线常选择肌肉比较丰厚部位的穴位,以背腰部及腹部穴最常用。如哮喘取肺俞,胃病取脾俞、胃俞、中脘等。选穴原则与针刺疗法相同,但取穴要精简,每次埋线 1～3 穴,可间隔 2～4 周治疗 1 次。

(二) 埋线方法

1. 传统埋线方法　传统埋线方法以穿刺针埋线法、埋线针埋线法、三角针埋线法、切开埋线法为代表,分别介绍如下。

(1) 穿刺针埋线法:常规消毒局部皮肤,取一段 1～2 cm 长的医用羊肠线,放置在腰椎穿刺针的前端,后接针芯。用一手拇指和食指固定拟进针穴位,另一只手持针刺入穴位,达到所需的深度,施以适当的提插捻转手法。当出现针感后,边推针芯,边退针管,将医用羊肠线埋置在穴位的皮下组织或肌层内,拔针后用无菌干棉球(签)按压针孔止血,针孔处覆盖无菌敷贴。

(2) 埋线针埋线法:常规消毒局部皮肤,以 2% 利多卡因做浸润麻醉,取一段约 1 cm 长的医用羊肠线,套在埋线针尖缺口上,两端

clamped with a hemostat. One hand holds the needle and the other holds forceps. The notch of the needle tip is pierced downward at an angle of 15°-45°. When the notch of the needle enters the intradermal, the hand holding the forceps loosens the vascular forceps, and the hand holding the needle continues to insert the needle until the thread is completely buried under the skin, then inserts the needle 0.5 cm, and then pulls the needle out(Fig. 16-6). Use sterilized dry cotton ball or gauze to pinch the needle to stop bleeding, and then apply the sterile dressing to cover the wound for 3-5 days.

用止血钳夹住。一手持针,另一手持钳,针尖缺口向下以 15°~45°角刺入,当针头缺口进入皮内后,持钳的手即将血管钳松开,持针的手持续进针直至线头完全埋入皮下,再进针 0.5 cm,随后把针退出(图 16-6)。用消毒干棉球或纱布压迫针孔止血,再用无菌敷贴敷盖保护创口 3~5 日。

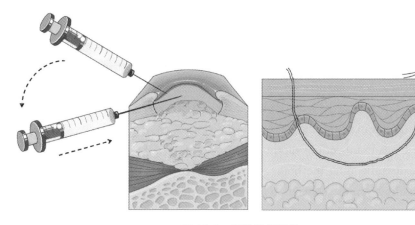

图 16-6 埋线针埋线法

③The triangle needle embedding method. It is used to mark the point of entry and exit points with iodophor at the distance from 1 to 2 cm on both sides of the catgut embedding points. After the skin is sterilized, 2% lidocaine is used as an intradermal anesthesia at the mark. On one hand the needle holder is used to clamp the triangular needle with a medical catgut, and on the other hand, the skin between the two sets of pocks is pinched, the needle is pierced from one side of the local point, through the subcutaneous tissue or the muscle layer below the acupoint, out through the contralateral local anesthesia point. Pinch the skin between the two pinholes. The ends of the thread should be cut with scissors closely attached to the skin. Relax the skin, and gently rub the part to make the medical catgut completely embedded in the subcutaneous tissue(Fig. 16-7). Use sterilized dry cotton ball or gauze to pinch the needle to stop bleeding, and then apply the sterilized dressing to cover the wound for 3-5 days.

（3）三角针埋线法:在距离埋线穴位两侧 1~2 cm 处,用碘伏做进出针点的标记。皮肤消毒后,在标记处用 2% 利多卡因做皮内麻醉,医者一手用持针器夹住穿有医用羊肠线的三角针,另一手捏起两局麻点之间的皮肤,将针从一侧局麻点刺入,穿过穴位下方的皮下组织或肌层,从对侧局麻点穿出,捏起两针孔之间的皮肤,紧贴皮肤剪断两端线头,放松皮肤,轻轻揉按局部,使医用羊肠线完全埋入皮下组织内(图 16-7)。用消毒干棉球或纱布压迫针孔止血,再用无菌敷贴敷盖保护创口 3~5 日。

④Incision and embedding method. Routinely disinfect the local skin and 2% lidocaine is used for infiltration anaesthesia. Prick the skin 0.5-1 cm with the tip of the knife. Probe the vascular forceps into the depths of the acupoints first, massage the sensitive points through the superficial fascia to the muscular layer for a few seconds, and rest for 1 to 2 minutes. Then 4-5 medical catgut with

（4）切开埋线法:常规消毒局部皮肤,用 2% 利多卡因做浸润麻醉,用刀尖刺开皮肤 0.5~1 cm,先将血管钳探到穴位深处,经过浅筋膜达肌层探找敏感点按摩数秒钟,休息 1~2 分钟。然后用 0.5~1

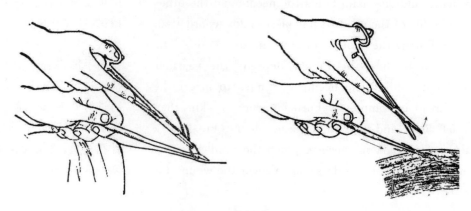

图 16-7　三角针埋线法

length between 0.5-1 cm should be embedded in the muscle layer. The medical catgut line should not be buried in the fat layer or too shallow to prevent the difficulty of absorption or infection. Incision should be sutured with a silk thread to suture and covered with a sterile dressing and the silk should be removed in 5-7 days.

（2）Modern clinical thread-embedding method.

Modern clinical thread-embedding methods are represented by simple acupoint embedding and special embedding needle embedding, which are introduced as follows:

①Simple acupoint embedding. This method is commonly used in clinic. Use a disposable No. 7 injection needle as a cannula, cut off the tip of a disposable 30-gauge 2-cun long acupuncture needle as a needle core, and put a 3-0 gauge medical catgut with a length of 0.8-1 cm into the tip of the injection needle. Routinely disinfect the local skin. Tighten or pinch the skin around the acupuncture point with the thumb and index finger of one hand, and hold the needle in the other hand（do not hold the needle vertically to prevent the needle core from squeezing the thread）, pierce the acupoint to the required depth, and apply appropriate lifting and twisting technique. When the needle sensation appears, push the needle core while retracting the injection needle, and embed the thread in the muscular layer or subcutaneous tissue of the acupoint. If there is no bleeding after the injection, no treatment is required.

②Special embedding needle embedding. The special embedding needle is based on the principle of lumbar puncture needle. It's mostly disposable. Routinely disinfect the local skin, take a piece of sterile medical catgut of 1-2 cm. Place the catgut at the front end of the special embedding needle tube, and then connect the needle core, tighten or pinch the skin around the acupoint with the thumb and index finger of one hand, and pierce the acupoint with the needle in the other hand to reach the required depth, and apply appropriate lifting-thrusting and twirling method. When a needle

cm 长的医用羊肠线 4～5 根埋于肌层内。医用羊肠线不能埋在脂肪层或过浅，以防止不易吸收或感染。切口处用丝线缝合，盖上无菌敷贴，5～7 日后拆去丝线。

2. 现代临床埋线方法　现代临床埋线方法以简易穴位埋线、专用埋线针埋线为代表，分别介绍如下。

（1）简易穴位埋线：此法为临床所常用。用一次性 7 号注射针头作套管，将一次性 30 号 2 寸长的针灸针剪去针尖作针芯，将长度为 0.8～1 cm 的 3-0 号医用羊肠线放入注射针针头内。常规消毒局部皮肤，医者一手拇指、食指绷紧或捏起进针穴周皮肤，一手持针（不能垂直持针，以防针芯将线挤掉），刺入穴位，到达所需深度，施以适当的提插捻转手法；当出现针感后，边推针芯，边退注射针头，将线埋置在穴位的肌层或皮下组织内。出针后针孔如无出血，则无需处理。

（2）专用埋线针埋线：专用埋线针是根据腰椎穿刺针的原理改制而成，现多为一次性使用。常规消毒局部皮肤，取一段 1～2 cm 长的无菌医用羊肠线，放置在专用埋线针针管的前端，后接针芯，医者一手拇指、食指绷紧或捏起拟进针穴周皮肤，一手持针刺入穴位，到达所需深度，施以适当的提插捻转

sensation appears, push the needle core while withdrawing the needle tube, and embed the catgut in the muscle layer or subcutaneous tissue of the acupoint. When the needle is extracted, use a sterile dry cotton ball to press the needle hole to stop bleeding.

3. Clinical application

3.1 Indications

This method is widely used for the treatment of asthma, stomachache, diarrhea, constipation, urine, facial paralysis and sinusitis, impotence, dysmenorrhea, epilepsy, lumbar pain, insomnia, simple obesity, apoplexy sequelae, optic atrophy, neurodermatitis, poliomyelitis sequelae, neurosis, etc. It can also be used for the prevention and healthcare of diseases.

3.2 Postoperative reaction and treatment

(1) Within 1-5 days after operation, due to stimulation injury and the stimulation of the medical catgut, there may be such dermal responses as being red, swelling, hot, painful and other aseptic inflammatory response. In a few cases, the reaction is severe, and there is a small amount of exudation from the wound, which is normal and unnecessary to be dealt with. If the seepage is more prominent on the skin surface, squeeze out the milky white extrude, wipe it off with a 75% alcohol cotton ball, and cover the wound with sterile dressing.

(2) Local hematoma is usually treated by cold compress, and then hot compress is applied to eliminate stasis.

(3) A small number of patients may have systemic reactions, showing a rise in body temperature within 4-24 hours after burial, generally around 38 ℃, no infection, 2-4 days after the temperature returned to normal. If there is a high fever, it is necessary to administrate the anti-inflammatory and antipyretic drugs.

(4) Due to the long interval of thread-embedding therapy, patients with buried line should be followed up from time to time to understand the patient's reaction after embedding and provide the treatment plan in time.

(5) If the patient is allergic to the medical catgut, there will be local redness, swelling, itching, fever and other reactions after treatment. If it is serious, there will be fat liquefaction at the embedding site and catgut will expose, then anti-allergic treatment should be implemented, and the thread should be taken out if necessary.

(6) If sensory nerve injuries, it can cause feeling dysfunction

手法；当出现针感后，边推针芯，边退针管，将羊肠线埋置在穴位的肌层或皮下组织内。出针后用无菌干棉球（签）按压针孔止血。

三、临床应用

（一）适应范围

本法适应范围较为广泛，可用于哮喘、胃痛、腹泻、便秘、遗尿、面瘫、鼻渊、阳痿、痛经、癫痫、腰腿痛、失眠、单纯性肥胖症、中风后遗症、视神经萎缩、神经性皮炎、脊髓灰质炎后遗症、神经官能症等，也可用于防病保健。

（二）术后反应及处理

（1）在术后 1～5 日内，由于刺激损伤及医用羊肠线的刺激，埋线局部可能出现红、肿、热、痛等无菌性炎症反应，少数病例反应较重，伤口处有少量渗出液，此为正常现象，一般不需处理。若渗液较多凸出于皮肤表面时，可将乳白色渗液挤出，用 75% 酒精棉球擦去，覆盖无菌敷贴。

（2）局部出现血肿一般先予以冷敷止血，再行热敷消瘀。

（3）少数患者可有全身反应，表现为埋线后 4～24 小时内体温上升，一般在 38 ℃ 左右，局部无感染现象，持续 2～4 日后体温恢复正常。如出现高热不退，应酌情给予消炎、退热药物治疗。

（4）由于埋线疗法间隔较长，宜对埋线患者进行不定期随访，了解患者埋线后的反应，及时给出处理方案。

（5）若患者对医用羊肠线过敏，治疗后出现局部红肿、瘙痒、发热等较为严重的反应，甚至埋线处脂肪液化，线体溢出，应适当做抗过敏处理，必要时切开取线。

（6）若感觉神经损伤，会出现

around nerve distribution area; if motor nerve is injured, its dominating muscle will be paralyzed, such as injury of sciatic nerve and sural, which can cause foot drop and failure of big toe dorsiflexion. If such a phenomenon occurs, the catgut should be drawn out in time and treatment follows appropriately.

3.3　Precautions

(1) Strict aseptic operation to prevent infection. The thread must not be exposed to the skin. The operation should be light and accurate to prevent the breakage of the needle while applying the triangle needle embedding method.

(2) After the operation, the remained medical catgut can be soaked in 75% alcohol, or sterilized with bromogeramine, and then soaked with the saline solution when using. The solution should be safe, non-toxic, clean and sterile.

(3) According to different parts of the body, grasp the depth of the buried line, and do not damage the internal organs, large blood vessels and nerve trunks, do not ligate nerve and blood vessels directly, so as to avoid the dysfunction and pain.

(4) Do not bury the line when there is an infection or ulcer in the skin. It is not suitable for tuberculosis, bone tuberculosis, serious heart disease or pregnancy.

(5) Patients with hemorrhagic tendencies should be cautious in applying thread-embedding therapy, which should not be used for those who have dysfunction in the absorption and repair of skin and subcutaneous tissue caused by diabetes and other diseases.

(6) If multiple treatments are applied in the same acupoint the catgut should be deviated from the previous site, and the interval should be more than 2 weeks.

(7) For those people with mental strain, overstrain or hunger, such therapy should be forbidden or cautious to avoid the occurrence of acupuncture syncope reaction, in case of which, the treatment should be stopped immediately.

(8) After the operation, mild redness, heat pain, or mild fever are normal, which are unnecessary to be dealt with, and generally disappear in 4-72 hours. If there is high fever or local severe pain, redness, itching, bleeding, infection, dysfunction (sensory nerve and motor nerve injury), it should be handled in a timely manner. We should apply local heat application, anti-infection, anti-allergy treatment. Regarding serious cases, acupuncturists should draw out the catgut in time, and give symptomatic treatment.

神经分布区皮肤感觉障碍;若运动神经损伤,会出现所支配的肌肉群瘫痪,例如损伤了坐骨神经、腓神经,会引起足下垂和蹈趾不能背屈。若发生此种现象,应及时抽出羊肠线,并给予适当处理。

(三) 注意事项

(1) 严格无菌操作,防止感染。线不可暴露在皮肤外面。三角针埋线时操作要轻、准,防止断针。

(2) 医用羊肠线用剩后,可浸泡在75%酒精中,或用新洁尔灭处理,临用时再用生理盐水浸泡,应保证溶液的安全无毒和清洁无菌。

(3) 根据部位不同掌握埋线的深度,不要伤及内脏、大血管和神经干(不要直接结扎神经和血管),以免造成功能障碍和疼痛。

(4) 皮肤局部有感染或有溃疡时不宜埋线。肺结核活动期、骨结核、严重心脏病或妊娠期等均不宜使用本法。

(5) 有出血倾向的患者慎用埋线疗法。由糖尿病及其他各种疾病导致皮肤和皮下组织吸收和修复功能障碍者忌用埋线疗法。

(6) 在同一个穴位上做多次治疗时应偏离前次治疗的部位,并需间隔2周以上。

(7) 精神紧张、过劳或者过饥者,禁用或慎用埋线,避免晕针现象发生。若发生晕针应立即停止治疗,按照晕针的处理方法进行处理。

(8) 术后局部出现轻度红肿、热痛或轻度发热,均属于正常现象,无需处理,一般多在4～72小时自行消失。若出现高热或局部剧痛、红肿较甚、瘙痒、出血、感染、功能障碍(感觉神经、运动神经损伤)者,应及时做相应处理,如局部热敷、抗感染、抗过敏处理,严重者应及时抽出羊肠线,并给予对症处理。

Section 4　Acupoint Injection Therapy

Acupoint injection therapy is guided by the theory of Chinese and Western medicine, with a drug injected into the acupoints according to the effect of acupoints and the properties of drugs, so as to prevent and cure diseases. It is also called "Liquid needle". Point injection is based on the combination of acupuncture therapy and block therapy in modern medical. It organically combines needling stimulation with acupoint pharmacology and plays a synergistic effect in order to improve curative effect. This method has many advantages, such as simple operation, small dosage, wide indications, quick action, and so on.

1. Drugs of injection

1.1　Equipment

Sterile syringes and needles are used, and disposable syringes are widely used in clinic. Syringes and needles of different specifications are selected according to the dosage, acupoint location and needling depth. Generally, 1 mL, 2 mL and 5 mL syringes can be used, while 10 mL and 20 mL syringes can be used for muscle hypertrophy. No. 5-7 syringe needle are selected usually in clinical.

1.2　Drugs

There are three main types of liquid medicines.

(1) Chinese herbal medicine preparations such as compound angelica injection, salvia miltiorrhiza injection, ligustrazine injection, heartleaf houttuynia herb injection, silver yellow injection, radix bupleuri injection, radix isatidis injection, clematis root injection, paniculate swallowwort root injection, qingkailing injection, etc.

(2) Vitamin preparations such as vitamin B_1 injection, vitamin B_6 injection, vitamin B_{12} injection, vitamin C injection, vitamin D_2 and calcium colloid injection.

(3) Other commonly used drugs such as $5\% \sim 10\%$ glucose, physiological saline, water for injection, adenosine triphosphate, coenzyme A, nerve growth factor, placenta tissue fluid, atropine sulfate, anisodamine, galantamine, sterane, procaine hydrochloride lidocaine, chlorpromazine, etc.

2. Manipulation

2.1　The prescriptions of acupoints

Choose acupoints according to the principle of making

第四节　穴位注射法

穴位注射法是以中西医理论为指导，依据穴位作用和药物性能，在穴位内注入药物以防治疾病的方法，又称"水针"。穴位注射是在针刺疗法和现代医学封闭疗法相结合的基础上发展而来的。它将针刺刺激与穴位药理有机地结合起来，发挥协同效应，以提高疗效。本法具有操作简便、用药量小、适应证广、作用迅速等优点。

一、注射药物

（一）用具

使用无菌注射器和针头，现在临床多使用一次性注射器。根据使用药物和剂量大小、腧穴部位及针刺的深浅，选用不同规格的注射器和针头，一般可使用 1 mL、2 mL、5 mL 注射器，肌肉肥厚部位可使用 10 mL、20 mL 注射器。针头可选用 5～7 号普通注射针头。

（二）药物

常用药液有三类。

1. 中草药制剂　如复方当归注射液、丹参注射液、川芎嗪注射液、鱼腥草注射液、银黄注射液、柴胡注射液、板蓝根注射液、威灵仙注射液、徐长卿注射液、清开灵注射液等。

2. 维生素类制剂　如维生素 B_1 注射液、维生素 B_6 注射液、维生素 B_{12} 注射液，维生素 C 注射液，维丁胶性钙注射液。

3. 其他常用药物　如 $5\% \sim 10\%$ 葡萄糖、生理盐水、注射用水、三磷酸腺苷、辅酶 A、神经生长因子、胎盘组织液、硫酸阿托品、山莨菪碱、加兰他敏、强的松龙、盐酸普鲁卡因、利多卡因、氯丙嗪等。

二、操作方法

（一）选穴处方

可根据针灸治疗处方原则取

acupuncture prescriptions. In general, it is advisable to select the most muscular areas for acupoint injection, and choose a few acupoints, with moderation of 1-2 acupoints, and no more than 4 acupoints.

In clinical, the acupuncturists often combine meridian palpation method with acupoint palpation method to select the positive reaction points for treatment, often select Back-Shu point on the lower back, Front-Mu point on the chest or abdomen and some specific points of the limbs. Acupoint injection performed on the tenderness points, the treatment effect is better.

2.2 Manipulation

(1) According to the selected acupoint or site, dosage of medication, select appropriate syringe and needle. Take the appropriate dose of the liquid, drain the air inside the syringe and set aside.

(2) Explore the points by pressing, guessing, or massaging and clawing along the meridian before inserting the needle into the needle. After the routine disinfection of the local skin, the needle is quickly penetrated into the skin of the patient's acupoint. Then slowly push down or up and down, after arrival of qi, pull back, if there is no blood, inject the medicine, and observe the patient's reaction at any time.

(3) Push drugs. Generally, push drugs into the skin at moderate speed. For weak patients with chronic diseases, mild stimulant should be given, which means pushing the needle slowly into the skin. In acute and strong cases, doctors use strong stimulation, push medicine quickly in. If there is plenty of injection drug, the injection needle can be withdrawn from the deep layer upto the shallow layer, and the injection can be given with the needle withdrawn, or the syringe can be changed in different directions to inject the drug around the acupuncture point.

(4) After injection, the needle is slowly withdrawn and the site is compressed for 1-2 minutes with sterile cotton swab or sterile cotton ball.

2.3 Angle and depth of needle injection

According to the different requirements of acupoint location and pathological tissue, the acupuncture angle and injection depth can be determined. The acupoints on the head, face and distal extremities where the skin is shallow are mostly shallowly pricked, while the acupoints on the waist and muscular parts of the extremities can be deeply pricked. For example, those with trigeminal neuralgia have a tender point on the face, the drug can be injected into the skin to form a "pimple". The injury site of lumbar

穴。一般选取肌肉比较丰厚的部位进行穴位注射,选穴宜少而精,以1~2个腧穴为宜,最多不超过4个腧穴。

临床常结合经络、经穴触诊法选取阳性反应点进行治疗,常取背腰部的背俞穴、胸腹部的募穴和四肢部的某些特定穴,压痛点等部位进行穴位注射,往往效果较好。

(二) 操作

(1) 根据所选穴位或部位、用药剂量,选择合适的注射器及针头。抽吸相应剂量药液,排出注射器筒内空气,备用。

(2) 进针前先揣穴,用手指按压、揣摸或循切的方式探索穴位。局部皮肤常规消毒后,将针头迅速刺入患者穴位处皮肤,然后慢慢推进或上下提插,待针下有得气感后,回抽一下,若回抽无血,即可将药推入,并随时观察患者的反应。

(3) 一般使用中等速度推入药物。慢性疾病、体弱者用轻刺激,将药物缓慢轻轻推入;急性疾病、体强者用强刺激,将药物快速推入。如果注射药物较多时,可以将注射针由深部逐渐退至浅层,边退针边推药,或将注射器变换不同的方向进行穴位注射。

(4) 注射后缓慢出针,并用无菌棉签或无菌棉球压迫1~2分钟。

(三) 针刺角度及深度

根据穴位所在部位与病变组织的不同要求,决定针刺角度和注射的深浅。头面及四肢远端等皮肉浅薄处的穴位多浅刺,而腰部和四肢肌肉丰厚部位的穴位可深刺。如三叉神经痛于面部有触痛点,可在皮内注射形成"皮丘";腰肌劳损的部位多较深,故宜适当深刺

muscle is deep, so it is appropriate to inject deeply.

2.4 Medicine dosage

The dosage of acupoint injection depends on the injection site, the nature and concentration of the drug.

The routine injection volume of each acupoint in different parts: auricular points 0. 1-0. 2 mL, acupoints on the head and face 0. 1-0. 5 mL, acupoints on the abdomen, back and limbs 1-2 mL, acupoints on the waist and buttocks 2-5 mL.

For less irritating drugs such as glucose liquid, physiological saline, dosage can be larger. For example, 5%-10% glucose can be injected 10-20 mL each time. The dosage of stimulant drugs (such as ethanol) and specific drugs (such as antibiotics, hormones, atropine, etc.) are generally small, usually 1/10-1/3 of the routine dosage.

2.5 Course of treatment

Injections are given everyday or every other day. With a strong response after treatment, it can be injected at an interval of 2-3 days. The selected acupoints can be used alternately in groups. 10 times for a course of treatment, rest for 5-7 days after one course of treatment.

3. Clinical application

3.1 Indications

The application of acupuncture point injection is very wide, and can be used in all departments including internal medicine, surgery, gynecology and pediatric. It is applied to the diseases of motor system, such as periarthritis of shoulder joint, arthritis, lumbar muscle strain, bone hyperplasia, joint torsion and contusion, etc. Neuropsychiatric disorders such as trigeminal neuralgia, facial paralysis, sciatica, multiple neuritis, schizophrenia, epilepsy, neurasthenia, etc. Digestive diseases, such as gastroptosis, gastrointestinal neurosis, diarrhea, dysentery, etc. Respiratory diseases, such as acute and chronic bronchitis, upper respiratory tract infection, bronchial asthma, tuberculosis, etc. Cardiovascular diseases, such as hypertension, coronary heart disease, angina pectoris, etc. Dermatological diseases such as urticaria, acne, neurodermatitis, etc. Gynecological diseases, such as uterine prolapse, hysteresis; Pediatric diseases, such as pneumonia, infantile diarrhea, etc.

3.2 Precautions

(1) Strictly follow the aseptic operation rules to prevent

注射。

（四）药物剂量

穴位注射的用药剂量取决于注射部位、药物的性质和浓度。

不同部位每穴每次常规注射量：耳穴 0.1～0.2 mL，头面部穴位 0.1～0.5 mL，腹背及四肢部穴位 1～2 mL，腰臀部 2～5 mL。

刺激性较小的药物如葡萄糖液、生理盐水等用量可较大，如 5%～10% 葡萄糖每次可注射 10～20 mL；刺激性较大的药物（如乙醇）和特异性药物（如抗生素、激素、阿托品等）一般用量较小，每次用量多为常规的 1/10～1/3。

（五）疗程

每日或隔日注射 1 次，治疗后反应强烈的也可以间隔 2～3 日注射 1 次。所选腧穴可分组交替使用。10 次为 1 个疗程，休息 5～7 日后再进行下 1 个疗程的治疗。

三、临床应用

（一）适应范围

穴位注射的适用范围非常广泛，内、外、妇、儿等各科均可以运用。应用于运动系统疾病，如肩周炎、关节炎、腰肌劳损、骨质增生、关节扭挫伤等；神经精神系统疾病，如三叉神经痛、面神经麻痹、坐骨神经痛、多发性神经炎、精神分裂症、癫痫、神经衰弱等；消化系统疾病，如胃下垂、胃肠神经官能症、腹泻、痢疾等；呼吸系统疾病，如急慢性支气管炎、上呼吸道感染、支气管哮喘、肺结核等；心血管系统疾病，如高血压病、冠心病、心绞痛等；皮肤科疾病，如荨麻疹、痤疮、神经性皮炎等；妇科疾病，如子宫脱垂、滞产等；儿科疾病，如小儿肺炎、小儿腹泻等。

（二）注意事项

（1）严格遵守无菌操作规则，

infection.

(2) Patients should be informed of the characteristics of the treatment and the normal response after injection. For example, there will be a feeling of soreness, mild discomfort in 4-8 hours at the injection site, or the discomfort will persist for a long time, but generally not more than 1 day.

(3) Pay attention to drug performance, pharmacological action, dosage, compatibility and toxicity. Any drug that can cause allergy, such as penicillin, streptomycin, procaine, etc., must be tested regularly so as to exclude those who have a positive skin test. Drugs with more serious side effects should be used with cautions. Certain Chinese herbal medicines may also be responsive and should be noted when applied. Pay attention to the expiry date and don't use expired drugs. And pay attention to checking whether the liquid is precipitated or deteriorated, if it has gone bad, its usage should be stopped.

(4) The drug should not be injected into the articular cavity, intravascular and spinal cavity. If the drug strays into the joint cavity, it can cause swelling, fever and pain. Strumming the spinal cord, there is a possibility of damaging the spinal cord and even causing paralysis.

(5) Attention should be paid to avoid damaging the nerve trunk when acupoint injection is performed at the location where the main nerve trunk passes through. If the tip of the needle touches the nerve stem, there is a feeling of electric shock, the needle should be withdrawn in time, and the insertion should not be repeated blindly.

(6) When injecting on both sides of the back spine, the tip of the needle should be tilted to the spine to avoid the pneumothorax. The paramount organs of the body should not be punctured too deep.

(7) When injecting on auricular point, it is advisable to use easy-to-absorb and non-irritating drugs.

(8) For the elderly and infirm and those who are receiving treatment for the first time, it is best to take the supine position. The injection site should not be too much, the dosage may be reduced as appropriate, in order to avoid fainting during acupuncture treatment. Pregnant women's lower abdomen, lumbosacral, Hegu (LI4), Sanyinjiao (SP6) and some other acupoints should not be injected, so as not to cause abortion.

防止感染。

(2) 应向患者说明本疗法的特点和注射后的正常反应。如注射局部会出现酸胀感,4~8 小时内局部有轻度不适,或不适感持续较长时间,但是一般不超过 1 天。

(3) 注意药物的性能、药理作用、剂量、配伍禁忌及毒副作用。凡能引起过敏的药物,如青霉素、链霉素、普鲁卡因等,必须做常规皮试,皮试阳性者不可应用。副作用较严重的药物,使用时应谨慎。某些中草药制剂有时也可能有反应,应用时也要注意。要注意药物的有效期,不要使用过期药物。并注意检查药液有无沉淀、变质等情况,如已变质应停止使用。

(4) 药物不宜注入关节腔、血管内和脊髓腔。若药物误入关节腔,可致关节红肿、发热、疼痛;误入脊髓腔,有损伤脊髓的可能,严重者可导致瘫痪。

(5) 在主要神经干通过的部位做穴位注射时,应注意避开神经干,以免损伤神经。如针尖触到神经干,有触电样的感觉,应及时退针,更不可盲目地反复提插。

(6) 注射背部脊椎两侧穴位时,针尖斜向脊椎为宜,避免直刺引起气胸等。体内有重要脏器的部位不宜针刺过深,以免刺伤内脏。

(7) 耳穴注射时,应选用易于吸收、无刺激性的药物。

(8) 年老体弱及初次接受治疗者,体位最好取卧位,注射部位不宜过多,药量也可酌情减少,以免晕针。孕妇的下腹部、腰骶部及合谷、三阴交等穴,不宜做穴位注射,以免引起流产。

Part Two　Application
应　用　篇

Chapter 17 The Basic Skills of Filiform Needle Operation

In order to insert the needle into the skin quickly without pain, and move the needle freely, every acupuncturist must be proficient in the manipulation of the needles, practicing all kinds of techniques and regulating the meridian qi, which makes patients pleased with acupuncture and achieves a good clinical effect. The manipulation of the filiform needles is to train finger force and manipulate technique. The finger force means the strength of fingers exerted by the acupuncturists during puncturing. The manipulating technique is reflected on the flexibility of the fingers. Only with strengthening the training of the finger strength and flexibility, can we insert the needle successfully and perform various techniques skills of the needles including lifting, thrusting, rotating and so on. During the process of practicing needles repeatedly, we should adhere to the norms of movement, to keep wholly with fixed attention for strengthening the government of mind and experience the needle sensation.

1. Practice for finger force

Finger force refers to the strength of the finger and the ability to control the needle. A good finger force is the basis of mastering the acupuncture manipulations. The body of the filiform needle is thin and soft, and it is difficult to insert the needle smoothly and operate various techniques flexibly without a certain finger force. The finger force is often practiced in soft paper packet.

It is folded into a paper pad about 2 cm thick, 8 cm long and 5 cm wide with soft straw paper or rough edge paper, and tied tightly with cotton thread in the shape of Chinese character "Jing(井)" externally. The paper pad can be used to practice the finger force and twisting and twirling movement. When practicing, hold the paper pad in one hand and hold the needle like a pen in the other hand so that the needle body is perpendicular to the paper pad. When the tip of the needle is against the paper pad, twist the handle of the needle with the thumb, index finger and middle finger to insert the needle into the paper pad. At the same time, gradually apply a certain amount of pressure to the finger downward. After penetrating the back of the paper pad, twist the needle to withdraw the needle, and then needle again. When the needle body can be vertically pierced into the paper pad, and the needle body can not be bent, swayed, and the depth of advance and retreat is free, it indicates that the finger force has reached the basic requirements. Practice must be done step by step, starting with short needles and then with long needles(Fig. 17-1).

第十七章 毫针操作基本功

每一个针灸医者必须熟练掌握毫针操作，才能进针快，透皮不痛，行针自如，患者乐于接受，并且能够施行手法，调整经气，取得良好的临床疗效。毫针的操作练习，基本上是对医者指力和手法的锻炼。指力就是手指的力量，手法则体现在手指的灵活度。医者只有加强训练手指的力量和灵活度，才能顺利进针和随意进行捻转、提插等各种手法。在反复练针的过程中，还要坚持动作规范，心宁神聚，以加强治神和体验针感。

一、指力训练

指力是指手指的力度和控针的能力，良好的指力是掌握好针刺手法的基础。毫针针身细软，医者若无一定的指力很难顺利进针和灵活操作各种手法。常采用的是纸垫练针法。

用松软的细草纸或毛边纸，折叠成厚度约 2 cm，长和宽分别为 8 cm、5 cm 的纸垫，外用棉线将纸垫呈"井"字形扎紧。在此纸垫上可练习进针指力和捻转动作。练习时，医者一手拿住纸垫，另一手如执笔式持针，使针身垂直于纸垫上，当针尖抵于纸垫后，拇指、食指、中指捻转针柄，将针刺入纸垫内，同时手指向下渐加一定压力，待刺透纸垫背面后，再捻转退针，另换一处如前再刺。如此反复练习至针身可以垂直刺入纸垫，并能保持针身不弯、不摇摆、进退深浅自如时，说明医者指力已达到基本要求。练针必须循序渐进，先用短针，后用长针（图 17-1）。

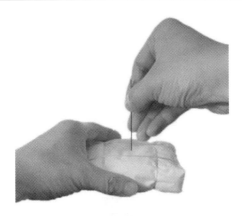

图 17-1 纸垫练针法

During practice, the needle can be inserted into the paper pad, and the needle handle can be alternately twisted back and forth between the thumb, index finger and middle finger. It is required that the angle of twisting and twirling is uniform, the application is flexible, and the speed can be twirling about 150 times per minute generally. At the beginning of needling with paper pad, 1-1.5 cun of short filiform needle can be used. After having a certain amount of finger force and basic skills of manipulation, 2-3 cun of filiform needle can be used. At the same time, it is necessary to practice acupuncture with both hands to meet the needs of continuous clinical acupuncture.

2. Practice for needling manipulation

Manipulation training refers to the standardization, coordination and flexibility of various acupuncture operations. More basic needling techniques, such as inserting, withdrawing, twisting, lifting and thrusting should be trained skillfully, which is the necessary conditions for needling in clinic. Cotton ball training acupuncture and self-training acupuncture are often used on the basis of finger strength training.

2.1 Cotton ball training acupuncture

Take some cotton wool, wind it with a cotton thread, and make it a ball tight outside and loose inside in 6-7 cm diameter, then wrap the ball with a layer of white cloth. As the cotton ball is soft, it is appropriate to practice various simulation operations such as lifting and thrusting, twirling, inserting, and withdrawing needles. When practicing lifting and thrusting, hold the needle just like holding a writing brush, insert the needle into the cotton ball, perform the movement of lifting and thrusting in the original place (Fig. 17-2). The depth should be appropriate, the amplitude should be uniform, and the manipulation frequency should be consistent, and to achieve coordinated movements, operation with dexterity, and skillful techniques.

做捻转练习时,可将针刺入纸垫后,在原处不停地来回做拇指与食指、中指的前后交替捻转针柄的动作。要求捻转的角度均匀,运用灵活,快慢自如,一般每分钟可捻转 150 次左右。纸垫练针初时可用 1～1.5 寸长的短毫针,待有了一定的指力和手法基本功后,再用 2～3 寸长的毫针练习。同时还应进行双手行针的练习,以适应临床持续运针的需要。

二、手法训练

手法训练是指各种针刺操作的规范性、协调性和灵活性。娴熟地进行速刺、捻转、提插手法的操作是针刺的必备条件。常在指力训练的基础上采用棉球练针法和自身练针法练习手法。

(一)棉球练针法

取棉絮一团,用棉线缠绕,外紧内松,做成直径为 6～7 cm 的圆球,外包白布一层缝制,即可练针。因棉球松软,可以练习提插、捻转、进针、出针等各种毫针操作手法的模拟动作。做提插练针时,医者以执毛笔式持针,将针刺入棉球,在原处做上提下插的动作,要求深浅适宜,幅度均匀,针身垂直(图17-2)。在此基础上,可将提插与捻转动作配合练习,要求提插幅度上下一致,捻转角度来回一致,操作频率快慢一致,达到动作协调、得心应手、运用自如、手法熟练的程度。

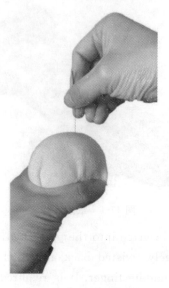

图 17-2　棉球练针法

2.2　Self-training acupuncture

After strong finger force and skillful needling techniques are made through the practice on the paper packed and cotton cushion, the practitioners can practice on their bodies so as to experience the strength of finger force, the sensation and the manipulation of acupuncture personally. During self-training acupuncture, Hegu (LI4), Quchi(LI11), Zusanli(ST36) and other acupoints can be selected. After standardized disinfection, the needling gradually achieved painless or slight pain, the needle body was inserted smoothly and without bending, manipulated freely, and the force was evenly. At the same time, carefully comprehend the relationship between finger force and needle insertion, manipulation and arrival of qi, as well as the feeling of holding the needle finger and the feeling of the punctured part.

3.　Practice for internal strength

The purpose of internal strength training is to train the mind and qi, combine the internal nourishment of mind and qi with the practice of finger strength, so that the mind can gather in the finger easily, the qi can transport to the finger easily, the mind and qi can accompany each other, the internal qi can be radiates outward and gained, and the curative effect can be improved. Qigong is the first recommended internal skill practice, followed by Taijiquan, Huatuo Wuqinxi, Yijinjing, etc. All of them need to be adjusted in heart, spirit and mind, and stress on consciousness, qi and strength. Long term practice makes people full of spirit and the internal qi can penetrate the feet. When acupuncture, it will be able to skillfully mobilize all aspects of the body's strength, so that it can reach the end of the finger and apply it under the needle.

（二）自身练针法

医者通过纸垫、棉球等物体练针,具有了一定的指力基础后,可以在自己身上进行试针练习,亲身体会指力的强弱、针刺的感觉、行针的手法等。在自身练针时,可选用自己的合谷、曲池、足三里等穴位,皮肤规范消毒后,逐渐做到进针无痛或微痛,针身挺直不弯,刺入顺利,提插、捻转行针自如,用力均匀,手法熟练。同时,要仔细体会指力与进针、手法与得气的关系,以及持针手指的感觉和受刺部位的感觉。

三、内功训练

内功训练旨在练意、练气,将内养意气与指力练习相结合,使神易聚于指,气易注于指,意气相随,内气外发,增强得气,提高疗效。内功练习首推气功,其次有太极拳、华佗五禽戏、易筋经等。其练习均需调心、调神、调意,讲究意到、气到、力到。长期习之,医者精力充沛,中气贯足,在针刺时必然能巧妙地调动全身各方面的力量,使之到达指端施于针下。

Chapter 18　Qi-Arrival by Needle Insertion and Method

1. An overview of needle insertion and arrival of qi

1.1　Needle insertion and arrival of qi

(1) Concept and indication of needle insertion and arrival of qi.

①Concept of arrival of qi. The word "arrival of qi" was first seen in the *Plain Questions—Lihe theory of truth and evil*, "[When the patient] inhales, insert the needle; do not let the [proper] qi revolt. Hold the needle calmly and let it remain [inserted] for a long time; do not let the evil [qi] spread. [When the patient] inhales,twist the needle to get a hold of qi. "Arrival of qi means that after the needle is inserted to a certain depth of point,and manipulated with certain kinds of needling techniques to get the sensation of meridian qi. The sensation of meridian qi under the needle is also called "arrival of qi" or "needling sensation". Clinically,it can be judged by both the patient's needling reaction and the acupuncturist's needling sensation, which shows that arrival of qi is the synchronous feeling of both the acupuncturist and the patient during the process of needling.

②Indication of arrival of qi. As recorded in *Song to Elucidate Mysteries*, If qi arrives, it will feel sluggish and tight under or around the needle, just like a fish swallows hook and bait when fishing;if it doesn't arrive,it will be felt like[the patient just stand in] a quiet and empty house, without any strange feeling. It was also recorded in *Miraculous Pivot—Nine needles and twelve Source* that "When the qi arrive, the effect shows. The effects are as reliable as the wind that blows away clouds;they are as clear as the appearance of a blue sky. That is all about the ways of needling theory. " Those are the ancient people's understandings of arrival of qi,which can be summarized to both the acupuncturist's feelings according to clinical experience and the patient's reactions.

• Subjective feeling aspect, also known as self-conscious indications,which refers to the subjective feelings and reactions of patients and acupuncturists in the process of needling,which are the main indications of arrival of qi. The patients have some special feeling, such as soreness, distension, numbness, heaviness, cool, heat,electric-shock,formication around the needle and pain under certain conditions,etc. The acupuncturist feels the changes of the senses of subsidence,astringency and tenseness under the needle.

第十八章　毫针得气与方法

一、针刺得气概述

(一) 针刺得气

1. 针刺得气概念与指征

(1) 得气概念。"得气"一词首见于《素问·离合真邪论》:"吸则内针,无令气忤,静以久留,无令邪布,吸则转针,以得气为故。"得气是指医者将毫针刺入腧穴一定深度后,施以一定的行针手法,使针刺部位产生经气感应,这种针下的经气感应又称"气至"或"针感"。临床上得气可以通过患者对针刺的反应与医者手下的感觉两方面加以判定。由此可见,得气是针刺过程中医患双方的同步感应。

(2) 得气指征。《标幽赋》中记载:轻滑慢而未来,沉涩紧而已至……气之至也,如鱼吞钩饵之沉浮,气未至也,如闲处幽堂之深邃。《灵枢·九针十二原》亦载:刺之要,气至而有效,效之信,若风之吹云,明乎若见苍天,刺之道毕矣。这些均是古人对得气的认识,结合临床可归纳为医患两方面的感觉及反应。

①主观感觉方面:又称自觉指征,是指接受针灸的患者与医者各自的主观感觉和反应,是判定得气的主要指征。患者方面的感觉主要有酸、麻、胀、重、凉、热、触电、蚁走以及特定条件下的疼痛等。医者方面的感觉主要指针下沉、涩、紧等感觉的变化。感觉的性质与

The nature of the feeling is closely related to the body's reactivity, the nature of the disease and the location of the needle.

· Objective representation aspect, also called others' indications, which refer some phenomena such as local muscles bulge by tension or muscles beats around acupoints, or skin rashes along the meridians observed by the acupuncturists or the patients. It is rare in clinical practice.

(2) Effect of arrival of qi. Arrival of qi is the key to the therapeutic effect of needling. It is an important basis for judging whether the acupuncturist's operation is correct or not, the prosperity and decline condition of patient's meridian qi, disease prognosis, and the presence or absence of clinical treatment effects. It is also the basis for further implementation of needling techniques.

①Arrival of qi is the basis for the effectiveness of acupuncture and moxibustion.

Miraculous Pivot—Nine Needles and Twelve Source pointed out: "When the qi arrive, the effect shows." It shows that the fundamental role of needling is to stimulate meridians qi, dredge the meridian, harmonize the yin and yang, reinforce deficiency and reduce excess by stimulating acupoints. The arrival of qi under the needle shows a condition of unimpeded meridian, harmonized qi and blood, with vitality going in and out freely.

②Arrival of qi is the prerequisite for the application of supplementation and draining manipulations. A discussion of the relationship between arrival of qi and needling manipulation methods was recorded in *Song to Elucidate Mysteries*, "When qi arrives, the needle is retained or quickly withdrawn according to cold and heat; when qi does not arrive, it is supposed to wait for qi according to deficiency and excess." *Compendium of Acupuncture and Moxibustion* pointed out, if qi fails to arrive, insert or withdraw the needle, induce the qi, and perform the supplementation and draining technique until qi reaching the acupoints. It also emphasized that awaiting qi is the priority of manipulating needle. *The Seventy-eighth Issue of Classic of Questioning* illustrated that after qi is obtained, pushing the needle downward means the supplementary method; moving the needle upward means the draining method, which indicates that arrival of qi is the prerequisite for the application of supplementation and draining manipulations.

③Arrival of qi is the basis for judging healthy qi from pathogenic factors. The speed of arrival of qi under the needle is an important basis for judging the ups or downs of the personal healthy qi and the severity of illness. As is said in the *Compendium*

机体反应性、疾病的性质和针刺部位密切相关。

②客观表象方面:又称他觉指征,是指医者或患者观察到的针刺腧穴局部紧张凸起、穴位处肌肉跳动、循经性皮疹等改变,临床上比较少见。

2. 针刺得气作用　得气是针刺产生治疗作用的关键,是判定医者针刺操作正确与否、患者经气盛衰、疾病预后转归、临床治疗有无效果的重要依据,也是针刺过程中进一步实施手法的基础。

(1) 得气是针灸起效的基础。《灵枢·九针十二原》指出:"刺之要,气至而有效。"表明针刺的根本作用在于通过针刺腧穴,激发经气、疏通经络、调整阴阳、补虚泻实。针下得气,说明经气通畅、气血调和,神气游行出入自如。

(2) 得气是应用补泻的前提。《标幽赋》中记载"既至也,量寒热而留疾;未至也,据虚实而候气"的操作方法,这是对得气反应与针刺操作手法关系的论述。《针灸大成》指出,气之未至,或进或退,或按或提,导之引之,候气至穴而方行补泻,并强调"用针之法候气为先"。《难经·七十八难》中有"得气,因推而内之,是谓补;动而伸之,是谓泻",这些都说明得气是应用补泻的前提。

(3) 得气是判定正邪的依据。针下得气的速度是判断机体正气盛衰和病情轻重的重要依据。《针灸大成》指出:针若得气速,则病易

of Acupuncture and Moxibustion, if the qi arrives fast, the body is easy to recover and the effect is rapid; if the qi arrives slowly, the body is difficult to recover, and the disease even cannot be cured. We can imagine that the healthy qi of those who obtain qi quickly are relatively sufficient, and their meridian qi are vigorous. With more sensitive reaction of the body, acupuncture effect works quickly and the prognosis is better. As is said in *Song to Elucidate Mysteries*, if qi arrives quickly, acupuncture effect will be shown quickly; otherwise, the diseases can hardly be cured. In contrast, if healthy qi is deficient, the meridian qi is weak, the body responses slowly with later arrival of qi, then the disease is difficult to heal, and the prognosis is poor. *Miraculous Pivot—Zhongshi* pointed out that when evil qi arrives,［the flow of qi］will be tense and swift. When grain qi arrives,［the flow of qi］will be slow and harmonious. *Compendium of Acupuncture and Moxibustion* pointed out that if the qi arrives, you should check the evil qi and the healthy qi, and distinguish the deficiency from the real, indicating that there supposed to be healthy qi or evil qi under the needle. Therefore, only on the basis of obtaining qi, can we distinguish healthy from evil, and use appropriate supplementation and draining method.

（3）Factors affecting the arrival of qi. Under normal circumstances, with proper locating acupoints, appropriate needling direction, angle and depth, qi sensation is easy to get. Otherwise, we should explore the root causes of failure to obtain qi and adopt appropriate methods to promote the arrival of qi as soon as possible. The factors that affect the arrival of qi mainly include the following aspects.

①Acupuncturists factors: It mainly includes the inaccuracy of acupoints location, unskilled needling techniques, improper grasp of needling angles, direction, depth and acupuncturists' lack of attention, which must be corrected in time.

②Patients factors: It mainly includes the individual's nature endowments, physical strength, and the body state. In general, people who recently got sick with a strong build would be sooner to obtain qi, and those who suffered from prolonged illness with a weak build would be slower to obtain qi. People with excess syndromes obtain qi faster than people with deficiency syndromes. Patients with excessive yang qi and sensitive spirit are easy to obtain qi, and can appear the sense of transmission along the meridians. For most patients whose yin and yang keep balance, qi and blood are moisten, and the functions of Zang-Fu organs coordinate with each other, needle sensation is neither dull nor sensitive, the qi comes timely and peacefully. If yin-qi is hyperactive

愈而效亦速也；若气来迟，则病难愈而有不治之忧。可见得气迅速者，正气相对充足，经气旺盛，机体反应灵敏，见效较快，预后较好。如《标幽赋》所云："气速至而速效，气迟至而不治。"反之，正气虚损，经气衰弱，机体反应迟缓，得气慢，则疾病缠绵难愈，且预后较差。《灵枢·终始》指出："邪气来也紧而疾，谷气来也徐而和。"《针灸大成》指出："若针下气至，当察其邪正，分清虚实。"说明针下之经气感应当有正邪之分。故只有在得气的基础上，才能分辨正邪，而有针对性地施用不同补泻方法。

3. 影响得气因素 一般情况下，取穴得当，针刺方向、角度、深浅适宜，多会出现得气感应。否则就应当探究未能得气的根源，采取相应的方法，以尽快促使得气。影响针刺得气的因素主要包括以下几个方面。

（1）医者因素：主要包括取穴失准，行针手法不熟练，针刺角度、方向、深浅把握不当，医者注意力不集中等因素，要及时加以纠正。

（2）患者因素：主要包括患者个体禀赋、体格强弱以及机体状态等因素。一般来说，新病、强壮者，得气较快；久病体衰者，得气较慢或较弱。实证得气较快，虚证得气较慢。有些患者阳气偏盛、神气敏感，容易得气，并可出现循经感传。机体阴阳之气无明显偏颇者，气血润泽通畅，脏腑功能较好，故针刺时感应既不迟钝，亦不过于敏感，得气适时而平和。属阴气偏盛者，多需经过一定的行针过程方有感

patients, it should be taken a certain period of time after needling to induce the meridian transmission, or there remains a sense of transmission after the needle was removed. Thus, the condition of obtaining qi varies from person to person.

③Environment factors: It mainly includes the solar terms of four seasons, rain or snow, cloudy or sunshine, cold or warm, damp or dry, ect. In general, It is easier to obtain qi when the weather is refreshing, the room temperature is appropriate and the humidity is moderate; otherwise, it is more difficult to obtain qi. Just as *Plain Questions-Bazheng Shenminglun* said, "When heaven is warm and the sun is bright, the people's blood is rich in fluid, and the defensive qi is on the surface. Hence, the blood can be drained easily and the qi can be made to move on easily. When heaven is cold and the sun is hidden, the people's blood congeals so that [its flow] is impeded, and the defensive qi is in the depth... It is said that one follows the seasons of heaven in regulating blood and qi."

1.2　Methods of promoting arrival of qi

(1) Qi arrives to local.

①Method of awaiting qi: It is a method of waiting for the arrival of qi after needling and it is also called retaining needle for qi. That is to say, if qi fails to come after the needle is inserted, leave the needle for a moment, which helps to obtain qi. It was said in *Lihe theory of truth and evil of Plain Questions* that, "[Hold the needle] calmly and let it remain [inserted] for long to have the qi arrive. As if one is waiting for someone of noble rank, one does not know whether [he will come during] daytime or in the evening." When waiting for qi, acupuncturist can wait for a long time quietly, or manipulate needles intermittently and apply a variety of manipulations of hastening qi till qi comes.

②Method of hastening qi: It is a method of hastening qi to gather around the needle after needle insertion through some needling manipulations. As is said in *Miraculous Effective Classic of Acupuncture*, hold the needle with the thumb and index finger of right hand, shake it carefully and twist the needle forward and backward. It's like shaking the hand, which is called qi stimulating.

③Method of keeping qi: It is a method of preventing qi from leaving after obtaining qi. This method allows the already acquired induction of qi to maintain a certain intensity and time. *Miraculous Pivot—Xiaozhenjie* explained that the outstanding [practitioner] guards the inner mechanism: he knows how to guard the qi. "The motion of the mechanism never leaves the enclosed empty space" that is [to say: one must] know about depletion and repletion of the qi, and about the slow and swift application of the needles. "The mechanism in the enclosed empty space is clear, calm, and subtle" is

应,或出针后针感仍然明显存在等。因此患者的得气状况是因人而异的。

(3) 环境因素:主要包括四时节气、雨雪阴晴、冷暖燥湿等因素。一般而言,天气清爽、室温适宜、干湿适度时针刺易于得气;反之得气较慢或不易得气。如《素问·八正神明论》所云:"天温日明,则人血淖液而卫气浮,故血易泻,气易行。天寒日阴,则人血凝泣而卫气沉……是以因天时而调血气也。"

(二) 促使得气方法

1. 局部得气

(1) 候气法:指针刺入腧穴后,留针等待经气而至的方法,又称留针候气法。即进针后经气不至,留针片刻,有候气、待气而至的作用。《素问·离合真邪论》说:"静以久留,以气至为故,如待所贵,不知日暮。"候气时,可以安静等待较长时间,也可以间歇地运针,施以各种催气手法,到气至而止。

(2) 催气法:指针刺入腧穴后,通过一些行针手法,催促经气速至针下的方法。如《神应经》载:用右手大拇指及食指持针,细细动摇进退搓捻,其针如手颤之状,是谓催气。

(3) 守气法:指针下得气之后使气留守勿去的方法。本法可使已经出现的得气感应保持一定的强度和时间。《灵枢·小针解》说:"上守机者,知守气也。机之动不离其空中者,知气之虚实,用针之徐疾也。空中之机清静以微者,针以得气,密意守气勿失也。"针灸临床也有"得气容易守气难"之说,得

[to say:] once the needle has came into contact with the qi, it is essential to aim at keeping qi lest it losts. It is said that it is easier to obtain qi than to keep qi in acupuncture clinical practice. It is easy to make the appeared qi induction disappear after the free change of the needle tip location or blindly lifting and thrusting, so the qi must be carefully observed and meticulously experienced. At this point, acupuncturists should not keep their hands free of needles, or use the thumb and index fingers to keep the needle still, keep the needle tip to the area where qi has arrived, or apply light needle techniques on the original position.

　　④Method of regulating qi: Broadly speaking, the purpose of acupuncture is to achieve yin and yang in a relative equilibrium by adjusting the qi of meridians. Therefore, *Plain Questions—Cijie theory of truth and evil* said, "For the application of needling, a regulation of the qi is decisive." *The Seventy-second issue of Classic of Questioning* said that acupuncture for regulating qi must also be based on yin and yang, and the relationship between the exterior and interior of the human body. Clinically, arrival of qi can make the blocked meridian qi flow smoothly, change "pain due to blocking" into "no pain due to unblocking". It also helps to reinforce deficiency and to reduce excess, reducing the redundant qi and reinforcing the deficient qi, as the saying goes, "obtaining qi means regulating qi".

　　In a narrow sense, the method of regulating qi refers to the specific method of adjusting the direction of meridian qi by twirling, massaging along meridian, needle-handle flicking, pressing, connecting the meridians qi just like dragon, tiger, turtle and phoenix, ect. As was referred in *Rhythm of Golden Needle* that for the method of regulating qi, first insert the needle to the deep level, then return to the middle level, at last the shallow level. Twist the needle rightward to draw qi up, while twist the needle leftward to induce qi downward.

　　（2）Focal arrival of acu-esthesia.

　　Focal arrival of acu-esthesia (Qi extending affected parts) refers to the induction of qi under the needle. Qi extending affected parts refers to make the qi induction expand and spread toward the direction of the lesion, eventually reaching the lesion by a certain acupuncture manipulation. Transmission of sensation along meridian is a kind of phenomenon that the needle sensation transmits along the meridian course after arrival of qi. Transmission of sensation along meridian and qi extending affected parts refers to the sense of needling is transmitted to the lesion location along the meridians, which is the mainly purpose of getting and promoting qi, also the best manifestation of obtaining qi, so as to balance yin-yang

气后若随意改变针尖部位或盲目提插，很容易使已出现的得气感应消失，故必须细心体察、密意守之。此时宜手不离针，或用拇、食两指持针不动，保证针尖不要偏离已得气的部位，或在原位施以轻巧的手法。

　　（4）调气法：从广义上讲，针刺的目的就是通过调整人体经络之气，使失去平衡的阴阳之气得到调理而归于平秘。故《灵枢·刺节真邪论》说："用针之类，在于调气。"《难经·七十二难》说："知其内外表里，随其阴阳而调之，故曰调气之方，必在阴阳。"临床上得气后可以使阻滞的经气流通，使"痛则不通"变为"通则不痛"，疼痛减轻或消失。得气之后可以补虚、泻实，使过盛之气复平，不足之气得助，所以有"得气即为调气"之说。

　　从狭义上讲，调气法是指应用捻转、循摄、搓弹、按压以及龙、虎、龟、凤通经接气等调整经气方向的具体方法。《金针赋》所说的"及夫调气之法，下针至地之后，复人之分，欲气上行，将针右捻，欲气下行，将针左捻"即属此法。

　　2. 气至病所　气至病所之气泛指经气，即针下的经气感应。气至病所是指通过一定的针刺手法，使针刺感应向着病变部位所在的方向扩延和传布，最终达到病变部位。循经感传是指针刺得气后，针感沿着经脉走行传导的现象。循经感传气至病所是针刺所得之经气沿着经脉走行传导到达病变部位，是得气、行气的主要目的，是得气的最佳表现，从而调整阴阳平衡，获得更好的临床疗效。循经感

to obtain better efficacy. The method of transmission of sensation along meridian and qi extending affected parts varies from person to person, depending on the body's reaction state, and should also be selected based on the experience of the operator. In case of trans-articular obstruction of meridian qi, the method of Qinglongbaiwei and the method of Baihuyaotou can be used, and the method of pressing along the meridian with fingers may be applied so as to let the meridian qi through the joint smoothly.

2. Regulation and concentration of the spirit

Regulation and concentration of the spirit includes both the acupuncturist and the patient aspects. On the one hand it refers to the acupuncturist being concentrated in the whole process of the acupuncture treatment. On the other hand it is the patient's devotion to complete the acupuncture treatment. Regulation and concentration of the spirit is the premise and foundation of acupuncture treatment. It runs through the entire acupuncture treatment process and directly affects the efficacy of acupuncture.

"Spirit" refers to the external manifestations of human activities and is a high degree of generalization of the human body's spiritual consciousness, thinking activities, and the external performance of Zang-Fu organs, qi and blood, and body fluids. *Plain Questions-The theory of maintaining life and physique* emphasized: For all piercing to be reliable, one must first regulate the spirit. *The Spiritual Pivot-Benshen* said, "All norms of piercing [require one] to consider the spirit as the foundation at first." *The Spiritual Pivot-Nine Needles and Twelve Source* pointed out, "Unrefined [practitioners] guard the physical appearance. Outstanding [practitioners] guard the spirit." It emphasized the role of "vitality" in acupuncture treatment. Regulation and concentration of the spirit not only affect the clinical efficacy of acupuncture, but also measure the level of acupuncturists.

2.1 To regulate the spirit for the purpose of obtaining qi

Acupuncture treatment is mainly implemented by concentrating the acupuncturist's thoughts and according to the patient's spirit, consciousness and general condition, so as to get qi. Meanwhile, the patient also needs to be on peace of mind, and his thoughts are required to focus on where the acupuncturist performs needling operation, prompting qi arrival under the needle and extending qi to affected parts. *Miraculous Pivot-the Official Acupuncture Guanneng* pointed out, "For applying the needles [successfully], it is important not to neglect the spirit." The regulation of the spirit should run through the whole process of acupuncture operation. The key to regulating the spirit is that the

传气至病所的方法因人因病而异，视机体反应状态灵活应用，同时也应根据施术者的经验来选择。若遇关节而经气阻涩者，可用青龙摆尾和白虎摇头等法，并施以循摄法，使经气通关过节。

二、治神与守神

治神与守神包括医者与患者两个方面。一是指医者专注于针刺治疗的全过程；二是指患者专心、认真配合完成医者的治疗。治神与守神是针刺治疗的前提与根本，贯穿整个针刺治疗过程，并且直接影响针刺疗效。

"神"是指人体生命活动的外在表现，是人体精神意识、思维活动以及脏腑、气血、津液活动外在表现的高度概括。《素问·宝命全形论》曰："凡刺之真，必先治神。"《灵枢·本神》曰："凡刺之法，先必本于神。"二者都明确指出治神的必要。《灵枢·九针十二原》中的："粗守形，上守神"，指出守神的重要性。针刺必须以"神"为根本，强调"神"在针刺治疗中的作用。治神与守神不仅影响针刺临床疗效，也是衡量针灸医者水平高低的标准。

（一）治神意在得气

医者意念集中，并且根据患者的精神、意识及全身情况进行施针，目的是得气。同时，患者也需要心平气和，思想集中于医者施术之处，促使针下得气甚而气至病所。《灵枢·官能》篇说："用针之要，勿忘其神。"治神要始终贯穿于针刺操作的全过程。治神的关键是医者认真审视患者机体强弱、病位深浅、邪正盛衰、气血虚实、阴阳平衡而决断用针之法，方能得气。

acupuncturist carefully examine the strength or weakness of the patient's body, the depth of the disease location, the prosperity or decline of vital qi and evil qi, the deficiency and excess of qi and blood, and the imbalance of yin and yang before determaining the needling methods so as to acquire a good efficacy.

2.2 To concentrate on the spirit for the purpose of maintaining qi

When qi has been obtained after needle insertion, acupuncturists need to maintain it, so as to enhance the efficacy of acupuncture. Concentration of the vitality covers both the acupuncturist and the patient aspects. For one, the acupuncturists are required to concentrate on the sensation from the needles and apply acupuncture techniques according to the changes of the patient's vitality. For another, the patients are asked to concentrate on the needling induction to coordinate with the acupuncturists' needle manipulation and to extend qi to affected parts, so as to achieve the purpose of enhancing the acupuncture efficacy. The *Plain Questions-The theory of maintaining life and physique* emphasized that one must be calm as if one looked down into a deep abyss, the hand must be strong as if it hold a tiger. The spirit should not be confused by the multitude of things. *Song to Elucidate Mysteries* has similar descriptions as following. The acupuncturists concentrate their thoughts and spirit, and are as calm and resolute as capturing a tiger; be as solemn and prudent as you are waiting for a noble man. The ancients emphasized that the acupuncturists need to be absorbed in the needling process. It is also said in *The Spiritual Pivot-Benshen* that, the fact is those who apply the needles, they observe a patient's condition to get to know whether his essence, spirit, hun soul and po soul are still present or have been lost, and whether he is subjected to a gain or loss. It is emphasized that the concentration of the vitality is that the acupuncturist observes the reaction of the patient, grasps the rise and fall of the essence and qi of the Zang-Fu organs, and applies the corresponding puncturing method at the appropriate time to maintain the qi under the acupuncture. *Plain Questions-Zhen Jie* said, "As for 'one must rectify his spirit', that is, one must look into the eyes of the patient and control his spirit, thereby letting the qi flow easily." In the process of needling treatment, the acupuncturist should quietly wait for qi to arrive, correctly feel the induction under the needle to discriminate properties of qi, accurately evaluate the condition of the body, reasonably adjust the depth, direction and manipulations of needling; It is supposed to guide the patient to concentrate on vitality, which helps the arrival of qi under the needle, and enhances the flow and smooth of qi.

（二）守神意在守住所得之气

当针刺已经得气后需要守气，勿使气散，以增强针刺疗效。守神包括医者和患者两个方面。其一，要求医者专心体会针下感应，并根据患者神气变化及时施以手法；其二，要求患者专心体会针刺感应，以配合医者行针，促使气至病所，达到增强疗效的目的。《素问·宝命全形论》说："如临深渊，手如握虎，神无营于众物。"《标幽赋》说："目无外视，手如握虎，心无内慕，如待贵人。"古人十分强调医者在针刺过程中需要全神贯注。《灵枢·本神》又说：是故用针者，察观病人之态，以知精神魂魄之存亡得失之意。即强调守神是医者通过观察患者的反应，掌握其脏腑精气的盛衰，把握适当的时机施以相应的针刺方法，以维系针下所得之气。《素问·针解》载：必正其神者，欲瞻病人目，制其神，令气易行也。针刺过程中，医者守神可静候气至，正确体会针下指感以辨气，准确判断机体状态，合理调整针刺深浅、方向和手法；引导患者守神则可意守病所，促使针下得气，使经气畅达。当经气已至，要慎守勿失，获得理想的调控效果。

When qi has arrived, be cautious not to lose it so as to get the ideal regulatory efficiency.

Modern acupuncturists propose that based on the "spirit" theory, the specific content of regulation and concentration of the vitality should be endowed to make it operational. In other words, when carrying out needle manipulations, the acupuncturist should guide the patient's activities of related site and (or) mental activities. By mobilizing the patient's own potential for recovering from the disease, the purpose of the treatment is achieved jointly.

现代医家提出,基于"神"的理论,应赋予治神与守神具体内容,使其具有可操作性。即医者在实施手法的同时,应指导患者活动相关部位和(或)进行精神活动。通过调动患者自身治疗疾病的潜能,共同达到治疗的目的。

Chapter 19 Unitary Reinforcing and Reducing Method

1. Rapid-slow reinforcing and reducing methods

It is mainly based on the speed of insertion, withdrawal the needle and the speed of pressing pinhole to distinguish the reinforcing or reducing needling methods.

Miraculous Pivot-Nine Needles and Twelve Source said, "[First] slowly and [then] fast, this will result in repletion. [First] fast and [then] slowly, this will result in depletion. " "The subtle secret of piercing lies in varying speeds" puts forward the basic operation requirements for rapid-slow reinforcing and reducing methods, "Xu" means slow and "Ji" means rapid. *Miraculous Pivot-Xiao Zhen Jie* said, "'[First] slowly and [then] fast, this will result in repletion' is to say: [the needle] is to be inserted slowly and to be withdrawn quickly. '[First] fast and [then] slowly, this will result in depletion' is to say: [the needle] is to be inserted quickly and to be withdrawn slowly. "

After the needle is inserted to the given depth and the arrival of qi is achieved in shallow layers, the reinforcing method is conducted by inserting the needle to the given depth slowly and lifting it rapidly, and repeatedly do it for required times. The reducing is performed by inserting the needle rapidly to the given depth in deep layer and lifting it slowly in a shallow layer and repeatedly do it for required times(Fig. 19-1).

第十九章 毫针单式补泻手法

一、徐疾补泻

主要依据针刺速度的快慢以及出针、按闭穴位的快慢以区分补泻的针刺手法。

《灵枢·九针十二原》说："徐而疾则实，疾而徐则虚。""刺之微在速迟"对徐疾补泻提出了基本术式要求，"徐"为缓慢之意，"疾"为快速之意。《灵枢·小针解》说："徐而疾则实者，言徐内而疾出也，疾而徐则虚者，言疾内而徐出也。"

进针后，浅层得气，随之缓慢进针至一定深度，再迅速退针至浅层，反复施行。快速进针至一定深度，得气后，随之缓慢退针至浅层，反复施行；重在徐出，是为泻法（图19-1）。

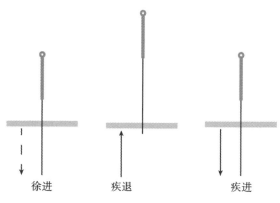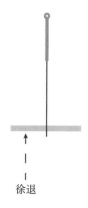

徐进　　疾退　　疾进　　徐退

图 19-1　徐疾补泻

2. Reinforcing and reducing by lifting and thrusting the needle

Mainly according to the change of the strength when conducting the lifting and thrusting methods, the reinforcing and reducing methods can be distinguished.

It was said in *The seventy-eighth issue of the Classic of*

二、提插补泻

主要依据实施提插手法时用力轻重的变化以区分补泻的针刺手法。

《难经·七十八难》说："得气，

Questioning that "after getting qi, to push the needle inward is called reinforcing; to move and pull the needle outward is called reducing. "As Li Chan said in the *Introduction to Medicine* , "All lifting and thrusting manipulations, rapid lifting and slow inserting as cold is reducing method; slow lifting and rapid inserting as hot is reinforcing method. " According to this, later physicians developed and evolved the lifting and thrusting methods into various operation methods.

After the needle is inserted to given depth and the qi arrives, the reinforcing method is conducted by lifting the needle gently, and thrusting it hard with a small amplitude, and repeatedly do it for required times, mainly by thrusting. The reducing is performed by thrusting the needle gently, and lifting it hard with a small amplitude, and repeatedly do it for required times, mainly by lifting (Fig. 19-2).

因推而内之，是谓补；动而伸之，是谓泻。"李梴《医学入门》说："凡提插，疾提慢按如冰冷，泻也；慢提紧按火烧身，补也。"后世医家根据此说，将提插补泻发展、演变成多种操作方法。

针刺得气后，在针下得气处反复施行小幅度的重插轻提手法，以下插用力为主，是为补法；针刺得气后，在针下得气处反复施行小幅度的轻插重提手法，以上提用力为主，是为泻法（图19-2）。

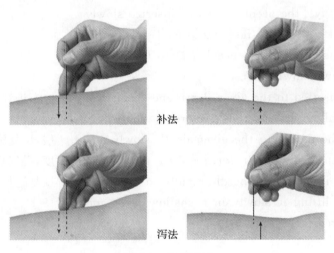

补法

泻法

图 19-2　提插补泻

3. Reinforcing and reducing by twirling and rotating the needle

Mainly according to the difference of the strength when twirling and rotating in different directions, the reinforcing and reducing methods can be distinguished.

Dou Hanqing's *Guide to the Acupuncture Classics* said, "Thumb and index finger are tied together, thumb upward, called left (reinforce); and thumb down ward, called right (reduce). " *Compendium of Acupuncture and Moxibustion* said, "Turning left belongs to yang, so can run yang; turning right belongs to yin, so can run yin. " These explanations above laid the foundation for reinforcing and reducing by twirling and rotating the needle.

After the needle is inserted to a certain depth and the qi arrives, it's called the reinforcing that the needle is rotated forcefully with the thumb forward (turn left) with finger force

三、捻转补泻

主要依据向不同方向捻转时用力轻重的不同来区分补泻的针刺手法。

窦汉卿《针经指南》中"以大指、次指相合，大指往上进，谓之左；大指往下退，谓之右"及《针灸大成》中"左转从阳，能行诸阳；右转从阴，能行诸阴"为捻转补泻奠定了基础。

针刺得气后，在针下得气处反复施行捻转手法，拇指向前捻转时用力重（左转），指力下沉，拇指向

sinking, and apply light force when the thumb restores backward. It's known as the reducing that the needle is rotated forcefully with the thumb backward (turn right) with finger force floating, and apply light force when the thumb restores forward (Fig. 19-3).

后还原时用力轻,是为补法。针刺得气后,在针下得气处反复施行捻转手法,拇指向后捻转时用力重(右转),指力上浮,拇指向前还原时用力轻,是为泻法(图 19-3)。

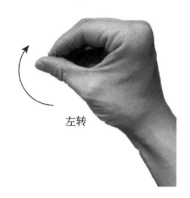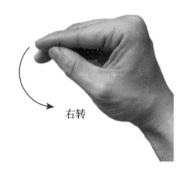

左转　　　　　　右转

图 19-3　捻转补泻

4. Directional supplementation and draining method

Mainly according to the forward and backward movement of needling direction and meridian qi and blood running direction, the reinforcing and reducing methods can be distinguished.

Miraculous Pivot-Zhongshi said, "Draining is to confront them. Supplementing is to pursue them. [Those who] know about confronting and pursuing, they are able to harmonize the qi." It is said in *The seventy-second issue of Classic of Difficult Issues*, "the so-called confront or follow is determined by the circulation of nutrient qi and defensive qi and the circulation of meridian qi. Go with it or go against it, that is confront or follow." According to this, later physicians developed and evolved the directional supplementation and draining.

When the needle inserting, the needle tip following the direction of meridian course means the reinforcing method; and against the meridian course means the reducing method.

5. Respiratory supplementation and draining method

Mainly according to the combination of insertion and withdrawal of needle and the patient's breathing state, the reinforcing and reducing methods can be distinguished.

The *Compendium of Acupuncture and Moxibustion* said, "when the reinforcing is needed, insert the needle when patients [exhale] and withdraw the needle when the patients [inhale]; when the reducing is needed, insert the needle when patients [inhale] and withdraw the needle when patients [exhale]." It is the key point of

四、迎随补泻

主要依据针刺方向与经脉气血运行方向的顺逆来区分补泻的针刺手法。

《灵枢·终始》说:"泻者迎之,补者随之,知迎知随,气可令和。"《难经·七十二难》说:"所谓迎随者,知荣卫之流行,经脉之往来也。随其逆顺而取之,故曰迎随。"后世医家多据此演化成迎随补泻方法。

进针时针尖随着经脉循行方向刺入为补法,针尖迎着经脉循行方向刺入为泻法。

五、呼吸补泻

主要依据针刺进退与患者呼吸状态的配合来区分补泻的针刺手法。

《针灸大成》中"欲补之时,气出针入,气入针出;欲泻之时,气入入针,气出出针",即呼吸补泻的操作要点。

respiratory breathing reinforcing and reducing.

Insert needle when patient breathes out deeply, and conduct the needle according to the method of breathing in and out after getting qi, withdraw needle when patient breathes in deeply, which is the reinforcing method; and insert needle when patient breathes in deeply, and conduct the needle according to the method of breathing in and out after getting qi, withdraw needle when patient breathes out deeply, which is the reducing method.

令患者深呼气时进针,得气后,依呼进吸退之法行针,患者深吸气时出针,是为补法;令患者深吸气时进针,得气后,依吸进呼退之法行针,患者深呼气时出针,是为泻法。

6. The open-closed supplementation and draining method

六、开阖补泻

Mainly according to whether the pinhole is pressed or closed when the needle is out, the reinforcing and reducing methods can be distinguished.

主要依据出针之时,是否按闭针孔来区分补泻的针刺手法。

Plain Questions-Ci Zhi Lun said, "In case [a needle] is inserted [to treat] repletion, the left hand opens the needle hole. In case [a needle] is inserted [to treat] depletion, the left hand closes the needle hole." It's the origin of reinforcing and reducing by keeping the pinhole open or closed.

《素问·刺志论》中"入实者,左手开针空也,入虚者,左手闭针空也",即是开阖补泻的由来。

It is a reinforcing method to withdraw the needle slowly and quickly press the pinhole for a moment after withdraw the needle, and it is a reducing method to quickly withdraw the needle and enlarge the pinhole without pressing.

缓慢退针,出针后迅速按压针孔片刻,是为补法;疾速出针,出针时摇大针孔且不加按压,是为泻法。

Chapter 20　The Comprehensive Reinforcing and Reducing Method

The comprehensive reinforcing and reducing method is a combination application of several unitary reinforcing and reducing methods. Its operation is relatively complicated, and it is mostly founded by acupuncturists after the Jin and Yuan dynasties, systematically recorded in *Rhythm of Golden Needle*. There are mainly methods such as mountain-burning fire (heat-producing needling), heaven-penetrating cooling(cool-producing needling), yin occluding in yang, yang occluding in yin, Zi-wu Daojiu needling, induction qi method and dragon-tiger fighting needling, qi-retaining method, Chou tian method, which are also called eight methods of treating diseases. On behalf of the comprehensive reinforcing and reducing method, mountain-burning fire and heaven-penetrating cooling are reinforcing and reducing in great degree. Reinforcing reducing method combined with needle manipulation are four groups of bionics methods, Dragon-tiger-tortoise-phenix. There are many operation steps of comprehensive reinforcing and reducing manipulation, some of which are standardized, and the approximate operation times are defined. That is to say, nine or six are taken as the cardinal number respectively. Generally, yang numbers of nine are used for reinforcing and yin numbers of six are used for reducing.

(1) Mountain-burning fire. The technique stems from *Plain Questions-the article of Zhen Jie*, "As for 'when piercing a depletion, then replenish it,' [that is, pierce until] there is heat below the needle. When the qi is replete, heat is present", while lacking of the specific operation method and name. *Needle Guide* contained the name of "cool-heat reinforcing and reducing method". The specific operation method can be found in *Rhythm of Golden Needle* and its needle sensation requirements have been defined.

The basic operation sequence of mountain-burning fire is shallow needling first, then deep needling, three times into and one back, that is three-step needling to the deep, one-step needling back to the shallow. The specific methods are mainly lifting and thrusting, breathing, opening and close, etc. It is the basic requirement to generate heat sensation under the needle. This method has the functions of promoting the body's yang qi to grow day by day, gradually generating heat sensation and removing cold from the body, and is suitable for the treatment of cold disorders of deficiency syndrome, such as stubborn numbness and cold

第二十章　毫针复式补泻手法

复式补泻手法是多种单式补泻手法的组合应用,操作较为复杂,多是金元时期以后的针灸医家所创立,系统地记载于《金针赋》之中,主要有烧山火、透天凉、阳中隐阴、阴中隐阳、子午捣臼、导气法与龙虎交战、留气、抽添法,又称为治病八法。复式补泻手法的代表烧山火、透天凉是大补大泻,补泻手法加上行气法是仿生学的四组手法:龙虎龟凤。复式补泻手法的操作步骤较多,其中一些动作还进行了规范化处理,明确了大致的操作次数。即分别以九或六作为基数,一般补法用九阳数,泻法用六阴数。

1. 烧山火　烧山火手法源于《素问·针解》中"刺虚则实之者,针下热也,气实乃热也",但缺少具体的操作方法与名称。《针经指南》载有"寒热补泻法"之名,具体操作方法见于《金针赋》,且明确了其针感要求。

烧山火手法的基本操作顺序是先浅后深、三进一退,具体手法以提插、呼吸、开阖等为主,针下产生热感为基本要求,具有使机体阳气日隆、热感渐生、阴寒自除的作用,适用于顽麻冷痹等虚寒之证。

syndrome.

Basic operation: First determine the designed puncture depth, then divide it into the shallow, middle and deep portions (the three parts of heaven, man and earth). Insert the needle to the shallow portion to get qi; then from shallow to deep, conduct heavy thrusting and slow lifting (reinforcing and reducing by twirling and rotating the needle) nine times portion by portion. After that lift the needle up directly from deep to shallow. The above is called one process (three times into and once back). Repeat this course until the heat sensation appears under the needle, then retain the needle in the deep portion.

The insertion and withdrawal of needle can be operated together with respiratory supplementation and draining and open-closed supplementation and draining. For example, insert and thrust the needle when the patient breathes out and lift and withdraw the needle when the patient breathes in, and press the pinhole quickly after needle withdrawal; when inserting the needle, use the pressing hand to assist in pressing (Fig. 20-1). All these will help to improve the success of manipulation.

基本操作:将腧穴的可刺深度分为浅、中、深三层(或天、人、地三部)。针至浅层得气;再先浅后深,逐层(部)施行紧按慢提法(或捻转补法)九数;然后一次将针从深层退至浅层,称之为一度(三进一退)。如此反复施术数度,待针下产生热感,即留针于深层。

进出针时可结合呼吸补泻、开阖补泻一同操作。如呼气时进针插针,吸气时退针出针,出针后迅速扪闭针孔;进针时还可以辅助使用押手重切(图 20-1)。这些均有助于提高手法操作的成功性。

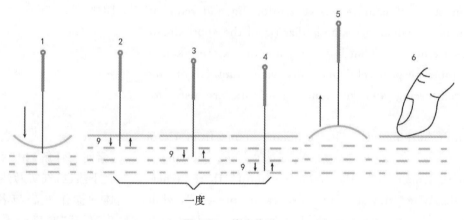

图 20-1　烧山火法

(2) Heaven-penetrating cooling. The technique stems from *Plain Questions-the article of Zhen Jie*, "As for 'when there is fullness, then discharge it,' [that is, pierce until] there is cold below the needle. When the qi is depleted, cold is present", but also lacking of the specific operation method and name. The specific operation method can be found in *Rhythm of Golden Needle* and its needle sensation requirements have been defined.

The basic operation sequence of heaven-penetrating cooling is first deep, then shallow, and then one into and three times back. The specific methods are mainly lifting and thrusting, breathing, opening and close, etc. It is the basic requirement to generate cool sensation under the needle. This method has the functions of strengthening the body's yin qi gradually, generating cool sensation

2. 透天凉　透天凉手法源于《素问·针解》"满而泄之者,针下寒也,气虚乃寒也",也缺少具体的操作方法与名称。具体操作方法见于《金针赋》,且明确了其针感要求。

透天凉手法的基本操作顺序是先深后浅、一进三退,具体手法以提插、呼吸、开阖等为主,针下产生凉感为基本要求,具有使机体阴气渐隆、凉感渐生、邪热得消的作用,适用于火邪热毒等实热之证。

and removing heat from the body, and is suitable for the treatment of hot disorders of excess type, such as fire and heat syndrome.

Basic operation: First determine the designed puncture depth, then divide it into the shallow, middle and deep portions (the three parts of heaven, man and earth). Insert the needle to the deep portion to get qi; then from deep to shallow, conduct heavily lifting and slow thrusting (or reducing by twirling and rotating the needle) six times portion by portion. After that thrust the needle directly from shallow into deep. The above is called one process (once into and three times back). Repeat this course until the cool sensation appears under the needle, then retain the needle there.

The insertion and withdrawal of needle can be operated together with respiratory supplementation and draining and open-closed supplementation and draining. For example, insert and thrust the needle when the patient breathes in, and lift and withdraw the needle when the patient breathes out, and when withdrawing the needle, shake and enlarge the pinhole without pressing the pinhole; when inserting the needle, use the pressing hand to assist in pressing (Fig. 20-2). All these will help to improve the success of manipulation.

基本操作：将腧穴的可刺深度分为浅、中、深三层(或天、人、地三部)。针至深层得气；再先深后浅,逐层(部)施行紧提慢按(或捻转泻法)六数；然后一次将针从浅层进至深层,称之为一度(一进三退)。如此反复施术数度,待针下产生凉感,即留针于此。

进出针时可结合呼吸补泻、开阖补泻一同操作。如吸气时进针插针,呼气时退针出针,出针时摇大其孔,不扪其穴；进针时控制押手轻压腧穴(图20-2)。这些均有助于提高手法操作的成功性。

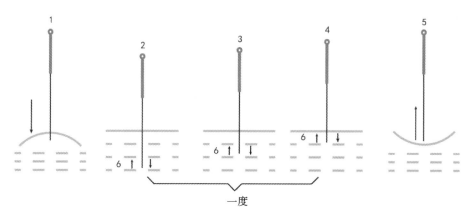

图 20-2　透天凉法

Precautions: The two methods of mountain-burning fire and heaven-penetrating cooling are mainly focused on rapid-slow reinforcing and reducing methods, performed as three times into and once back or once into and three times back. Taking reinforcing and reducing by lifting and thrusting the needle as the basic action, it is manifested as heavily thrusting and slowly lifting or heavily lifting and slowly thrusting. At the same time, combining with the nine-six technique theory, breathing, open-close reinforcing and reducing, etc. Only when the acupuncturist manipulates the techniques skillfully and canonically, can ideal effect of needling be achieved in clinic.

It is advisable to use the method of mountain-burning fire and heaven-penetrating cooling to choose acupoints with relatively rich

注意事项：烧山火与透天凉两法主要以徐疾补泻为技术核心,表现为三进一退或一进三退；以提插补泻手法为基本动作,表现为紧按慢提或紧提慢按；同时结合九六术数理论和呼吸、开阖等法。临床上操作熟练、规范才能取得相应的针刺效应。

应用烧山火或透天凉法,以选用肌肉比较丰厚处的穴位为宜；当

muscles. When the basic needle sensation is strong, the manipulation range should not be too large, and the number of repetition should not be too much. It should not be enforced strongly to avoid causing pain to patients. The grasping of basic needle sensation and the reasonable application of pressing hand are also the conditions to improve the success rate of manipulation.

In short, the specific operation methods of mountain-burning fire and heaven-penetrating cooling in clinic are slightly different among physicians, but their basic principles are all implemented according to *Rhythm of Golden Needle*.

基础针感较强时,手法操作幅度不宜过大,重复次数不宜太多;更不可强力施行,以免引起患者疼痛;基础针感的把握以及押手的合理应用也是提高手法操作成功率的条件。

总之,临床上烧山火和透天凉两法的具体操作方法,各医家虽略有不同,但其基本原则皆遵循《金针赋》施行。

Chapter 21　Penetration Needling Method

Penetration needling method is a method of needling two or more acupoints with a needle by changing the angle and direction of the acupuncture. It is also called acupoint penetration needling, or penetration acupuncture.

There are some descriptions about "Hegu needling" in *Miraculous Pivot-the Official Acupuncture*. Wang Guorui, a physicians of the Jin and Yuan Dynasties, illustrated the penetration needling method by which the needle is inserted from Sizhukong to Shuaigu backwards in the treatment of migraine and headache, from Dicang to Jiache to treat patients with facial paralysis in *Bianque's Classic of Yulong of Acupuncture and Moxibustion*. There are many descriptions of indications and operation methods of penetrating acupuncture in some literature of acupuncture and moxibustion such as *Guide to the Acupuncture Classics*, *Acupuncture Principles in Six Volumes*, *The Great Compendium of Acupuncture and Moxibustion*. Zhou Shudong, a doctor in the Qing Dynasty, also made a comprehensive discussion and summary of penetration needling method in "*Golden Needle and Plum Blossom Poetry Note*".

(1) Operation method.

①Direct penetration method: Select two acupoints which are relative in yin and yang. After the needle is inserted perpendicularly and qi arrives, pointing into another acupoint subcutaneously. This method is applicable to the acupoints on the four limbs.

②Obliquely permeable method: Two acupoints opposite to the exterior and interior of the yin and yang of the limbs are selected, and the needle is inserted obliquely from one acupoint, and then the needle is pricked subcutaneously to the other acupoint after getting qi; two acupoints on the same level of the limbs can also be selected, first directly insert one acupoint to obtain qi, and then obliquely insert to the other acupoint subcutaneously. It is more suitable for acupoints on limbs or the same meridian.

③Horizontal permeable method: Select two acupoints at the same level of the limb, and then insert the needle from one acupoint to the subcutaneous of the second acupoint after arrival of qi. It is suitable for acupoints on the head, face, chest, back and superficial muscle.

④Multidirectional penetration method: Select a part where

第二十一章　毫针透穴刺法

透穴刺法是针刺时借助不同的针刺角度、方向与深度的调整，以达到一针透达两个或更多穴位的针刺方法，又称为"透穴"或"透刺"。

《灵枢·官针》中已有"合谷刺"等类似针法的描述，金元时期的医家王国瑞所著《扁鹊神应针灸玉龙经》有"偏正头风最难医，丝竹金针亦可施，沿皮向后透率谷，一针两穴世间稀"及"口眼㖞斜最可嗟，地仓妙穴连颊车"等记载，即是透刺针法的具体应用。《针经指南》《针方六集》《针灸大成》等针灸文献，也记录了大量透穴刺法的适应证和操作方法。清代医家周树冬在《金针梅花诗钞》中也对透穴进行了全面的论述与总结。

1. 操作方法

（1）直透法：选择肢体阴阳表里相对的两个腧穴，从其一腧穴直刺进针，得气后，再刺达另一腧穴皮下的方法。适用于四肢部位的腧穴。

（2）斜透法：选择肢体阴阳表里相对的两个腧穴，从其一腧穴斜刺进针，得气后，再刺达另一腧穴皮下的方法；亦可选择肢体同一层面的两个腧穴，先在其一腧穴直刺进针，得气后，再斜向刺达另一个腧穴皮下。适用于四肢部位或同一经脉上的腧穴。

（3）平透法：选择位于肢体同一个层面的两个腧穴，从其一腧穴平刺进针，得气后，刺达另一个腧穴皮下的方法。适用于头面部、胸背及肌肉浅薄部位的腧穴。

（4）多向透刺法：选择腧穴较

acupoints are concentrated, after the needle is inserted obliquely or perpendicularly, inserting into others acupoints one by one until arrival of qi. It is suitable for acupoints in muscular parts.

(2) Clinical applications. Penetration needling method is provided with few quantity of needles, large amount of acupoints, strong sensation of needling, wild scope of application. This method can reduce needle insertion pain and improve the efficacy resulting from the synergistic effect of multi-acupoints. This method is used for headache, facial nerve paralysis, apoplexy hemiplegia, gastroptosis, uterus prolapse, periarthritis of shoulder, injury of soft tissue, psychosis, neurosis and so on.

(3) Precautions.

①Be familiar with the anatomical structure of the acupoints and prevent the possible accidents in puncturing.

②Take arrival of qi as the suitable degree for piercing, and it's unsuitable to penetrate the contralateral skin.

③The strength of needling manipulation should not be too strong.

④Generally, the needle retention time is 20-30 minutes.

为密集的部位,以其中任一腧穴为进针点,或直刺或斜刺进针,得气后,将针依次刺向其他腧穴。适用于肌肉丰厚部位的腧穴。

2. 临床应用 透穴刺法具有用针数量少、刺激穴位多、针刺感应强、适应范围广等特点。既可减少进针疼痛,又有利于多穴位协同增效。适用于针灸临床诸如头痛、面神经麻痹、中风偏瘫、胃下垂、子宫下垂、肩关节周围炎、软组织损伤、精神病、神经官能症等多种疾病。

3. 注意事项

(1)熟悉腧穴的解剖结构,防止针刺的异常情况发生。

(2)以针刺得气为度,不宜刺透对侧腧穴皮肤。

(3)透刺过程中的行针手法不宜过强。

(4)透穴刺法留针时间一般为20～30分钟。

Chapter 22　Multi-needle Method

Multi-needle method is a needling method that uses multiple needles, different combinations and arrangements, and stimulates lesions or points at the same time so as to enhance the efficacy through the synergistic effect of multi-needle.

Proximal needling, triple needling, centro-square needling in *Miraculous Pivot-the Official Acupuncture*, and modern clinical surrounding puncture method are all part of multi-needle method.

(1) Proximal needling method. Local lesion or acupoint is the center of proximal needling. First, one needle is inserted perpendicularly, then the other needle is inserted obliquely in the vicinity of this acupoint. This method is originated from *Miraculous Pivot-the Official Acupuncture*, "proximate needling: one [needle] each is to be inserted straight into and sideways to [the location of the disease]. This serves to cure blockages remaining at one and the same location for a long time."

①Operation method: Local lesion or acupoint is the center of proximal needling. First, one needle is inserted perpendicularly, after the qi arrival, and the other needle is inserted obliquely at 0.5-1 cun in the vicinity of this acupoint. The depth of the two needles is same(Fig. 22-1).

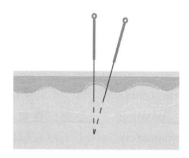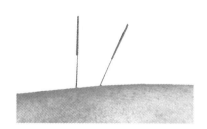

图 22-1　傍针刺法

②Clinical applications: The method is suitable for the diseases with long course, and fixed pain spot with obvious pressing pain. Such as headache, arthralgia, backache, heel pain, lumbar hyperplasia, myositis.

(2) Triple needling method. The local pathology or acupoint is the center, one needle should be inserted perpendicularly, then the other two needles are inserted obliquely in the vicinity of this acupoint, and three needles should be used together, so it is called

第二十二章　局部多针刺法

局部多针刺法是指针刺时使用多支毫针，以不同的组合与排列方式，同时刺激病变局部或者腧穴，以达到多针协同增效的针刺方法。

《灵枢·官针》记载的"九刺""五刺""十二刺"等刺法中的傍针刺、齐刺、扬刺以及现代临床常用的围刺法等均属于此范畴。

1. 傍针刺法　以病变局部或腧穴为中心，直刺一针，再于其近旁斜向加刺一针，正傍配合，故称傍针刺法。此法源于《灵枢·官针》"傍针刺者，直刺、傍刺各一，以治留痹久居者也"。

（1）操作方法：一般以痛点或某一腧穴为中心，直刺一针，得气后，再在其旁 0.5～1 寸处斜向刺入一针，针尖靠近直刺的毫针针尖，两针的针刺深度大致相同（图22-1）。

（2）临床应用：适用于痛点固定、压痛明显、病程日久的病证。如头痛、关节痛、腰背痛、足跟痛、腰椎增生症、肌纤维组织炎等。

2. 齐刺法　以病变局部或腧穴为中心，直刺一针，再于其两旁各刺一针，三针齐用，故称齐刺法。此法源于《灵枢·官针》中的"齐刺

triple needling method. This method comes from the description in the chapter of the *Miraculous Pivot-the Official Acupuncture*, "triple needling:one [needle] is inserted straight [into the location of the disease];two [needles] are inserted sideways. This serves to cure cold qi that is present in small quantities in the depth. It is also called triple piercing, which serves to cure blockage qi that is present in small quantities in the depth. "

①Operation method:The local pathology or acupoint is the center,one needle should be inserted perpendicularly,then the other two needles are inserted obliquely at 0. 5-1 cun in the vicinity of this acupoint. The two needles are close to the perpendicular needle,and the needling depth of the three needles is approximately the same(Fig. 22-2).

者,直入一,傍入二,以治寒气小深者。或曰三刺,三刺者,治痹气小深者也"。

(1) 操作方法:一般以痛点为中心,直刺一针,得气后,再在其两旁(或上下,或左右)0.5~1 寸处斜向刺入两针。针尖靠近直刺的毫针针尖,三针的针刺深度大致相同(图 22-2)。

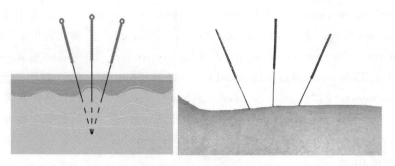

图 22-2　齐刺法

②Clinical application:It's similar to the proximal needling method.

(3) Centro-square needling method. After the needle is inserted to the center of diseased region,stab four needles around the position dispersedly, so it's called. This method comes from *Miraculous Pivot-the Official Acupuncture*, "shallow surround needling:one [needle] is inserted straight [into the location of the disease]. Four [needles] are inserted sideways superficially. This serves to cure massively pounding cold qi. "

①Operation method:After one needle is inserted to the center of diseased region, stab four needles around the position dispersedly. The needling depth of the five needles is approximately the same(Fig. 22-3).

②Clinical applications:It is suitable for the diseases with large pathological area,shallow pathological position and cold pathogenic stagnation, such as rheumatism pain, dermatoneuritis, soft tissue injury. In modern times,the tapping of plum-blossom needle is the evolution of Centro-square needling.

(4) Surrounding puncture method. Surrounding puncture is a multi-needle method,which means after one needle is inserted to the center of diseased region,stab multi needles around the position

(2) 临床应用:与傍针刺的临床应用相近。

3. 扬刺法　在病变之中心部位直刺一针,然后在其四周各浅刺一针,刺的部位较为分散,故称扬刺法。此法源于《灵枢•官针》中的"扬刺者,正内(纳)一,傍内(纳)四而浮之,以治寒气之博大者也"。

(1) 操作方法:选取病变之中心部位直刺一针,得气后,再于其上下左右(即病变部位的周边)向病变中心各斜刺一针,五针的针刺深度大致相同(图 22-3)。

(2) 临床应用:适用于病变范围大、病变位置较浅、以寒邪凝滞为主的病证。如风湿痛、皮神经炎、软组织损伤等。近代梅花针叩刺法即为扬刺法的演变。

4. 围刺法　以病变部位为中心,在其边缘多针直刺或平刺,形成包绕病变之势的多针刺法。围

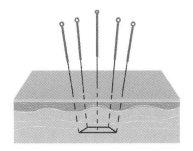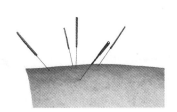

图 22-3　扬刺法

dispersedly or perpendicularly. Surrounding puncture method is developed by Centro-square needling, with broader application scope.

①Operation method：According to the size and depth of the pathological region，the appropriate length of filiform needle should be selected，and inserted obliquely or horizontally around the periphery of the lesion area，The depth and direction of the needling can be determined by the nature of the disease and size and depth of the position.

②Clinical applications：This method is suitable for nodules，numbness，and other skin lesions，such as soft tissue injuries of the extremities，external epicondylitis，urticaria，herpes zoster.

刺法由扬刺法发展而来，应用更为广泛。

（1）操作方法：根据病变之大小深浅，选择长短适宜毫针，围绕病变区域周边斜刺或平刺数针，进针深浅与针刺方向可根据病变性质和病灶大小调整。

（2）临床应用：适用于结节、麻木等病证以及部分皮肤病变，如四肢关节软组织损伤、肱骨外上髁炎、荨麻疹、带状疱疹等。

Chapter 23　Kinetic Acupuncture

Kinetic acupuncture therapy refers to a method by which the patients can move the affected area or related parts, when the acupuncturists implement the acupuncture technique on the basis of obtaining qi. The acupuncturist cooperates with the patient so as to improve the clinical efficacy. The characteristic of this method is the emphasis on the coordination of patients' movements in the needling process, so this method is also known as the interactive acupuncture method.

(1) Operation method.

①Acupuncture method: After needles are inserted and obtaining qi conventionally, the acupuncturist continues to carry out the lifting, thrusting and rotating technique methods for 1-2 minutes. At the same time, acupuncturist guides patients to do related functional activities, once every 5-10 minutes for 2-3 times. The strength of needle manipulation operation should be weak at first and gradually increased, and the reaction of patients should be observed closely to prevent excessive pain or faint.

②Exercise mode: Different parts of the disease have different ways of performing functional activities. The movement of joints is mainly composed of flexion and extension, rotation, such as walking, lifting arms, rocking arm, even loading arms, finger fine movements. The movement of the five sense organs and nine orifices, is dominated by their physiological activities, such as swallowing, teeth massaging, anus contraction and pronunciation. The movement of viscera, chest and abdomen, is mainly breathing activities. For example, patients with the side stitch and chest tightness usually make a chest or abdominal deep breathing.

No matter which type of exercise the patient is doing, the speed of movement should be from slow to fast and the range of movement should be from small to large, and reach the physiological limit gradually. Exercise can be performed intermittently, and for some diseases, activities can be gradually strengthened in a clear direction towards where pain is obvious.

③Principle of acupoint selection: Take acupoints remotely. Normally, select acupoints in the lower body to treat diseases in the upper body. Selecting acupoints in the upper part of the body to treat diseases in the lower body. If the disease is in the left half, select acupoints in the right half; if the disease is in the right part, select acupoints in the left part; if the disease is in the middle part,

第二十三章　运动针刺法

运动针刺法是指在针刺得气的基础上,医者实施行针手法的同时,令患者活动患处或相关部位,医患配合,提高临床疗效的针刺方法。本法的特点在于针刺过程中强调患者的运动配合。因其强调医者和患者间的配合互动,又称互动式针刺法。

1. 操作方法

(1) 针刺方法:常规针刺操作得气后,医者继续实施提插或捻转或提插捻转手法1～2分钟,同时指导患者做相关的功能活动,每隔5～10分钟施行1次,实施2～3次为宜。实施行针手法应由弱到强,并注意观察患者反应,防止过于疼痛或晕针发生。

(2) 运动方式:患病部位不同,患者进行功能活动的方式也有所不同。关节部位的运动方式以屈伸、旋转形式为主,如做行走、举臂、摇臂甚或负重举臂、手指精细动作等;五官九窍等部位的运动方式以其生理活动为主,如做吞咽、叩齿、缩肛、发音等动作;内脏或胸腹部的运动方式以呼吸活动为主,例如岔气、胸闷等病证的患者以做胸式或腹式深呼吸为主。

无论患者做何种运动,其速度都应由慢到快,幅度由小到大,渐至生理活动极限;可以间歇进行,某些病证可逐步向疼痛明显的方向去强化活动。

(3) 选穴原则:以远道取穴为主。一般是病在上取之下,病在下取之上;病在左取之右,病在右取之左;病在中,取之外。

select acupoints outside.

（2）Clinical applications. It is suitable for movement disorders, such as acute lumbar sprain, periarthritis of shoulder, soft tissue injury, apoplexy and hemiplegia.

（3）Precautions. The position of the patients should be suitable for the exercise of affected extremity and helpful to maintain the relative stabilization of the needling site. Considering the need of repeated manipulation for acupuncturists and the need of activities for the patients, sticking or bending needles should be avoided.

2. 临床应用　适用于急性腰扭伤、肩关节周围炎、软组织损伤、中风偏瘫等运动障碍性疾病。

3. 注意事项　患者的体位要适合活动患处，并有助于保持针刺部位的相对稳定。因需反复施行手法，加之患者的活动，要防止滞针或弯针。

Chapter 24　Moxibustion Sensation

Moxibustion sensation generally refers to the patient's self feeling during moxibustion. Like acupuncture sensation, moxibustion sensation not only has the local sensation of the moxibustion site, but also has the sensation of transmitting to the distance or along the meridians. There are different forms of local heat sensation: ① surface heat sensation, that is, only surface heat sensation; ② deep thermal sense, that is, the surface is not hot or slightly hot, but the deep is hot; ③ diathermy sense, that is, the surface heat gradually penetrated into the deep tissue; ④ the sense of heat expansion, that is, the sense of heat gradually diffuses around the moxibustion site; ⑤ heat transferring sense, that is, local heat sense can conduct to the distance; ⑥ the transmission of sensation along meridians refers to the conduction of heat sensation along meridians. However, it should be noted that the transmission of sensation along meridians of moxibustion is sometimes not the conduction of heat sensation, but the sensation similar to that of meridian qi conduction of acupuncture. In addition, there is a special phenomenon of moxibustion sensation, that is, the local part of moxibustion is not hot or slightly hot, but the far part is hot, or the viscera and organs related to the acupoints are hot.

The appearance or different manifestations of moxibustion sensation can be affected by many factors, such as moxibustion methods, initial temperature, temperature duration and stimulation degree, and the patient's condition, constitution and sensitivity to thermal stimulation. Generally speaking, the difference of moxibustion methods and stimulation degree are important factors to produce moxibustion sensation, but even if the same moxibustion method and stimulation degree, due to the patient's condition, constitution and sensitivity to thermal stimulation, there will be different moxibustion sensation. In recent years, some scholars have put forward the "theory of heat sensitivity" and "method of heat sensitive Moxibustion". They believe that, those who have moxibustion sensation of heat penetration, heat expansion, heat transfer, sensation transmission along the meridian, local non heat or slight heat but far heat are more sensitive to the heat stimulation of moxibustion, and their moxibustion effect is relatively significant.

第二十四章　灸感的表现形式

灸感一般是指施灸时患者的自我感受。与针感一样，灸感既有施灸部位的局部感觉，也有向远处传导或循经感传的感觉。局部的热感有不同的表现形式：①表热感，即仅表面有热感；②深热感，即表面不热或微热而深部较热；③透热感，即表面的热感逐步透达组织深部；④扩热感，即热感以施灸部位为中心向周围逐渐扩散；⑤传热感，即局部的热感可向远处传导；⑥循经感传，即热感沿着经脉传导，但需注意的是，灸法的循经感传有时不是热感的传导，而是类似针法经气传导的感觉。除此之外，还有比较特殊的灸感现象，即施灸局部不热或微热而远部较热，或与所灸经穴相关的脏腑、器官热。

灸感的出现或不同的表现形式可受多方面因素影响，如施灸方法、施灸起始温度、温度持续时间、刺激程度和患者病情、体质及其对热刺激的敏感度等。一般而言，施灸方法与刺激程度的不同，是产生灸感强弱的重要因素，但即使同样的施灸方法与刺激程度，由于患者病情、体质和对热刺激的敏感度不同也会有不同的灸感出现。近年来有学者提出"热敏学说"和"热敏灸法"，认为在施灸中，凡能够出现透热、扩热、传热、循经感传、局部不热或微热而远部较热等灸感者，多属于对灸法的热刺激较为敏感者，其灸效果也相对显著。

Chapter 25 Calculation of Moxibustion Quantity

Moxibustion quantity refers to the stimulation intensity generated by the burning moxibustion fire on the skin where moxibustion is applied, and the accumulation of thermal stimulation applied within a certain unit of time. The quantity of moxibustion is closely related to the curative effect. Reaching a certain amount of moxibustion will produce a certain moxibustion effect. Moxibustion effect is the result of different moxibustion methods cooperate with different moxibustion quantity.

In ancient moxibustion, although there was no word "moxibustion quantity", but there was a saying of "raw moxibustion and ripe moxibustion". Raw moxibustion means less moxibustion, while ripe moxibustion means more moxibustion. Moxibustion quantity is based on the comprehensive factors of the patient's age, severity of illness, constitution, moxibustion site and so on. The number of cone and cumulative number of cone are different each time. However, the ancients stressed that moxibustion has to reach a certain degree of warmth and produce a certain moxibustion sensation. Only skin surface has heat sensation, which often fails to achieve the purpose of treatment. As the *Yizong Jinjian* said, "When moxibustion is used to treat a disease, it is necessary to make sure the moxibustion quantity is enough to get moxibustion sensation, then the disease can be cured." In ancient literature, the records of moxibustion in the hundreds of cone referred to the cumulative number of moxibustion treatment for many times.

Clinically, there are different calculation methods for the moxibustion quantity. Generally, the unit that moxa-cone moxibustion is quantified by the size and amount of moxa cones; while moxa roll moxibustion and moxa-burner moxibustion is quantified by time and Taiyi miraculous moxa roll and thunder-fire miraculous moxa roll are quantified by the number of ironing moxibustion. There is also the cumulative amount of moxibustion, that is, the total amount of moxibustion in the course of treatment.

It is generally believed that the amount of moxibustion should be small for children and teenagers, and large for the middle-aged and the old; for head, limbs, chest, back and other places with thin skin and less muscles, moxa cone should be small and less; for waist, abdomen, buttocks, limbs and other places with thick skin and more muscles, moxa cone should be large and more. To solve the symptoms of superficial pathogenic factors, such as cold wind at the beginning, or the diseases of upper excess and lower deficiency,

第二十五章 灸量的计算

灸量,即施灸的刺激量,是指施灸时,燃烧的灸火对施灸部位所产生的刺激强度,及其在一定的施灸时间范围内产生的累积刺激量。灸量与疗效密切相关,达到一定的灸量就会产生一定的灸效。灸效是不同的灸法与不同的灸量协同产生的灸治效果。

古代灸法中,虽然没有"灸量"一词,但有"灸之生熟"之说,生,即少灸,熟,即多灸。少灸与多灸根据患者的年龄大小、病情轻重、体质、施灸部位等综合因素来确定,每次施灸的壮数及累积的壮数是不同的。但古人强调施灸时必须达到一定的温热程度,产生一定的灸感,仅皮表有热感,往往达不到治疗目的,如《医宗金鉴》所说:凡灸诸病,必火足气到,始能求愈。古代文献中灸百壮记载,是指多次灸治的累积数。

临床上不同的施灸方法有不同的灸量计算方法。一般艾炷灸以艾炷的大小和壮数来定,艾条灸、温灸器多用时间计算,太乙神针、雷火神针则以熨灸的次数计算。还有累积施灸的量,即疗程的总灸量。

现普遍认为,小儿、青少年灸量宜小,中老年人灸量宜大;头面、四肢、胸背等皮薄肉少处,艾炷均宜小而少;腰腹、臀和四肢皮厚肉多处,可大炷多壮。若治初感风寒等邪气轻浅之证,或上实下虚之疾,欲解表通阳,祛散外邪,或引导气血下行时,不过三、五、七壮已

to relieve the exterior, dredge yang, dispel external evil, or guide the downward flow of qi and blood, even 3 Zhuang, 5 Zhuang, 7 Zhuang are enough, and the moxa cone should not be too big. For the syndrome of chronic cold and exhaustion of the vital qi, it is necessary to moxibustion with large amount of big moxa cones. Especially for the critical syndrome, moxibustion can not stop till the recovery of yang and pulse returns(Tab. 25-1).

足,艾炷亦不宜过大;但对沉寒痼冷、元气将脱等证,须扶助阳气、温散寒凝时,则须大炷多壮,尤其对危重证,甚至不计壮数,灸至阳回脉复为止(表 25-1)。

Tab. 25-1　The Grasp of Moxibustion Quantity(表 25-1　灸量的掌握)

Conditions（条件）	Large amount of moxibustion（灸量大）	Small amount of moxibustion（灸量小）
Age（年龄）	The middle-aged and the old（中老年）	Children and teenagers（小儿、青少年）
Constitution（体质）	Strong (large amount in single treatment with short course)（体实（单次灸量大,但疗程宜短））	Weak (small amount in single treatment with long course)（体弱（单次灸量小,但疗程宜长））
Position（部位）	Waist, abdomen and four limbs with thick muscles（腰腹、臀和四肢的皮肉深厚处）	Head, chest and four limbs with thin skin and few muscles（头面、胸背、四肢的皮肉浅薄处）
Disease condition（病情）	Exhaustion of the vital qi, chronic diseases（元气欲脱,沉寒痼冷）	Light and shallow pathogenic factor, excess in the upper and deficiency in the lower（邪气轻浅,上实下虚）

The length of treatment course is another aspect of moxibustion quantity, which is flexible according to the disease condition. The treatment course of acute disease is short, it can be carried out once a day for 2-3 days or 2-3 times a day; while the treatment course of chronic disease is long, which can last for months or even more than one year. When moxibustion is used at first, once a day, changed to once every 2-3 days after 3 times.

The key influencing factors of moxibustion quantity include: ①The moxibustion fire: the moxibustion fire is the factor that determines the amount of moxibustion produced in unit time. ②The moxibustion time: the longer the moxibustion time is, the more energy spectrum and chemical active substances release during moxibustion are absorbed by the body, that is, the greater the moxibustion quantity produced. ③The moxibustion distance: moxibustion distance refers to the distance between moxibustion fire and skin when moxibustion with moxa stick and moxa burner. The moxibustion distance determines the local temperature of moxibustion and the absorption of chemical active substances released from the burning of moxibustion materials. ④Frequency of moxibustion: moxibustion frequency is not only related to the accumulation of moxibustion quantity, but also directly related to the effect of moxibustion. Understanding the key factors affecting

关于施灸疗程的长短,可根据病情灵活掌握。急性疾病疗程较短,可每日 1 次,连灸 2～3 日,亦可每日灸 2～3 次;慢性疾病疗程较长,可灸治数月乃至 1 年以上。一般初灸时,每日 1 次,3 次后改为2～3 日 1 次。

影响灸量的关键因素:①灸火的大小;灸火的大小是单位时间内产生灸量的决定因素。②施灸时间的长短:灸法与用药一样有量的积累,施灸时间越长,施灸时释放的能谱和化学活性物质被机体吸收越多,即灸量越大。③灸距的大小:灸距是指艾条灸、温灸器灸时灸火与皮肤之间的距离,灸距决定了施灸局部温度的高低和灸材燃烧释放的化学活性物质吸收的多少。④施灸频度:施灸频度不仅影响灸量的积累,而且也直接关系到灸法的疗效。了解影响灸量的关键因素,对能否恰当地控制灸量,

the moxibustion quantity is of great significance for properly controlling the amount of moxibustion, exploring the application rules of moxibustion quantity for different diseases, improving the effect of moxibustion, and standardizing the operation of moxibustion.

探索不同病证灸量的应用规律,提高灸疗效果,以及灸法操作规范化有着重要的意义。

Chapter 26   Selection of Cupping Method and Cupping Skin Marks

1. Selection of cupping method

Types of cupping method such as flash-fire cupping, retained cupping, moving cupping, pricking-cupping bloodletting method, needle cupping and medicated cupping, are commonly used in clinic practice, among which pricking-cupping bloodletting method and moving cupping method are relatively effective.

1. 1   Selection according to experience

(1) Pain. For pain syndrome, pricking-cupping bloodletting method is often used. For example, in patients with primary trigeminal neuralgia, miliary or oval pink positive reaction points may be found in the back of T1-T2 skin, and pricking-cupping bloodletting method is used for the positive reaction points. For facial paralysis patients with pain behind the ear, take the point 1 cun below Yifeng(TE17) on the affected side to get effect. Acute tonsillitis and acute laryngitis are treated by pricking-cupping bloodletting at Dazhui (GV14). For patients with functional headache, pricking-cupping bloodletting can be applied at Tianzong (SI11). Pricking-cupping bloodletting can be applied on tenderness points, Huantiao(GB30), Weizhong(BL40), Yanglingquan(GB34), Kunlun (BL60) for the treatment of sciatica. Pricking and bloodletting around Weizhong(BL40)combined with cupping at lumbar pain point are used to treat acute lumbar sprain. Bloodletting at the most painful point, combined with cupping and electro-acupuncture at affected areas are used to treat postherpetic neuralgia. Acute gouty arthritis is treated with plum-blossom needle with tapping plus cupping, and combine with Chinese herbal medicine.

(2) Chronic diseases. Chronic diseases are mainly treated by moving cupping. For example, take moving cupping therapy along the sides of the spine combined with needling to treat insomnia, and back acne. Needling plus moving cupping at range from Fengfu (GV16), Fengchi(GB20) and Jing-jiaji points to the sixth cervical vertebra is used to treat cervical spondylosis of vertebral artery type. The treatment of ankylosing spondylitis with moving cupping of erector spinae muscle plus western medicine. The treatment of irritable bowel syndrome with moving cupping from Dazhui (GV14) to Guanyuanshu (BL26) on the back.

(3) Others. Chronic urticaria is treated with pricking-cupping

第二十六章　罐法选择与罐斑诊治

一、临床罐法的选择

闪火法、留罐、走罐、刺血拔罐法、留针拔罐、药罐等是临床常用罐法，其中刺血拔罐法和走罐法疗效相对突出。

（一）依据经验选择

1. 痛证　痛证多选用刺血拔罐法，如：在背部 T1～T2 范围内寻找粟粒状或卵圆形呈粉红色阳性反应点，采用刺血拔罐法治疗原发性三叉神经痛；取患侧翳风穴下 1 寸处治疗面瘫耳后疼痛症；大椎穴刺血拔罐治疗急性扁桃体炎及急性喉炎；取天宗穴刺血拔罐治疗功能性头痛；取压痛点、环跳、委中、阳陵泉、昆仑穴刺血拔罐治疗坐骨神经痛；委中穴周围点刺放血，配合腰部疼痛点拔罐治疗急性腰扭伤；最痛点针刺放血并辅以拔罐、电针法治疗带状疱疹后遗神经痛；病灶处皮肤针叩刺出血拔罐配合中药治疗急性痛风性关节炎等。

2. 慢性病　治疗慢性病以走罐法为主，如：沿脊柱两侧采用背部走罐法结合针刺治疗失眠、背部痤疮，针刺加风府、风池、颈夹脊穴至第 6 颈椎之间走罐治疗椎动脉型颈椎病，背部竖脊肌走罐加西药治疗强直性脊柱炎，背部大椎穴至关元俞穴走罐治疗肠易激综合征。

3. 其他　刺血拔罐肺俞、肝

bloodletting at Feishu(BL13), Ganshu(BL18) and Pishu(BL20), which is often combined with flash-fire cupping at Shenque(CV8). Red eye is treated by pricking-cupping bloodletting at Dazhui (GV14). Intensive cupping on the back is used for the treatment of chronic fatigue syndrome. Facial shallow needling combined with flash-fire cupping can treat chloasma and so on.

1.2　Selection according to the function of cupping method

The effects of cupping method vary with different application methods as follows. Retained cupping is mainly used to treat accumulation of severe pathogenic cold. Flash-fire cupping is mainly used to dispel wind and relax sinews. Moving cupping is mainly used to release the exterior and eliminate the pathogenic factors, free the collateral vessels and activate blood. And a mild suction is often used to external contraction and skin impediment disease, while a heavy suction is often used to disorders of some meridians or/and Zang-Fu organs. Multi-cups cupping is suitable for the diseases with larger lesion range, while one-cup cupping is suitable for the diseases with smaller lesion range. The main function of cupping in rows is reducing excess; cupping with boiling water method is to warm meridians and disperse cold. Pricking-cupping bloodletting is mainly used to expel blood stasis and remove stagnation, and to relieve obstruction and unblock knot. The combination of needle and cupping produces various effects due to different needling methods.

2. The effect of cupping skin marks and the stimulation amount of cupping

The effect of cupping skin marks and the stimulation amount of cupping are the keys to the effective use of the cupping methods. Mr. Cheng Dan'an suggested that the appearance of the cupping skin marks could enhance the efficacy to some extent, and had proposed that cupping to "seeing purplish and red is better". Modern acupuncture believes that the cupping skin marks are produced by the pressure inside the cup and the local tissue congestion, the edema and bleeding in various skin layers, so that capillary permeability and tissue gas exchange are enhanced, the superficial capillaries are dilated, and then capillary rupture occurs due to blood spilling into the tissue space. It is used by practitioners for the aided diagnosis of various ailments through the observation of the syndrome reflected by the cupping skin marks, which characterizes the clinical use of the cupping methods.

In general, the parts of the darker cupping marks are the places where the disease is located. A disease of the corresponding organ is indicated, for example, by the presence of a dark cupping marks on

俞、脾俞穴,配合神阙穴闪罐法治疗慢性荨麻疹;大椎穴刺血拔罐治疗红眼病;背部密集排罐治疗慢性疲劳综合征;面部浅刺配合闪罐法治疗黄褐斑等。

(二)依据罐法功能选择

拔罐法的作用随着应用方法的不同而有所侧重和区别,如:留罐主治阴寒痼冷,闪罐主祛风疏筋;走罐主宣卫祛邪,通络活血,轻吸快推常用于外感、皮痹等证,重吸快推常用于某些经脉、脏腑功能失调的疾病;多罐适用于病变范围较大的病证,单罐则适用于病变范围较小的病证;排罐法以泻实为主,水罐法以温经散寒为主;刺血拔罐法以逐瘀化滞、解闭通结为主;针罐结合则因选用的针法不同可产生多种效应。

二、罐斑效应和罐法刺激量

罐斑效应和罐法刺激量是罐法有效运用的关键。承淡安先生认为罐斑的出现可以在一定程度上提高疗效,并曾提出拔至"见紫红色为佳"。现代针灸认为,罐斑的形成是由于拔罐致机体局部组织充血、水肿,使毛细血管通透性与组织气体交换增强,浅表的毛细血管扩张,进而毛细血管破裂,血液溢入组织间隙而发生瘀血。通过罐斑反映证候、协助诊断是罐法临床运用的特色。

一般而言,罐斑越深的部位乃病邪所在之处。例如在背部走罐时出现深色罐斑即表明相应部位

the back after moving cupping performed. Cupping skin marks or cupping sha is turned shallow from deep, which shows that healthy qi recovers and the pathogen gradually is driven out. If the patient has a shallow cupping skin marks at the beginning of cupping therapy, the patient is weak and deficient in qi and blood. The more easily blistering of the skin at the treated site in a patient after cupping therapy indicates that the condition of the patient is due to deficiency of yang qi, flooding with water, or dampness accumulation.

The stimulation amount of cupping is closely related to the formation of the cupping skin marks, which are induced by the pressure, the time, the speed, the strength, the site of cupping and so on. According to the China Academy of Chinese Medical Sciences, in general, the negative pressure value for clinical practical applications is 0.04 MPa. Cupping by both the fire-insertion cupping and flash-fire cupping, results in phase approximations of strong limits of negative pressure, up to 0.05 MPa, whether pottery or glass cups, whether large or small cups are used. The larger negative pressure suction, the larger stimulation intensity, and vice versa. In clinical practice, light and gentle cupping makes the nerve to be restrained, strong and acute cupping causes nerve excitation; reinnervate when too strong to excess suction pull. Some scholars also propose that retained cupping belongs to suppression therapy according to modern medical theory, the flash-fire cupping belongs to the excitement therapy, the moving cupping is a benign bidirectional conditioning therapy. Slowly moving the cups weighs on adjusting the Zang-Fu function, while rapidly moving the cups is strong in activating blood circulation and eliminating stasis. Moving cups along the starting and ending points of muscles treats diseases that are in a hyperexcitable state, conversely promoting the site of the lesion in a suppressed state to recover.

的脏器有疾患。罐斑或罐痧由深变浅,表现病邪去,正气恢复。若患者在罐疗开始时罐斑就浅,则患者正气较虚弱,气血衰少。若罐疗时易产生罐泡,则患者性质为阳气虚衰,水湿泛滥或停聚。

拔罐的刺激量与罐斑的形成密切相关,压力、时间、速度、力度、施罐部位等均是影响因素。据中国中医科学院报道:临床实际应用的负压值一般为 0.04 MPa。用投火法和闪火法拔罐,无论陶罐还是玻璃罐,无论大号罐还是小号罐,都能获得近似的负压强极限值,其值高达 0.05 MPa。负压吸拔力越大,刺激强度就越大,反之则越小。临床实践中,轻而缓的拔罐,可使神经受到抑制;强而急的拔罐,则使神经兴奋;过强过重的吸拔又使神经受到抑制。有学者根据现代医学理论还提出留罐属于抑制类疗法;闪罐属于兴奋类疗法;走罐则是一种良性的双向调节疗法。缓缓走罐重在调整脏腑功能,快速走罐则强在活血化瘀;沿着肌肉起止点的走罐疗法可治疗处于过度兴奋状态的疾病,反之则促进处于抑制状态的病变部位恢复正常。

Chapter 27　Auricle Diagnosis

Auricle is an important part of human body, which is considered to be a unique micro world that can reflect the whole physiological and pathological state of human body. When disorders occur in the internal organs or other parts like limbs of the body, various positive reactions may appear at the corresponding areas of the auricle, such as the changes of pain threshold and auricular cutaneous electric resistance at the related areas of the auricle will be found in some acute diseases, while morphological changes in some chronic diseases. And the common clinical diagnosis methods of auricle are auricle inspection and auricle palpation.

1. Auricle inspection

During the inspection, the doctor holds patient's ear with his thumb and index fingers, and carefully observes the auricle from top to bottom and from inside to outside in a good light. When suspicious positive reactants are found, it is advisable to lift them from the back of the ear with fingers, so that the suspicious positive reactants are tightened first, then slowly relaxed, and then slowly tightened, and then relaxed, so as to carefully observe their position, size, color, hardness, etc. When a positive reactant is found in one ear, it must be compared with the same part of the opposite ear to identify its authenticity and nature. The shape, size, hardness and mobility of the reactants should be determined when they are found to be protuberant, nodular and striped. When observing the triangle fossa, auricular concha and other parts, it should be expanded with a stick or matchstick to fully expose the inspection parts.

Discoloration accounts for more than half of the positive reactions, morphological change accounts for about 20% of the positive reactions, papules, desquamation and vascular malformation account for about 10% of the positive reactions respectively. There is a certain regularity between the types of positive reaction found in auricle inspection and disease reactions. Acute inflammation is often seen in sheet congestion ruddy, some white in the middle while red edge, with telangiectasia, bright red color and seborrheic luster. In chronic organic diseases, the discoloration is mostly white or gray, and the deformation is mostly bulge or depression, or swelling, with dot or flake white bulge or depression as the most common deformation, generally without seborrhea and luster. Skin diseases often present furfural-like desquamation, papules, skin thickening, rough. Nodular protuberances or spots, dark gray flakes, no luster are often seen in tumor diseases. The scar after trauma or operation can be seen as white or gray

第二十七章　耳郭诊察法

耳郭是人体的一个重要组成部分,其被认为是一个能反映人体整体生理、病理状态的独特微观世界。当人体脏腑、组织器官、四肢发生疾病时,耳郭相应的部位会出现各种不同的阳性反应,如急性病证时相关耳穴以痛阈和电阻值的改变为主,而慢性病证时相关耳穴则以形态改变为主。临床常用的耳郭诊断方法主要是耳郭视诊和耳郭触诊法。

一、耳郭视诊法

视诊时,医者两眼平视,以拇、食二指捏住耳郭,对准光线,由上而下、由内而外地顺着解剖部位仔细观察。发现有可疑阳性反应物时,宜用手指从耳背顶起,使可疑阳性反应物处先绷紧,再慢慢放松,然后慢慢绷紧,再放松,以仔细观察其位置、大小、色泽、硬度等。当发现一侧耳郭有阳性反应物时,必须与对侧耳郭的同一部位进行对比观察,以鉴别其真伪和性质。发现隆起、结节及条索状等一类反应物时,应确定反应物的形状、大小、硬度、活动度等。在三角窝、耳甲等部位视诊时,要用探棒或火柴棍等扩开,以充分暴露视诊部位。

视诊所见阳性反应以变色所占的比重最大,占一半以上,变形约占二成,丘疹、脱屑、血管变化各约占一成。耳郭视诊的阳性反应类型与疾病反应有一定的规律。急性炎症多见片状充血红润,有的中间发白、边缘红润,毛细血管扩张,色泽鲜红,有脂溢性光泽。慢性器质性疾病时,变色多为白色或灰色,变形则多为隆起或凹陷,或见肿胀,以点、片状白色隆起或凹陷为较常见,一般无脂溢及光泽。皮肤病多呈现糠皮样脱屑、丘疹,皮肤增厚、粗糙。肿瘤疾病常见结节状隆起或点、片状黯灰色,无光

scar changes of local line shape or half moon shape.

2. Auricle palpation

Auricle palpation is a method of disease diagnosis based on the decrease of pain threshold and morphological changes of auricular points related to the disease when the human body is sick, and then touch the auricular points through the probe to find the sensitive points of tenderness and whether there are indentation and morphological changes. When searching for the sensitive points of tenderness, the doctor gently holds the back of the ear with his left hand, holds the probe with his right hand, and evenly presses each area of the auricle to observe the patient's expression and pain reaction, and compares the degree of sensitivity of each acupoint, area and point to touch and press the pain. When the shape of the auricular points is changed, the doctor can gently hold the auricle with his left hand, place his right thumb-pulp on the auricular points to be tested, sets his index finger against the opposite part of the back of the ear, and touch the two finger-pulp together to feel whether the auricular points corresponding to the disease have swelling, depression, edema or other changes.

When palpating the auricle, we usually touch the anatomic part of the auricle in the order of first up and then down, first inside and then outside, first right and then left. On the basis of systematically touching all parts of the auricle, the right ear mainly touches the areas of liver, gallbladder, stomach, duodenum and appendix; the left ear is mainly used to touch the areas of heart, lung, pancreas, small intestine and large intestine. Punctate eminence of auricle is more common in headache and tracheitis, cord-like eminence is more common in uterine leiomyoma and vertebral hyperplasia, round nodules are seen in tumor diseases. Linear depression is more common in duodenal ulcer, linear depression is more common in coronary heart disease, flaky depression is more common in chronic colitis, dizziness, etc.

泽。外伤或手术后瘢痕可见局部线条状或半月形的白色或灰色瘢痕改变。

二、耳郭触诊法

耳郭触诊法是根据人体患病时,与疾病相关部位的耳穴出现痛阈降低及形态改变,进而通过探棒探触耳穴,寻找压痛敏感点及有无压痕和形态改变以诊断疾病的一种方法。当寻找压痛敏感点时,医者用左手轻扶耳背,右手持探棒,均匀按压耳郭各穴,观察患者的表情与痛觉反应,比较各穴、区、点触压疼痛敏感的程度。当探触耳穴的形态改变时,医者可左手轻扶耳郭,右手拇指腹放在被测耳穴上,食指衬于耳背相对部位,两指腹互相配合进行触摸,以感触与疾病相应的耳穴是否有隆起、凹陷、水肿等变化。

耳郭触诊时,一般按先上后下、先内后外、先右后左的顺序,顺着耳郭解剖部位进行探触。在系统探触耳郭各部位的基础上,右耳以探触肝、胆、胃、十二指肠、阑尾穴为主;左耳以探触心、肺、胰腺、小肠、大肠穴为主。耳郭有点状隆起多见于头痛、气管炎,条索状隆起多见于子宫肌瘤、脊椎增生,圆形结节见于肿瘤疾病,有点状凹陷多见于十二指肠溃疡,线状凹陷多见于冠心病,片状凹陷多见于慢性结肠炎、头目眩晕等。

Chapter 28　Needling Methods on Different Parts of the Human Body

In the clinical applications of acupuncture，syndrome differentiation and individual treatment are necessary. Selecting acupoints and needling methods properly according to the specific situation of the patient's condition and disease symptoms is necessary. It is more helpful to be familiar with the anatomical characteristics of the acupuncture site and choose a more appropriate acupuncture angle，direction and depth，so as to improve the therapeutic effect of acupuncture and prevent the occurrence of acupuncture accidents.

In general，the acupoints with similar sites are also similar in terms of acupuncture methods. In combination with the knowledge related to human anatomy，it is necessary to describe the routine acupuncture methods in various parts of the body.

1. Acupuncture at head，face and neck

1.1　Acupuncture at acupoints of head

（1）Manipulation. Acupoints on the head are needled 0.1-0.2 cun perpendicularly，or 0.5-1.5 cun obliquely. Rapid penetration methods are used commonly.

While needling obliquely，the direction of acupuncture can be chosen according to the direction of the meridians moving towards obverse and reverse. It's punctured from the convenience of operation，or from the upward to the downward，or from the anterior to the posterior. Insert the needle at 30° angle to the scalp，and the tip of the needle reaches the lower layer of epicranial aponeurosis，by twisting of the needling manipulation mainly.

（2）Precautions. The head is rich in blood collaterals，and the punctured acupoints should be pressed to avoid bleeding after the withdrawal of the needles. Xinhui（GV22）should not be needled when the fontanel of infant is not closed.

1.2　Acupuncture at acupoints of ocular area

（1）Manipulation. While needling Chengqi（ST1），Jingming（BL1），Qiuhou（EX-HN7）and others，the patient is asked to close eyes and the eyeball is pushed gently by doctor's pressing hand to emerge the acupuncture site adequately. The needle is slowly penetrated 0.3-0.7 cun along the inner edge of the orbit，not more than 1.5 cun and not be lifting and thrusting，generally with the light manipulation.

（2）Precautions. The blood vessels of the ocular area are rich

---

第二十八章　特殊部位腧穴操作

针刺要辨证施治,结合患者病情、病证等具体情况,合理选择腧穴与刺法。但具体操作时,熟悉针刺部位的解剖特点,选择更为恰当的针刺角度、方向与深度,更有助于提高针刺治疗效果,防止针刺意外的发生。

一般而言,部位相近的腧穴,其针刺方法也相近,下面结合人体解剖学相关知识,择要阐述身体各部位的常规针刺方法。

一、头、面、颈项部腧穴刺法

（一）头部腧穴刺法

1. 一般刺法　头部腧穴,可直刺 0.1～0.2 寸,或斜刺 0.5～1.5寸。多选用快速刺入的方法。

斜刺时,针刺方向可以按照顺逆经脉循行方向来选择,或从操作便利的角度,或从上往下,或从前往后进行针刺,针体与头皮约成30°角进针,针尖抵达帽状腱膜下层,行针手法以捻转为主。

2. 注意事项　头部血络丰富,出针后要多加按压,以防出血。小儿囟门未闭时禁刺囟会穴。

（二）眼部腧穴刺法

1. 一般刺法　针刺承泣、睛明、球后等穴时,嘱患者闭目,用押手轻推眼球,以充分暴露针刺部位,针沿眼眶内缘缓慢刺入 0.3～0.7寸,不宜超过 1.5寸。一般不行提插手法,手法要轻。

2. 注意事项　眼区血运丰

and the tissue is loosen with high blood vessel mobility, it's easier to cause bleeding using the lifting and thrusting or other manipulations, so that patients should be treated with caution. If it is needled deeply, optic nerve is impaired more easily. The patient would feel headache and dizzy, then flickering in the eyes and even nausea and vomiting.

Withdraw the needle immediately, and if deep needling continues, the tip of the needle penetrates through superior orbital fissure into the cavernous sinus. It causes intracranial hemorrhage and acute headache, nausea and vomiting, and severe cases can lead to shock and death. If it is close to the needle inserting or not pushed by the pressing hand, the eyeball will be stabbed easily.

1.3　Acupuncture at acupoints of auricle area

（1）Manipulation. The patient should be asked to open the mouth slightly to relax while needling Ermen(TE21), Tinggong (SI19) and Tinghui (GB2), and they are needled 0.5-1 cun perpendicularly or obliquely backwards. At Wangu(GB12), it's needled obliquely downwards 0.5-0.8 cun; at Yifeng(TE17), it's needled perpendicularly 0.8-1 cun or is punctured obliquely and medially downwards 0.5-1 cun.

（2）Precautions. When the needle is retained, the patient should be asked to relax the mouth naturally. The deeper site of Yifeng(TE17) is the place where the facial nerve perforates the stylomastoid foramen, so the needle shouldn't be inserted too deep lest the facial nerve be impaired.

1.4　Acupuncture at facial acupoints

（1）Manipulation. Acupoints on the frontal and temporal regions are needled horizontally 0.3-0.8 cun. Cuanzhu (BL2) is needled downwards to Jingming(BL1) for the treatment of ocular diseases and externally to Yuyao(EX-HN4) for the treatment of facial paralysis which is not able to frown; Yintang (GV29) is generally needled horizontally downwards 0.3-1 cun; they are horizontally needled backwards 1-1.5 cun at Sizhukong(TE23), Tongziliao(GB1) and Taiyang(EX-HN5); Sibai(ST2) is needled perpendicularly or obliquely downwards 0.2-0.5 cun; Shuigou (GV26) and Suliao (GV25) are inserted obliquely upwards; Yingxiang(LI20) is needled perpendicularly or obliquely upwards along the nose; avoid arteries when needling Daying(ST5); Dicang (ST4)-through-Jiache(ST6) for the treatment of peripheral facial paralysis.

（2）Precautions. It's extremely easy to stab and cause bleeding because Sibai(ST2) is in the depression at the infraorbital foramen including the infraorbital arteries and veins. As *Tong-ren Shu-xue Zhen-jiu Tu-jing* (*Illustrated Manual of Acupuncture Points of the Bronze Figure*) said, when needling this point, the needle should

富,且组织疏松,血管移动性大,提插等手法更易导致针刺出血,要慎重使用。针刺过深,又易伤及视神经,患者会感到头痛、头晕,继而感觉眼内有火光闪烁,甚至伴恶心、呕吐等。

此时应立即退针。若继续深刺,则针尖透过眶上裂至海绵窦,造成颅内出血,引起剧烈头痛、恶心、呕吐,严重者会导致休克、死亡。如进针时贴近眼球或眼球未用押手固定,则容易刺中眼球。

(三)耳部腧穴刺法

1. 一般刺法　针刺耳门、听宫、听会三穴,须嘱患者微微张口放松,直刺或稍向后斜刺0.5～1寸。针刺完骨穴,宜向下斜刺0.5～0.8寸;针刺翳风穴直刺0.8～1寸,或向内下斜刺0.5～1寸。

2. 注意事项　留针期间,口颊自然放松。翳风穴深部正当面神经从颅骨穿出处,故进针不宜过深,以免损伤面神经。

(四)面部腧穴刺法

1. 一般刺法　额区及颞部腧穴横刺0.3～0.8寸,攒竹向下可透睛明,治疗目疾,向外透鱼腰,治疗面瘫不能皱眉;印堂穴多向下平刺0.3～1寸;丝竹空、瞳子髎、太阳穴多向后平刺1～1.5寸;四白穴多直刺或向下斜刺0.2～0.5寸;水沟、素髎穴多向上斜刺;迎香穴多直刺或沿鼻向上斜刺;大迎穴针刺时要避开动脉;地仓、颊车可相互透刺治疗面瘫。

2. 注意事项　四白穴直对眶下孔(内含眶下动、静脉),极易刺伤,造成出血。《铜人腧穴针灸图经》云:"凡用针稳审方得下针,若针深即令人目乌色。"所以此穴不

be inserted after careful consideration. If the needle is inserted too deep to make patient's eyes get black, it shouldn't be needled deep and the punctured acupoint should be pressed to avoid bleeding after the withdrawal of the needle.

1.5　Acupuncture at nape acupoints

(1) Manipulation. Yamen(GV15), Fengfu(GV16) and other points are generally needled 0.5-1 cun toward the mandible. Fengchi(GB20)is needled 0.5-1 cun toward the apex of the nose.

(2) Precautions. Medulla oblongata will be punctured if Yamen(GV15), Fengfu(GV16) and Fengchi(GB20) are needled too deep and the angle is not proper, so it is necessary to control the angle and depth of needling strictly(Fig. 28-1,28-2).

When needling, such as the posterior atlantooccipital membrane, the resistance under the needle increases; when the needle enters the subarachnoid space,there is a sense of loss. When the needle enters the medulla oblongata, there is a soft feeling under the needle. At the same time, the patient has a sense of electric shock like feeling that spreads to the extremities, accompanied by nerve abnormalities such as near death. Mild cases may be accompanied by head pain, nausea and vomiting, dizziness, palpitation, sweating, apathy or drowsiness. In severe cases, there may be dyspnea,coma,convulsion,paralysis and even death.

可深刺,出针后亦需按压针孔,防止出血。

（五）项部腧穴刺法

1. 一般刺法　针刺哑门、风府等穴多向下颌方向刺入 0.5～1 寸,风池穴可向鼻尖方向刺入 0.5～1 寸。

2. 注意事项　针刺哑门、风府以及风池穴过深、角度不当,会刺伤延髓,故要严格控制针刺角度和深度（图 28-1、图 28-2）。

针刺时,当针刺至寰枕后膜时,阻力感增大;当针进入蛛网膜下腔时,则有落空感。当针刺入延髓时,针刺为松软感,同时患者有触电样感向肢端放散,伴有濒死样感觉等神经异常。轻者可伴头项强痛、恶心呕吐、头晕、眼花、心慌、出汗、表情淡漠或嗜睡等症,重者还可见呼吸困难,神志昏迷、抽搐、瘫痪甚至死亡等延髓出血现象。

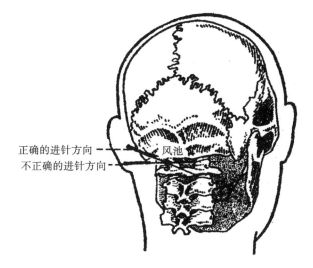

图 28-1　风池穴解剖与针刺（1）

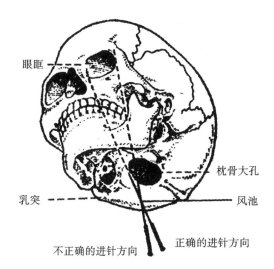

图 28-2　风池穴解剖与针刺（2）

1.6　Acupuncture at neck acupoints

(1) Manipulation. These points are usually punctured slowly, perpendicularly and superficially 0.3-0.8 cun,avoiding the arteries of the neck. It is advisable to use less needle manipulation,and the handle -scraping method or trembling method is appropriate for supplementary needle manipulation.

The common carotid artery is touched by the left hand when

（六）颈部腧穴刺法

1. 一般刺法　多直刺、浅刺,深度在 0.3～0.8 寸,要避开颈部动脉,进针宜缓,少行手法,辅助手法以刮法、震颤法为宜。

人迎穴针刺时先用押手扪住

Renying(ST9)is needled 0.2-0.8 cun along the inside of the artery. Tiantu（CV22）is needled perpendicularly 0.2-0.3 cun into subcutaneous tissue and then slowly downwards 0.5-1 cun along the gap between sternal manubrium and trachea(Fig. 28-3).

搏动的颈总动脉，刺手沿动脉内侧刺入 0.2～0.8 寸；天突穴先直刺入皮下 0.2～0.3 寸，再沿胸骨柄与气管之间向下缓慢刺入 0.5～1 寸（图 28-3）。

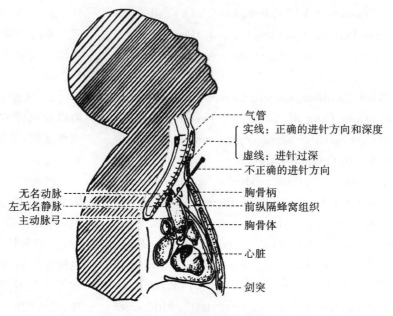

图 28-3　天突穴解剖与针刺

（2）Precautions. It's helpful to ensure the needling safety by confirming the locations of sternocleidomastoid and carotid artery on the neck acupoints. The tissue of the neck is loose and the feeling under the needle is soft. Stop needling in case of other abnormal feelings lest the accident occurs.

If the needling sensation under the finger is soft and flexible, and the pulse is obvious, it reflects stab injury to the artery. If puncturing the vagus nerve, it can slow down the heart rate and cause coronary vasoconstriction, and the patient feels chest tightness, shortness of breath, palpitations and so on, which seriously endangers patient's life. If the tip of needle meets tough and elastic resistance, the patient feels itchy in the throat, it indicates that the trachea is being stabbed.

2. Acupuncture at chest and abdomen

2.1　Acupuncture at chest acupoints

（1）Manipulation. The acupoints on the chest are mainly needled obliquely or horizontally 0.5-0.8 cun. The acupoints on the Conception Vessel are mostly needled horizontally. Danzhong (CV17)is generally needled horizontally downwards, but externally for the treatment of the breast diseases. Ruzhong(ST17),which is just the symbol of the anchor points,can't be used for acupuncture

2. 注意事项　颈部腧穴须确定胸锁乳突肌以及颈动脉位置等才有助于保证针刺安全。颈部内组织松弛，针感多为松软感，如有其他异样感觉应停止针刺，以防意外发生。

若针下柔软有弹性，搏动明显，则说明刺中动脉；若刺中迷走神经，患者心率减慢，冠状血管收缩，患者感到胸闷、气短、心悸等，严重时危及生命；若针下遇到坚韧而有弹性的阻力，患者感觉喉中发痒，说明刺中气管。

二、胸腹部

（一）胸部腧穴刺法

1. 一般刺法　胸部腧穴多以斜刺或平刺为主，刺入 0.5～0.8 寸为宜。其中任脉所属腧穴多平刺。膻中穴一般向下平刺，治疗乳房疾病则向外平刺。乳中穴不针不灸，仅作为定位标志。位于肋间

or moxibustion. The acupoints on spatium intercostales are generally needled obliquely or horizontally outwards along the rib spaces. Rugen(ST18)is needled horizontally upwards.

(2) Precautions. The chest contains heart, lungs and other important organs, so the depth should not be deep into the thorax, whatever needling obliquely or horizontally. The angel of acupuncture is less than 25° in most cases.

2.2 Acupuncture at hypochondriac region acupoints

(1) Manipulation. The acupoints are mostly needled obliquely downwards or outwards 0.5-0.8 cun. Zhangmen(LR13), Jingmeng(GB25) and other acupoints could be needled perpendicularly and shallowly.

(2) Precautions. The liver and spleen are in this region and it shouldn't be needled deeply, especially for the patients with hepatosplenomegaly.

2.3 Acupuncture at abdomen acupoints

(1) Manipulation. The acupoints on the abdomen are generally needled perpendicularly 0.5-1.5 cun. Acupoints on the upper and lower abdomen are needled shallowly or obliquely downwards. Shenque(CV8) is conducted by moxibustion, mainly insulated by salt or moxa roll. The points around the navel could be needled more deep. Needling manipulation are mainly based on a small amount of lifting and thrusting, rotating or trembling methods.

(2) Precautions. Deeply needling acupoints on the upper abdomen may easily hurt the liver and cause hepatic hemorrhage. If the stomach is stabed, plusing a wide range of lifting, trusting and rotating to bring stomach contents into the abdominal cavity, may cause peritonitis, especially when the stomach is overfilled. When needle at the acupoints of the lower abdomen, such as Qugu(CV2), Zhongji(CV3), Henggu(KI11), Guanyuan(CV4) and others, the patient should be advised to empty the bladder before acupuncture. Needle manipulation should not be excessively large to prevent stabbing of the intestinal wall. The abdomen acupoints shouldn't be needled for pregnant women.

3. Acupuncture at the back and lumbosacral region

3.1 Acupuncture at back acupoints

(1) Manipulation. Due to the spinous process of the thoracic vertebrae arranged in the form of imbricate, needling at Governor Vessel obliquely generally upwards 0.5-1 cun along the spinous process space. The acupoints on the first side line of Bladder Meridian are needled shallowly or obliquely 0.5-0.8 cun to the spine, for those on the second line are needled obliquely downwards

隙中的腧穴,一般沿肋骨间隙向外斜刺或平刺,乳根穴多向上方平刺。

2. 注意事项 胸部含心、肺等重要脏器,无论斜刺、平刺,其深度均不宜深入胸廓。针刺角度也多小于 25°。

(二) 胁肋部腧穴刺法

1. 一般刺法 多向下或外侧方向斜刺 0.5～0.8 寸。章门、京门等穴可浅刺。

2. 注意事项 胁肋部内有肝、脾等重要脏器,故不宜深刺,对于肝脾肿大者更应注意。

(三) 腹部腧穴刺法

1. 一般刺法 腹部腧穴大多可直刺 0.5～1.5 寸。上、下腹部宜浅刺,或向下斜刺;神阙穴多选用灸法,以隔盐灸或艾卷灸为主;脐周腧穴可适当深刺。腹部行针手法以小幅度提插捻转或震颤法等为主。

2. 注意事项 上腹部腧穴深刺易伤及肝,引起肝出血;刺中胃,再加上大幅度提插捻转,将胃内容物带入腹腔,可能引发腹膜炎,尤其是胃过度充盈时;针刺下腹部曲骨、中极、横骨、关元等腧穴时,应嘱患者排空膀胱后针刺。腹部行针不宜幅度过大,防止刺破肠壁。孕妇禁用或慎用。

三、背、腰骶部

(一) 背部腧穴刺法

1. 一般刺法 胸椎棘突呈叠瓦状向下排列,故针刺督脉腧穴,多沿棘突间隙向上斜刺,刺入 0.5～1 寸。针刺膀胱经第一侧线的腧穴,多浅刺,或向脊柱斜刺 0.5～0.8寸;针刺膀胱经第二侧线的腧

or horizontally 0. 5-0. 8 cun along the scapular margin. The angel of needle is less than 25° while needling obliquely.

(2) Precautions. Locate according to the bony landmarks such as spinous process and scapula. When needling the acupoints of Governor Vessel, if it is too deep, there will be a sense of loss under the needle, suggesting that the puncture should be stopped immediately, otherwise the spinal cord may be injured. While needling the acupoints of Bladder Meridian, it is essential to ensure that it does not penetrate into the thorax.

3. 2　Acupuncture at lumbar acupoints

(1) Manipulation. The spinous process of lumbar vertebrae is vertical plate. Therefore, acupoints of Governor Vessel are needled perpendicularly 0. 5-1. 5 cun. Those on the Bladder Meridian are mainly based on needling perpendicularly or shallowly.

(2) Precautions. When needling the acupoints of Governor Vessel, if it is too deep, there will be a sense of loss under the needle, suggesting that the puncture should be stopped immediately, otherwise the spinal cord may be injured. The acupoints on the both sides of the spine shouldn't be needled too deep or outward deeply to prevent hurting kidneys, such as Weishu (BL21), Sanjiaoshu(BL22), Shenshu(BL23), Zhishi(BL52) and others.

3. 3　Acupuncture at sacral acupoints

(1) Manipulation. While needling Shangliao(BL31), the needle tip should slightly point medially downwards to the public symphysis in order to the posterior sacral foramen and the depth is generally 1-1. 5 cun. It is advisable to puncture perpendicularly into the posterior sacral foramen when needling Ciliao (BL32), Zhongliao(BL33) and Xialiao(BL34). Changqiang(GV1) and Yaoshu (GV2) are needled obliquely upwards 0. 5-1 cun.

(2) Precautions. When needling the Changqiang(GV1), the needle tip is parallel upwards to the coccyx and is inserted between the rectum and the coccyx to avoid infection due to penetrating the rectum. The lower end of the subarachnoid space lies on the second lumbar plane. The Yaoshu(GV2) cannot be needled too deep to avoid causing subarachnoid hemorrhage.

4.　Acupuncture at the limbs

4. 1　Acupuncture at upper limbs acupoints

(1) Manipulation. The points of the forearm such as Jianyu (LI15), Binao (LI14) and Jianliao (TE14) can be needled perpendicularly or obliquely, and the depth should be 0. 8-1. 5 cun. Jianjing(GB21) is needled horizontally forwards or outwards, not

穴,多浅刺,或沿肩胛骨缘向下斜刺或平刺0.5～0.8寸;斜刺时针刺的角度以小于25°为宜。

2. 注意事项　通过棘突和肩胛骨等骨性标志进行定位。针刺督脉腧穴过深,会出现落空感,提示刺入脊髓腔,应立即停止进针,否则可伤及脊髓。针刺膀胱经腧穴时,以避免刺入胸廓内为基本要求。

(二)腰部腧穴刺法

1. 一般刺法　腰椎棘突呈垂直板状,故针刺督脉腧穴,多直刺0.5～1.5寸。膀胱经腧穴针刺以直刺、浅刺为主。

2. 注意事项　针刺督脉腧穴过深,会出现落空感,提示刺入脊髓腔,应立即停止进针。脊柱两侧的腧穴,如胃俞、三焦俞、肾俞、志室等,不可深刺或向外侧深刺,以防伤及肾脏。

(三)骶部腧穴刺法

1. 一般刺法　针刺上髎穴时针尖应稍向内下即耻骨联合方向进针,易刺及骶后孔,针刺深度多为1～1.5寸。次髎、中髎、下髎直刺以刺达骶后孔为宜。长强、腰俞穴均向上斜刺0.5～1寸。

2. 注意事项　针刺长强穴时针尖向上与尾骨平行,在直肠与尾骨之间刺入,避免刺穿直肠引起感染。蛛网膜下腔的下端止于第2腰椎平面,针刺腰俞穴不可过深,以免引起蛛网膜下腔出血。

四、四肢部

(一)上肢部腧穴刺法

1. 一般刺法　上臂肩髃、臂臑、肩髎等穴均可直刺或斜刺,深度以0.8～1.5寸为宜;肩井穴宜向前、外方向平刺,不低于锁骨深

less than the depth of the clavicle, or punctured into the direction of the scapula. The points of the forearm are mainly needled perpendicularly 0. 5-1. 2 cun. Pianli (LI6), Yanglao (SI6) and other points on the bone edge are generally needled along the bone edge. Jing-well Point, Shixuan (EX-UE11) and Sifeng (EX-UE10) are pricked to cause bleeding. Jiquan (HT1) is needled obliquely upwards 0. 5-1 cun.

(2) Precautions. Jiquan(HT1)should not be punctured deeply, avoiding the iliac artery. Taiyuan(LU9)should be needled to avoid the arteries. Hegu (LI4), Houxi (SI3) and other points should be prevented from hurting deep arcus palmaris profundus when piercing. The direct puncture at Jianjing(GB21)should prevent the injury of the pleura and lung, it shouldn't be needled for pregnant women. There is a median nerve in the deep part of the acupoint of pericardium passing through the forearm. If there is an electric shock like feeling to release to the middle finger during acupuncture, suggesting that the median nerve was stabbed. If the needle is lifted and thrusted in a large range, the median nerve will be injured.

4.2　Acupuncture at lower limbs acupoints

(1) Manipulation. The points on the lower limbs are needled perpendicularly 1-3 cun. The muscles of the thighs are quite rich, and they are usually punctured perpendicularly 1-3 cun. When needling Huantiao(GB30), the patient is required to lie on his side, bend the knee and hip, that is, the lower leg is straight, while the upper leg is flexing. Then doctor holds a needle to puncture 2-3 cun perpendic-ularly, and the manipulation makes the local part feel heaviness and distention. At the same time, the needle sensation radiates to the heel, and the effect is better. The points on the leg are generally needled perpendicularly 0. 5-2 cun. When needling Dubi(ST35), the patient is required to bend the knee, and the doctor holds the needle to puncture to the medial and upward, or penetrate 0. 5-1. 5 cun to the Neixiyan(EX-LE4). Jing-well Point on the feet and Bafeng(EX-LE10)are pricked to cause bleeding. Others are needled perpendicularly or obliquely and the depths are generally less than 1 cun.

(2) Precautions. Needling Qichong(ST39), Chongmen(SP12), Jimen(SP11), Yinlian(LR11), Jimai(LR12), Chongyang(ST42)and other points should protect the arteries from being hurt. The intensity and frequency of stimulation should be controlled when needling nerve stem.

部为宜,或向肩胛骨方向针刺。前臂腧穴以直刺为主,深度为0.5~1.2寸。骨缘的偏历、养老等穴以沿骨缘针刺为多。井穴、十宣、四缝等多点刺放血。针刺极泉穴以向上斜刺为宜,深度为 0.5~1 寸。

2. 注意事项　极泉穴当注意避开腋动脉,且不宜深刺。太渊穴应避开动脉针刺,合谷、后溪等穴透刺时应防止伤及掌深弓。肩井穴直刺宜防止伤及胸膜、肺脏,孕妇亦当禁用。心包经前臂的腧穴,其深部有正中神经,针刺时如有触电样感觉向中指放散,是刺中了正中神经,此时如进行大幅度提插,会损伤正中神经。

(二) 下肢部腧穴刺法

1. 一般刺法　下肢多直刺,深度为1~3寸。大腿部的肌肉较为丰厚,一般直刺 1~3 寸。环跳穴取侧卧屈膝屈髋位,下面的腿伸直,上面的腿屈曲,直刺 2~3 寸,使局部有胀重感,同时针感向足跟部放射效果较好。小腿部腧穴一般直刺 0.5~2 寸。针刺犊鼻穴时,患者取屈膝位,向内上方针刺,或向内膝眼穴透刺 0.5~1.5 寸。足部井穴、八风等可点刺出血,其余穴位均可直刺或斜刺,针刺深度多在 1 寸以内。

2. 注意事项　针刺气冲、冲门、箕门、阴廉、急脉、冲阳等穴应防止伤及动脉。针刺神经干时应控制刺激强度和刺激次数。

Chapter 29 Prevention and Management of Possible Accidents

Safe and effective as it is, acupuncture may sometimes cause some possible accidents such as fainting, sticking of needle, bending of needle, abnormal sensation after needling, injury of internal organs, traumatic pneumothorax in clinic due to the careless manipulation, violation of acupuncture contraindications, unsuitable needling techniques or lack of an overall understanding of anatomy of human body. In case of any abnormal situation, effective treatment shall be carried out immediately. The common abnormal situations of needling are as follows.

1. Fainting during needling

This term means the patient goes off in a faint during acupuncture treatment.

[Symptoms] Sudden abnormal expression on the face, dizziness and nausea, etc. Even pallor, palpitation, short of breath, perspiration, cold extremities, deep and thready pulse. In severe cases, even sudden fall without consciousness, cyanosis of lips and finger nails, sweating, urinary and fecal incontinence, and faint pulse.

[Causes] Faintness is mostly observed in those who receive acupuncture treatment for the first time and who are afraid of needling and pain with nervous tension. It can be caused during needling or needle retaining due to such factors as the patient's nervous tension, weak constitution, fatigue, hunger, excessive perspiration, serious diarrhea and massive hemorrhage; or improper position, the operator's forceful manipulations, the consulting room is too muggy or too cold, etc.

[Management] Stop needling immediately and pull out all the needles. Help the patients lie down, with his/her head a little bit lower. Release their clothes and belts. It is advised to keep him/her warm and ask him/her to have a rest and drink a little hot water or sugar water(be cautious when it may affect the patient's own pre-existing disease) in order to help him/her recover, and ensure proper ventilation indoors. In severe cases, needling or press with the finger nail on such acupoints as Shuigou (DU26), Suliao (DU25), Neiguan(PC6), Hegu(LI4), Taichong(LR3), Yongquan (KI1)and Zusanli(ST36), or apply moxibustion to Baihui(GV20), Qihai(CV6) and Guanyuan(CV4), etc. Generally, the patients will recover in a few minutes. If the patients don't respond to the above measures, still being unconsciousness, weak breathing, and

第二十九章 异常情况预防与处理

针刺治病是一种既简便又安全有效的治疗方法，但如操作不当、疏忽大意，或犯针刺禁忌，或对人体解剖部位缺乏全面了解，也可能出现晕针、滞针、弯针、折针，针后异常感，损伤内脏，造成创伤性气胸等异常情况。一旦出现异常情况，应立即进行有效的处理。常见的针刺异常情况有以下几种。

一、晕针

晕针是指在针刺过程中患者发生晕厥的现象。

【现象】在针刺过程中，患者突然出现神情异常、头晕目眩、恶心欲吐等；甚至面色苍白、心慌气短、出冷汗、四肢厥冷、脉沉细等；严重者出现神志昏迷、唇甲青紫、大汗淋漓、二便失禁、脉微欲绝等。

【原因】晕针多见于首次接受针刺，恐针、畏痛、情绪紧张者。患者在施针过程中精神过度紧张；或素体虚弱，或劳累过度，或空腹，或大汗、大泻、大出血后；或体位不当，或针刺激手法过强，或诊室闷热，或过于寒冷等。

【处理】立即停止针刺，迅速全部出针。患者平卧，头部放低，松解衣带，保暖；轻者静卧片刻，给予温开水或糖水之后即可恢复。服用糖类饮料或制品（可能影响患者自身原有疾病者慎用）或温开水，保持空气流通。重者在行上述处理后，可选指压或针刺水沟、素髎、内关、合谷、太冲、涌泉、足三里等穴，亦可灸百会、气海、关元等穴，一般患者可逐渐恢复正常。若见不省人事、呼吸微弱、脉微欲绝者，必要时可配合西医学的急救措

pulseless, other emergency measures in western medicine should be taken. If the patient faints after the needle is removed, he should be asked to rest, closely observed and treated accordingly. After the dizziness was relieved, the patient still need to have a rest, he/she can leave only when his/her situation is stable.

[Prevention] For the first time to receive acupuncture treatment, especially for those patients with mental tension, explanations should be given beforehand so as to dispel his or her worries. For those with weak constitution, sweating, diarrhea and bleeding, it is better to choose less acupoints, gentle needle manipulation, and the lying position. For those who are hungry or over tired, the treatment should be postponed for a while, waiting for their physical strength recovered or after they have eaten something. Meanwhile, a comfortable and endurable posture should be chosen for the patients with the lying posture being the best. In the process of treatment, the operator should concentrate upon the manipulation, focus his or her attention on patient's expression and inquire about the patient's feeling whenever necessary so that emergency measures can be taken in time once the indications of the fainting appear.

2. Sticking of needle

This term means that during the manipulation or retaining, the acupuncturist feels the needle stuck and firmly held, which makes it difficult to twirl, lift and thrust and withdraw the needle. At the same time, the patient may suffer from great pain.

[Phenomenon] It is difficult for the practitioner to twirl, lift and thrust, and withdraw the inserted needle with the needle under the skin of acupoints. If doing it by force, the pain will be too intense for the patient to endure.

[Causes] If the patient is in a nervous or painful state, the insertion of the needle into the point may cause the strong spasm of the local muscle. The case may be caused by the patients' changing posture or improper manipulation, e. g. excessively twirling the needle in one direction, which may cause the muscle fiber to twine the needle body. Sometimes the case may be caused by the overtime retaining.

[Management] If stuck needle is caused by temporary muscle spasm resulting from nervousness, explanation before needling should be made to eliminate the patient's tension. If the stuck needle is caused by the changing of posture, the original one should be returned and then withdraw the needle. If the needle is stuck due to excessive rotation in one direction, the condition will be released when the needle is rotated in the opposite direction or pressing the

施。如出针后患者有晕针现象，应嘱其休息，密切观察并做相应处理。患者晕针缓解后，仍需适当休息待情况稳定后离开。

【预防】对晕针要重视预防，对于初次接受针刺治疗，特别是精神紧张者，要先对其做好解释工作，消除其恐惧心理；对体质虚弱、大汗、大泻、大出血等患者，取穴宜精，手法宜轻，尽量采用卧位；对于饥饿或过度疲劳者，应推迟针刺时间，待其体力恢复、进食后再行针刺。注意患者体位的舒适自然，尽可能选取卧位。注意室内空气流通，消除过热、过冷因素。医者在施术过程中，应守神入微，密切观察患者的神态，随时询问其感觉，如有不适立即处理。

二、滞针

滞针是指在行针时或留针后出针时，医者感觉针下滞涩，行针困难的现象，捻转、提插、出针均感困难，且患者感觉疼痛或疼痛加剧的现象。

【现象】针在穴位内，在行针或出针时，医者捻转、提插和出针均感困难，若强行捻转、提插，患者痛不可忍。

【原因】针刺时，由于患者紧张或疼痛，针刺入腧穴后引起局部肌肉痉挛；或进针后患者移动体位；或医者向单一方向捻针太过，肌纤维缠绕于针身；或若留针时间过长，也可出现滞针等。

【处理】精神紧张而致肌肉痉挛者，针刺前医者需耐心做好解释工作，消除其紧张情绪；体位移动者，需帮助其恢复原来体位；单向捻转过度者，需向反方向捻回转；或用手指亦可在滞针邻近部位做循按手法，或弹动针柄，或在针刺

skin around the point or flipping the handle of needle or inserting another needle nearby to disperse the qi and blood, and to relieve the spasm.

[Prevention] Explanations should be given to the nervous patient beforehand to dispel unnecessary worries and nervousness. Choose a more comfortable needling position for the patient during treatment, and avoid moving the position randomly when the needle is retained. In spastic diseases, the needling technique should be light and the twist angle should not be too large. If using the rubbing method, care should be taken to prevent the needle from getting stuck.

3. Bending of needle

This term means that needle body is bent in the body during the process of insertion, manipulation and retention.

[Phenomenon] The direction and angle of the needle are changed when the needle is inserted or retained, which is different from the original ones. For acupuncturist, it is difficult to lift, thrust and withdraw the needle. And The patient feels pain in the inserted position.

[Causes] This may be resulted from unskillful manipulation with too much force or great speed, or the needle tip touches hard tissues or organs, the change of patient's posture during the insertion or retention, or some external force press and collide on the needle handle, or the inserted site in a state of spasm, or improper treatment of stuck needles, etc.

[Management] When it happens, no more manipulations (lifting, thrusting and twirling) should be allowed. Lifting needle with excessive force and withdrawing the needle fiercely are forbidden to avoid needle broken and bleeding, etc. If the case is caused by the change of patient's posture, the patient should return slowly back to the original posture, and only when the local muscle of patient relaxes can the needle be withdrawn slowly along the angle of bend as usual. If it is bent slightly, the needle maybe withdrawn slowly. And if it is bent severely, the needle may be withdrawn through shaking and withdrawing slightly along the course of bend until it is withdrawn totally. If the needle body is bent in more than one place, it must be pulled out one by one in accordance with the twisting and tilting direction of the needle handle. Do not pull it sharply to prevent the needle from breaking.

[Prevention] The practitioner should insert the needle skillfully and gracefully, avoid inserting the needle too forcefully or too rapidly. The patient should take the proper position (and not change his/her position during the treatment. The needling area and

邻近部位再刺一针,以宣散邪气、解除滞针。

【预防】对于初诊患者和精神紧张者,要做好针刺前解释工作,消除其顾虑及紧张情绪。针刺时选择患者较舒适的针刺体位,避免留针时患者随意移动体位。痉挛性疾病行针时手法宜轻巧,捻转角度不可过大。若用搓法时,应注意防止滞针。

三、弯针

弯针是指进针、行针或留针时,针身在患者体内出现弯曲的现象。

【现象】进针时或留针时针的方向和角度发生了改变,医者提插、捻转和出针均感困难,或患者感觉针刺部位疼痛。

【原因】医者手法不熟练,进针用力过猛、过速,或针下碰到坚硬组织;进针后患者改变了体位;或外力碰击或压迫针柄;或针刺部位处于痉挛状态;或滞针处理不当等。

【处理】出现弯针后,不得再行手法,切忌强拔针、猛退针,以防引起折针、出血等。若体位移动所致,须先恢复原来体位,局部放松后退针。若针身弯曲度较小,可按一般的起针方法,随弯针的角度将针慢慢退出。若针身弯曲度较大,可顺着弯曲的方向轻微地边摇动边退针直至将针完全退出。如针身弯曲不止一处,须结合针柄扭转倾斜的方向逐次分段退出,切勿急拔猛抽,以防断针。

【预防】医者手法要熟练、轻巧,避免进针过猛、过速。患者的体位选择要舒适且适当,留针期间不可改变体位。避免针刺部位和

the needle handle should be protected from impact or external force. In addition, the acupuncturist should be cautious when needling the spasmodic position.

4. Hematoma

This term implies the swelling and pain caused by subcutaneous bleeding at punctured area.

[Phenomenon] Local bleeding, swelling, and pain, even the skin cyanotic occurs after the withdrawal of the needle.

[Causes] The hook of the tip of the needle impairs the skin and muscle, or blood vessels are injuried by mistake in the process of needling, or the patient's coagulation mechanism is impaired.

[Management] For patients with pinhole bleeding, use a sterilized dry cotton ball to press for a long time until the bleeding stop. If there is a small amount of subcutaneous bleeding and local small pieces of cyanosis, it generally do not have to be dealt with, for it will disappear by itself. If local swelling and pain are severe, and the hematoma is large, it may affect the activity function, cold compress should be used to stop bleeding within 24 hours, and then hot compress or local massage should be used after 24 hours, so that the local blood stasis can be absorbed and dissipated.

[Prevention] Before operation, check needles carefully, be familiar with the anatomical structure of acupoints, and avoid needling vascular. Avoid excessive needling manipulation and ask the patient not to move the body position at will. Delay needle withdrawal in layers. When the needle is withdrawn, immediately press the needle hole with a sterilized dry cotton ball. More attention should be paid when puncturing points around eye area, and the pressing time can be extended appropriately. People with bleeding tendency should be paid cautious when needling.

5. Abnormal sensation

This term implies the uncomfortable feeling, such as pain, heaviness, numbness, soreness, distension and other discomfort left at the acupuncture site after the withdrawal of the needle.

[Phenomenon] After the withdrawal of the needle, the patient cannot change his or her posture; or has such unwell feeling at the punctured area as ache, distension, heaviness, numbness and soreness, etc; or the original symptoms worsen, and hinder the normal life of patients; or pinhole bleeding, or cyanosis, nodules, etc. show on needle skin

[Causes] If the limb movement is inconvenient, it may caused by a needle left behind, not completely out, or improper position selection during needling, the patient moves the position or something presses the needle handle. Acupuncturists are not

针柄受外力碰压。另外,针刺呈痉挛状态的部位时,宜慎重。

四、血肿

血肿是指针刺部位因皮下出血而肿痛的现象。

【现象】出针后针刺部位出血或肿胀疼痛,甚至皮肤呈青紫等现象。

【原因】针尖带钩,使皮肉受损,或针刺时误伤血管,或者因个别患者凝血机制障碍所致。

【处理】针孔出血者,可用消毒干棉球进行长时间按压止血。当微量的皮下出血而出现局部小块青紫时,一般不必处理,可自行消退。若局部肿胀疼痛较剧,青紫面积大而且影响到活动功能时,在24小时内先冷敷止血,24小时之后,再做热敷或在局部轻轻按揉,促使局部瘀血吸收消散。

【预防】术前仔细检查针具,熟悉腧穴解剖结构,避开血管针刺。针刺时避免针刺手法过重,并嘱患者不可随意改变体位。分层延时出针,出针时立即用消毒干棉球按压针孔,眼区腧穴针刺更应注意,可适当延长按压时间。有出血倾向者,针刺时要慎重。

五、针后异常感

针后异常感是指患者针刺后,针刺部位遗留疼痛、沉重、麻木、酸胀等不适感觉。

【现象】出针后患者不能改变体位;或患者被针刺的局部或肢体遗留酸痛、沉重、麻木、酸胀等不适感;或原有症状加重,并妨碍患者的正常生活;或针孔出血,或针处皮肤出现青紫、结节等。

【原因】患者肢体不能挪动,可能是有针遗留、出针未完全,或针刺时体位选择不当、患者移动体位或外物碰压针柄;医者手法不熟

proficient in manipulation, too heavy manipulation and too long needle retention time. The original symptoms worsened, mostly because the manipulation is contrary to the condition. Before the needling, the inspection of the needles hasn't been done, and the tip of the needle has a hook, which damages the skin and flesh. Some cases may be caused by coagulation dysfunction.

[Management] If there is a needle left behind, the needle should be put out immediately. After withdrawing the needle, let the patient rest for a while, and don't let him/her leave in a hurry. If there are discomfort feelings such as soreness and swelling remain in the local area, the acupuncturists should use fingers to rub the area up and down in the mild cases, and perform massage or press on the puncturing area of the patient, then residual sensation can disappear or ameliorate after massage. If the residual sensation is obvious, other methods such as moxibustion, hot compress and magnetotherapy can be applied to eliminate the discomfort feelings. If the original symptom worsens, we should find out the causes, adjust the treatment principles and manipulations, and implement targeted needling methods. Local bleeding, cyanosis, cotton ball can be used to press for a moment; if hematoma and cyanosis are obvious, acupuncturists should first apply cold compress and then hot compress.

[Prevention] Check the needle carefully before needling. The technique should be skillful, the needle should be inserted quickly, and the needling technique should be appropriate, not too strong. Ask the patient not to change the position at will to prevent something from touching the needle handle. The needle retention time should not be too long. The number of needles should be counted after withdrawal to avoid omission. The needling technique shouldn't be carried out with large force and the needle retention time shouldn't be too long. For common symptoms, massage along the meridian should be carried out after withdrawing the needle to avoid the occurrence of abnormal sensation. Clinical treatment should be carried out according to syndrome differentiation, with refined acupoints selection and appropriate reinforcing and reducing methods.

6. Traumatic pneumothorax

Traumatic pneumothorax caused by improper needling is a kind of pneumothorax caused by the needle penetrating into the chest, damaging the pleura and air entering the pleural cavity.

[Phenomenon] The patient suddenly felt chest tightness, chest pain, palpitation, shortness of breath, poor breathing, irritative dry cough, and in severe cases, dyspnea, cyanosis, cold sweat, irritability, mental tension may occur, and even blood pressure

练,行针或手法过重,留针时间过长等。原有症状加重,多因手法与病情相悖等。针前未检查针具,针尖带钩,使皮肉受损,个别可能由患者凝血功能障碍引起。

【处理】如有遗留未出之针,应随即出针。退出针后让患者休息片刻,不要急于离开。若局部遗留酸胀等不适感,轻者用手指在局部上下揉按,在患者针刺局部做循按或推拿手法,后遗感即可消失或改善;重者可加用艾灸温灸,或用热敷、磁疗等方法加以消除。对原有症状加重者,应查明原因,调整治则和手法,另行针治;局部出血、青紫者,可用棉球按压片刻;血肿青紫明显者,应先冷敷再热敷。

【预防】针前要仔细检查针具。医者手法要熟练,进针要迅速,行针手法要适当,不可过强。嘱患者不可随意改变体位,防止外物碰压针柄。留针时间不宜过长。退出针后应清点针数,避免遗漏。针刺手法不宜过重,留针时间不宜过长。一般病证,出针后可做上下揉按,避免异常感出现;临诊时要认真辨证施治,处方选穴精炼,补泻手法适度。

六、气胸

针刺引起的创伤性气胸是指针刺入胸腔,使胸膜破损,空气进入胸膜腔所造成的气胸。

【现象】针刺后患者突感胸闷、胸痛、心悸、气短、呼吸不畅、刺激性干咳,严重者呼吸困难、发绀、出冷汗、烦躁、精神紧张,甚至出现

drop, shock and other critical phenomena.

Physical examination: the rib space of the affected side is widened, the chest is full, the drum sound is found on the percussion side, the breath sound is weakened or disappeared on the auscultation side, and the trachea is shifted to the healthy side on palpation.

Imaging examination shows that the affected lung tissue is compressed.

Some patients do not have symptoms immediately after withdrawing the needle, but gradually feel chest tightness, pain, dyspnea after a certain period of time.

[Causes] When puncturing the points at or nearby the chest and the back, the needle is inserted too deep or in a wrong direction that injury the chest, then air enter the pleural cavity causing pneumothorax.

[Management] In case of pneumothorax, the needle should be taken out immediately. Patients should rest in semi-reclining position, avoid breath holding, exerting and shouting, calm down and try to reduce postural turnover. Generally, for the mild condition, it can be absorbed on their own naturally. If there are accompanying symptoms, symptomatic treatment should be given, such as antitussive, anti-inflammatory drugs, in order to prevent the expansion of the hole due to cough, and to avoid aggravation and infection. In severe cases, such as dyspnea, cyanosis, shock and other phenomena, rescue should be organized immediately.

[Prevention] Choose proper position for the patient. For acupoints at or nearby the chest and the back, the angle, direction and depth of needling should be strictly controlled according to the patient's body shape, and the range of lifting and thrusting manipulation should not be too large.

7. Injury of the nervous system

This term implies the injury of brain, spinal cord, visceral nerve and nerves near acupoints caused by improper needling manipulation.

7.1　Injury of the central nervous system

[Phenomenon] When injuring the medulla, headache, nausea, vomiting, convulsions, dyspnea, shock and coma may occur, even life-threatening. When injuring the spinal cord, there may be a electric shock like sensation radiating to the extremities, temporary limb paralysis and so on, which may sometimes endanger life.

[Causes] When needling acupoints on nape, if the direction and depth of needling are not appropriate, it is easy to damage the

血压下降、休克等危急现象。

体格检查:视诊可见患侧肋间隙变宽、胸廓饱满,叩诊患侧呈鼓音,听诊患侧呼吸音减弱或消失,触诊或可见气管向健侧移位。

影像学检查可见患侧肺组织被压缩。

部分患者,出针后并不立即出现症状,而是过一定时间才逐渐感到胸闷、疼痛、呼吸困难等。

【原因】针刺胸部、背部及其邻近穴位不当,刺伤胸膜,空气聚于胸腔而造成气胸。

【处理】一旦发生气胸,应立即出针;嘱患者采取半卧位休息,避免屏气、用力、高声呼喊,应平静心情,尽量减少体位翻转。一般轻者可自然吸收;如患者有症状,医者可对症处理,如给予镇咳、镇痛、抗感染、消炎等对症药物,防止因咳嗽扩大创孔,避免症状加重和感染。重者,如出现呼吸困难、发绀、休克等现象,应立即组织抢救。

【预防】为患者选择合适体位。对于胸部、背部及邻近腧穴,根据患者体型,严格掌握针刺的角度、方向和深度,施行提插手法的幅度不宜过大。

七、刺伤神经系统

针刺不当,可刺伤脑、脊髓、内脏神经,以及穴位附近的神经等。

(一)刺伤中枢神经

【现象】刺伤延脑时,可出现头痛、恶心、呕吐、抽搐、呼吸困难、休克和神志昏迷等,甚至危及生命。刺伤脊髓时,可出现触电样感觉向肢端放射、暂时性肢体瘫痪等,有时可危及生命。

【原因】针刺项部穴位时,若针刺的方向及深度不当,容易伤及

medulla oblongata, resulting in brain tissue damage, and in severe cases, causing brain hernia and other serious consequences. When puncturing thoracolumbar and interspinous acupoints, if the depth of the needle insertion is too deep or the manipulation is too strong, the spinal cord may be injured by mistake.

[Management] The needle should be taken out immediately. In mild cases, pay close attention to the patient's condition and let him/her have a rest quietly and wait for recovery. The patients with severe symptoms should be treated in time with modern medical measures.

[Prevention] When needling acupoints at the Governor Vessel, on the head, the back and the lumbar, especially like Fengfu (GV16), Yamen (GV15), Fengchi (GB20) and so on, it is not allowed to needle upward or too deep. Acupuncturists should strictly control the angle, direction and depth of needle insertion. Pay attention to the patient's sensation at any time, choose the twirling method, and try to avoid the manipulation like lifting-thrusting method.

7.2 Injury of the peripheral nervous system

[Phenomenon] When peripheral nervous system is injured by mistake, there may be a electric shock like radiation sensation immediately, and even the sensory abnormalities such as numbness, heat and pain along the nerve distribution route, or the movement disorder and muscle atrophy of different degrees can occur.

[Causes] When puncturing the acupoints near the nerve trunk or main branches, the acupuncturists still lift or/and insert the needle in a large range, or carry out strong manipulation with the thick needle, or the needle is kept for a long time, or needling one point for several times after the patient feels electrifying, which may injured the peripheral nervous.

[Management] Treatment should be taken immediately after the injury. Massage can be used for mild cases. Patients should be instructed to strengthen functional exercise. B vitamins can be used for treatment. For example, B vitamins injection is injected into corresponding meridians and acupoints. The severe cases should be treated with means of modern medicine.

[Prevention] When puncturing the acupoints near nerve trunk, the manipulation should be mild. When an electric shock like sensation appears, lifting-thrusting and twirling method shouldn't be carried out. The stimulation time and needle retention time shouldn't be too long and the frequency should be controlled.

8. Injury of internal organs

This term implies the injury of heart, liver, spleen, kidney and

延髓，造成脑组织损伤，严重者出现脑疝等严重后果。针刺胸、腰段，以及棘突间腧穴时，针刺过深，或手法太强，可误伤脊髓。

【处理】立即出针。轻者，加强观察，安静休息，能逐渐恢复；重者应配合西医学措施进行及时救治。

【预防】凡针刺督脉腧穴，头项及背腰部的腧穴，特别是风府、哑门、风池等穴时，不可向上针刺，也不可刺之过深。医者应认真掌握进针深度、方向和角度。行针中必须随时注意患者感觉，选用捻转手法，尽量避免提插等手法。

（二）刺伤周围神经

【现象】针刺误伤周围神经，患者可立即出现触电样的放射感觉，甚至出现沿神经分布路线发生麻木、热、痛等感觉异常，或有程度不等的运动障碍、肌肉萎缩等。

【原因】在有神经干或主要神经分支分布的腧穴上，针刺或使用粗针强刺激出现触电感后仍然大幅度提插，或留针时间过长，或同一腧穴反复针刺等。

【处理】应该在损伤后立即采取治疗措施，轻者可做按摩，嘱患者加强功能锻炼，可应用B族维生素类药物治疗。如在相应经络腧穴上进行B族维生素类穴位注射；重者应配合西医学措施进行处理。

【预防】针刺神经干附近的腧穴时，手法宜轻，出现触电感时，勿继续提插捻转。刺激时间不宜过长，刺激次数不宜过多，留针时间不宜过长。

八、刺伤内脏

针刺引起内脏损伤是指针刺

some other organs due to improper needling at acupoints on chest, abdomen and back.

[Phenomenon] Impairment of heart by puncture: In mild cases, the patients may have strong stabbing pain in the chest. In severe cases, the patients feel severe tearing pain, which caused extracardiac hemorrhage, resulting in immediate shock and death.

Impairment of liver or spleen by puncture: It can cause internal bleeding, patients may feel liver or spleen pain, or radiation to the back. If the bleeding is massive, abdominal pain, tension of the abdominal muscles, abdominal tenderness and rebounding pain may be accompanied.

Impairment of kidneys by puncture: There may be lumbago, tenderness and percussion pain in the renal area, or hematuria. In severe cases, blood pressure drops and shock occurs due to massive bleeding.

Impairment of gallbladder, bladder, stomach, intestine and other cavity organs: There may be local pain, abdominal muscle tension, tenderness and rebound pain.

[Causes] The acupuncturists lack the anatomical knowledge, or fail to grasp correct angel, direction and depth of the needle insertion.

[Management] Patients with mild injury can generally recover after rest in bed. If the injury is serious or the bleeding sign is obvious, the hemostatic drugs and other symptomatic treatment should be applied. Closely observe the condition and blood pressure changes. If the injury is serious, bleeding with a large amount, hemorrhagic shock occurs, practitioner must quickly carry out blood transfusion and other emergency or surgical treatment.

[Prevention] Have a sound anatomical knowledge, and make clear the organs and subcutaneous tissues under the local of acupoints clear in mind. The angle, direction and depth of needling, especially the depth, should be paid more attention in patients with enlargement of liver, spleen, gallbladder, and heart and filling of bladder, and also in the the place around the organ and where large blood vessels and nerve trunks locates.

胸、腹和背部相关腧穴不当，引起心、肝、脾、肾等内脏损伤而出现的各种症状。

【现象】刺伤心脏时，轻者可出现胸部强烈的刺痛；重者有剧烈的撕裂痛，引起心外射血，导致休克，甚至死亡。

刺伤肝、脾时，可引起内出血，患者可感到肝区或脾区疼痛，或向背部放射；如出血过多，可出现腹痛、腹肌紧张、压痛以及反跳痛等症状。

刺伤肾脏时，可有腰痛、肾区压痛及叩击痛，或见血尿；严重时血压下降、休克。

刺伤胆囊、膀胱、胃、肠等空腔脏器时，可引起局部疼痛、腹肌紧张、压痛及反跳痛等症状。

【原因】医者缺乏腧穴解剖学知识，或未能掌握正确的进针角度、方向和深度。

【处理】损伤轻者，卧床休息后，一般即可自愈。如果损伤严重或出血征象明显，应用止血药等进行对症处理。密切观察病情及血压变化。若损伤严重，出血较多，出现失血性休克时，则必须迅速进行输血等急救或外科手术治疗。

【预防】熟悉腧穴解剖学知识，明确腧穴下的脏器组织。凡脏器组织、大血管、神经干处，肝、脾、胆囊、心脏扩大，以及膀胱充盈的患者，其相应部位的穴位，都应注意针刺的角度、方向和深度，特别是针刺的深度。

Appendix 附 录

Appendix A Introduction to the Basic Imaginary Points, Lines and Divisions of the Auricle

1. Designation of basic marking line on the auricle(Fig. A-1)

Medial edge of the helix: The boundary between the helix and other parts of the auricle; a fold line formed by the helix, scapha, crura of the antihelix, triangular fossa, and concha.

Fold line of the concha: The boundary between the flat part and the prominent part of the concha.

Line of the antihelix spine: A connecting line, formed by the highest prominence stretching from the bifurcation to the body of the antihelix.

Line of the groove of the scapha: A line at the deepest depression of the scapha.

Boundary of the antihelix and the scapha: The midline between the antihelix(including the superior antihelix crus) spine and the groove of the scapha.

The posterior edge of the triangular fossa: The lower border of the triangular fossa.

(The following see Fig. A-2)

Boundary of the antihelix and the triangular fossa: The midline between the spines of antihelix crus and posterior edge of triangular fossa.

附录 A 耳郭基本标志点、线的划定及耳郭分区说明

一、耳郭基本标志线的划定（图 A-1）

耳轮内缘：耳轮与耳郭其他部分的分界线，即耳轮与耳舟，对耳轮上、下脚，三角窝及耳甲等部的折线。

耳甲折线：耳甲内平坦部与隆起部之间的折线。

对耳轮脊线：对耳轮体及其上、下脚最凸起处的连线。

耳舟凹沟线：沿耳舟最凹陷处所作的连线。

对耳轮耳舟缘：对耳轮与耳舟的分界线，即对耳轮（含对耳轮上脚）脊与耳舟凹沟之间的中线。

三角窝凹陷处后缘：三角窝内较低平的三角形区域的后缘。

（以下见图 A-2）

对耳轮三角窝缘：对耳轮上、下脚与三角窝的分界线，即对耳轮上、下脚脊与三角窝凹陷处后缘之间的中线。

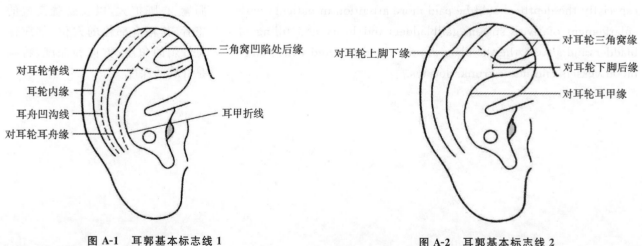

图 A-1 耳郭基本标志线 1　　　　图 A-2 耳郭基本标志线 2

The concha edge of the antihelix: The midline between the spine of antihelix (including the inferior antihelix crus) and the anatomical border between the antihelix and the concha.

The inferior edge of the antihelix: The boundary between the superior antihelix crus and the body of the antihelix formed by a line extending vertically from the bifurcation of the antihelix to the boundary of the antihelix and the scapha.

The posterior edge of the antihelix: The boundary between the inferior antihelix crus and the body of the antihelix formed by a line extending vertically from the bifurcation of the antihelix to the concha edge of the antihelix.

(The following see Fig. A-3)

The superior line of the ear lobe (also used as the boundary between the antihelix-ear lobe edge and the helix-ear lobe edge): It refers to the straight line to divide ear lobe between screens and other parts of auricle. That refers to the straight line made by the cut between tragus-antitragus notch and the helix-ear lobe notch.

The concha edge of the antitragus: The boundary between the medial rim of the antihelix and the concha. It refers to the fold line between the inner side of the tragus and the concha.

The anterior edge of the tragus: The boundary between the anterior of the tragus and the cheek. It refers to the straight line along the front groove of the tragus.

The anterior edge of the helix: The boundary between the helix and the cheek. It refers to the straight line along the front of the helix.

The anterior edge of the ear lobe: The boundary between the ear lobe and the cheek. It refers to the straight line along the front groove of the ear lobe.

2. Imaginary points and lines on the auricle (Fig. A-4)

Imaginary point A is located at the medial edge of the helix at the junction between the middle and upper 1/3 of the line from the notch of helix crus and the inferior edge of the inferior antihelix crus.

Imaginary point B is located at the junction of the middle and posterior 1/3 of the line extending from the end of the helix crus to point D.

Imaginary point C is located at the junction of upper 1/4 and lower 3/4 of the posterior edge of the orifice of the external auditory meatus.

Imaginary point D is located at where a level line drawn from the end of the helix crus crosses the concha edge of the antihelix.

Line AB is a curved line extended from point A to point B that

对耳轮耳甲缘:对耳轮与耳甲的分界线,即对耳轮(含对耳轮下脚)脊与耳甲折线之间的中线。

对耳轮上脚下缘:对耳轮上脚与对耳轮体的分界线,即从对耳轮上、下脚分叉处向对耳轮耳舟缘所作的垂线。

对耳轮下脚后缘:对耳轮下脚与对耳轮体的分界线,即从对耳轮上、下脚分叉处向对耳轮耳甲缘所作的垂线。

(以下见图 A-3)

耳垂上线(亦作为对耳屏耳垂缘和耳屏耳垂缘):耳垂与耳郭其他部分的分界线,即过屏间切迹与轮垂切迹所作的直线。

对耳屏耳甲缘:对耳轮与耳甲的分界线,即对耳屏内侧面与耳甲的折线。

耳屏前缘:耳屏外侧面与面部的分界线,即沿耳屏前沟所作的直线。

耳轮前缘:耳轮与面部的分界线,即沿耳轮前沟所作的直线。

耳垂前缘:耳垂与面颊的分界线,即沿耳垂前沟所作的直线。

二、耳郭标志点、线的设定(图 A-4)

A点:在耳轮的内缘上,耳轮脚切迹至对耳轮下脚间中、上 1/3 交界处。

B点:耳轮脚消失处至 D 点连线中、后 1/3 交界处。

C点:外耳道口后缘上 1/4 与下 3/4 交界处。

D点:在耳甲内,由耳轮脚消失处向后作一水平线与对耳轮耳甲缘相交点处。

AB线:从 A 点向 B 点作一条

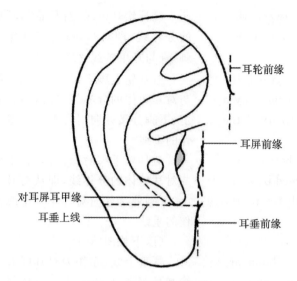

图 A-3　耳郭基本标志线 3

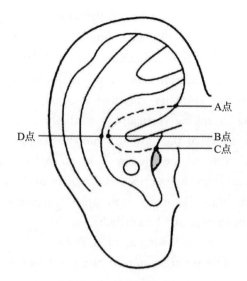

图 A-4　耳郭标志点

mirrors the concha edge of the antihelix.

Line BC is a curved line extended from point B to point C that mirrors the inferior edge of the helix crus.

Line BD is a line between point B and point D.

3. Partition and auricular points of helix(Fig. A-5, Tab. A-1)

There are 13 points in 12 areas in helix.

The helix crus is HX_1 (area 1 of the helix).

The part of the helix from helix notch to the upper edge of the inferior antihelix crus is equally divided into three parts, HX_2, HX_3 and HX_4, counting from below to above.

HX_5 is the area between the upper edge of the inferior antihelix crus and the front edge of the superior antihelix crus.

HX_6 is the area between the front edge of the superior crura of antihelix crus and ear apex.

HX_7 is the area between the ear apex and the upper edge of the helix tubercle.

HX_8 is the area between the upper edge of the helix tubercle and the lower edge of the helix tubercle.

The region from the lower edge of the helix tubercle to the helix lobe notch is equally divided into four areas, HX_9, HX_{10}, HX_{11}, and HX_{12}, from above to below respectively.

与对耳轮耳甲艇缘弧度大体相仿的曲线。

BC线：从 B 点向 C 点作一条与耳轮脚下缘弧度大体相仿的曲线。

BD线：B 点与 D 点之间的连线。

三、耳轮部分区与耳穴（图 A-5,表 A-1）

耳轮部分为 12 区，共有13 穴。

耳轮脚为耳轮1 区。

耳轮脚切迹到对耳轮下脚上缘之间的耳轮分为三等份，自下而上依次为耳轮 2 区、耳轮 3 区、耳轮 4 区。

对耳轮下脚上缘到对耳轮上脚前缘之间为耳轮 5 区。

对耳轮上脚前缘到耳尖之间为耳轮 6 区。

耳尖到耳轮结节上缘为耳轮7 区。

耳轮结节上缘到耳轮结节下缘为耳轮 8 区。

耳轮结节下缘至轮垂切迹之间的耳轮分为四等份，自上而下依次为耳轮 9 区、耳轮 10 区、耳轮 11区和耳轮 12 区。

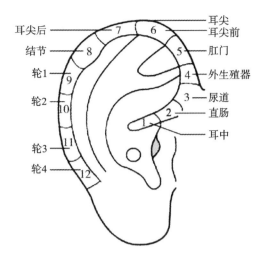

图 A-5　耳轮部分区与耳穴

Tab. A-1　Acupoints on the helix crus and helix(表 A-1　耳轮穴位)

Acupoint name （穴名）	Location （定位）	Indications （主治）
Ear Center(HX$_1$) （耳中(HX$_1$)）	On the helix crus （在耳轮脚处，即耳轮 1 区）	Hiccup,urticaria,pruritus,hemoptysis （呃逆，荨麻疹，皮肤瘙痒，咯血）
Rectum(HX$_2$) （直肠(HX$_2$)）	On the helix anterior to the spine of the helix crus （在耳轮脚棘前上方的耳轮处，即耳轮 2 区）	Constipation,diarrhea,rectal prolapse,hemorrhoid （便秘，腹泻，脱肛，痔疮）
Urethra(HX$_3$) （尿道(HX$_3$)）	It is located on the helix superior to Rectum(HX$_2$) （在直肠上方的耳轮处，即耳轮 3 区）	Enuresis,micturition,urgency,pain of urination,retention of urine （遗尿，尿频，尿急，尿痛，尿潴留）
External Genitals(HX$_4$) （外生殖器(HX$_4$)）	On the helix at the level with the upper border of the inferior antihelix crus （在对耳轮下脚前方的耳轮处，即耳轮 4 区）	Orchitis, epididymitis, vaginitis, pruritus vulvae （睾丸炎，附睾炎，阴道炎，外阴瘙痒）
Anus(HX$_5$) （肛门(HX$_5$)）	On the helix anterior to the triangular fossa （三角窝前方的耳轮处，即耳轮 5 区）	Hemorrhoid and anal fissure （痔疮，肛裂）
Anterior Ear Apex(HX$_6$) （耳尖前(HX$_6$)）	It is located anterior to the ear apex （在耳尖的前部，即耳轮 6 区）	Fever and conjunctivitis （发热，结膜炎）
Ear Apex(XH$_{6,7i}$) （耳尖(HX$_{6,7i}$)）	It is the apex formed when the auricle is folded anteriorly at the juncture of HX$_6$ and HX$_7$ （在耳郭向前对折的上部尖端处，即耳轮 6、7 区交界处）	Fever, hypertension, acute conjunctivitis, hordeolum,pain syndrome,rubella,insomnia （发热，高血压，急性结膜炎，麦粒肿，痛证，风疹，失眠）
Posterior Ear Apex(HX$_7$) （耳尖后(HX$_7$)）	It is posterior to the ear apex （在耳尖的后部，即耳轮 7 区）	Fever,conjunctivitis （发热，结膜炎）
Node(HX$_8$) （结节(HX$_8$)）	It is located on the helix at the helix tubercle （在耳轮结节处，即耳轮 8 区）	Dizziness,headache,hypertension （头晕，头痛，高血压）

Acupoint name （穴名）	Location （定位）	Indications （主治）
Helix$_1$（HX$_9$） （轮 1（HX$_9$））	It is located on the helix inferior to the helix tubercle （在耳轮结节下方的耳轮处，即耳轮 9 区）	Tonsillitis, upper respiratory tract infection, fever （扁桃体炎，上呼吸道感染，发热）
Helix$_2$（HX$_{10}$） （轮 2（HX$_{10}$））	It is located on the helix inferior to HX$_1$ （在轮 1 区下方的耳轮处，即耳轮 10 区）	Tonsillitis, upper respiratory tract infection, fever （扁桃体炎，上呼吸道感染，发热）
Helix$_3$（HX$_{11}$） （轮 3（HX$_{11}$））	It is located on the helix inferior to HX$_2$ （在轮 2 区下方的耳轮处，即耳轮 11 区）	Tonsillitis, upper respiratory tract infection, fever （扁桃体炎，上呼吸道感染，发热）
Helix$_4$（HX$_{12}$） （轮 4（HX$_{12}$））	It is located on the helix inferior to HX$_3$ （在轮 3 区下方的耳轮处，即耳轮 12 区）	Tonsillitis, upper respiratory tract infection, fever （扁桃体炎，上呼吸道感染，发热）

4. Partition and auricular points of scapha (Fig. A-6,Tab. A-2)

There are 6 points in 6 areas in scapha.

The scapha is divided into 6 equal areas. From above to below, they are SF$_1$ (area 1 of the scapha), SF$_2$, SF$_3$, SF$_4$, SF$_5$ and SF$_6$.

四、耳舟部分区与耳穴（图 A-6，表 A-2）

耳舟部分为 6 区，共有 6 穴。

耳舟部自上而下依次分为六等份，分别为耳舟 1 区、2 区、3 区、4 区、5 区、6 区。

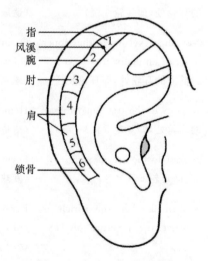

图 A-6 耳舟部分区与耳穴

Tab. A-2 Acupoints on the scapha(表 A-2 耳舟穴位)

acupoint name （穴名）	Location （定位）	Indications （主治）
Finger(SF$_1$) （指（SF$_1$））	At the top of the scapha （在耳舟上方，即耳舟 1 区）	Paronychia, numbness, pain, stiffness of the fingers （甲沟炎，手指疼痛、麻木和僵硬）

续表

acupoint name （穴名）	Location （定位）	Indications （主治）
Wrist(SF_2) （腕（SF_2））	In the area inferior to SF_1 （在指区的下方处，即耳舟 2 区）	Wrist spain （腕部疼痛）
Windstream($SF_{1,2i}$) （风溪（$SF_{1,2i}$））	In the area anterior to the helix tubercle at the juncture of SF_1 and SF_2 （在耳轮结节前方，指区与腕区之间，即耳舟 1、2 区交界处）	Urticaria, pruritus, allergic rhinitis, asthma （荨麻疹，皮肤瘙痒，过敏性鼻炎，哮喘）
Elbow(SF_3) （肘（SF_3））	In the area inferior to SF_2 （在腕区的下方处，即耳舟 3 区）	External humeral epicondylitis, elbow pain （肱骨外上髁炎，肘部疼痛）
Shoulder($SF_{4,5}$) （肩（$SF_{4,5}$））	In the area inferior to SF_3 （在肘区的下方处，即耳舟 4、5 区）	Periarthritis of shoulder, shoulder pain （肩关节周围炎，肩部疼痛）
Clavicle(SF_6) （锁骨（SF_6））	In the area inferior to $SF_{4,5}$ （在肩区的下方处，即耳舟 6 区）	Periarthritis of shoulder （肩关节周围炎）

5. Partition and auricular points of antihelix (Fig. A-7, Tab. A-3)

There are 14 points in 13 areas in antihelix.

The superior antihelix crus is divided into three equal parts. The lower third is AH_5 (area 5 of the antihelix). The middle third is AH_4, and the upper third is divided horizontally into two equal subparts, of which the lower half is AH_3. The upper half is once again divided perpendicularly into two: the posterior half is AH_2 and the anterior half is AH_1.

The inferior antihelix crus is divided into three equal parts. From the anterior to the posterior, the first two-thirds are AH_6; the posterior third is AH_7. The body of the antihelix from its bifurcation to the antihelix-antitragus notch is divided into five equal parts from the superior to the inferior, and once again it is divided into the anterior (one fourth) and the posterior (three fourths) paralleling to the boundary of the antihelix and the concha. In this way, the body of the antihelix is divided into ten parts. The anterior superior two parts are AH_8; the posterior superior two parts are AH_9; the anterior intermediate two parts are AH_{10}; the posterior intermediate two parts are AH_{11}; the anterior inferior part is AH_{12}; the posterior inferior part is AH_{13}.

五、对耳轮部分区与耳穴（图 A-7，表 A-3）

对耳轮部分为 13 区，共有 14 穴。

对耳轮上脚分为上、中、下三等份，下 1/3 为对耳轮 5 区，中 1/3 为对耳轮 4 区；再将上 1/3 分为上、下两等份，下 1/2 为对耳轮 3 区，再将上 1/2 分为前后两等份，后 1/2 为对耳轮 2 区，前 1/2 为对耳轮 1 区。

对耳轮下脚分为前、中、后三等份，中、前 2/3 为对耳轮 6 区，后 1/3 为对耳轮 7 区。将对耳轮体从对耳轮上、下脚分叉处至轮屏切迹分为五等份，再沿对耳轮耳甲缘将对耳轮体分为前 1/4 和后 3/4 两部分，前、上 2/5 为对耳轮 8 区，后、上 2/5 为对耳轮 9 区，前、中 2/5 为对耳轮 10 区，后、中 2/5 为对耳轮 11 区，前、下 1/5 为对耳轮 12 区，后、下 1/5 为对耳轮 13 区。

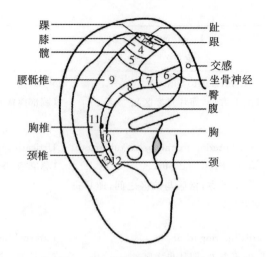

图 A-7　对耳轮部分区与耳穴

Tab. A-3　Acupoints on the antihelix(表 A-3　对耳轮穴位)

Acupoint name （穴名）	Location （定位）	Indications （主治）
Heel(AH_1) （跟（AH_1））	Medial and superior angle of the superior antihelix crus （在对耳轮上脚前上部，即对耳轮 1 区）	Heel pain （足跟痛）
Toe(AH_2) （趾（AH_2））	Lateral and superior angle of the superior antihelix crus （在耳尖下方的对耳轮上脚后上部，即对耳轮 2 区）	Paronychia, numbness and pain in the toes （甲沟炎，足趾部麻木疼痛）
Ankle(AH_3) （踝（AH_3））	Inferior to Heel(AH_1)and Toe(AH_2) （在趾、跟区下方处，即对耳轮 3 区）	Ankle sprain and ankle arthritis （踝关节扭伤，踝关节炎）
Knee(AH_4) （膝（AH_4））	On the middle 1/3 of the superior antihelix crus （在对耳轮上脚中 1/3 处，即对耳轮 4 区）	Knee joint pain （膝关节肿痛）
Hip(AH_5) （髋（AH_5））	On the lower 1/3 of the superior antihelix crus （在对耳轮上脚的下 1/3 处，即对耳轮 5 区）	Hip pain, sciatica and lower back pain （髋关节疼痛，坐骨神经痛，腰骶部疼痛）
Sciatic Nerve(AH_6) （坐骨神经（AH_6））	On the anterior 2/3 of the inferior antihelix crus （在对耳轮下脚的前 2/3 处，即对耳轮 6 区）	Sciatica and paralysis of the lower limbs （坐骨神经痛，下肢瘫痪）
Sympathetic Nerve(AH_{6a}) （交感（AH_{6a}））	The terminal of the inferior antihelix crus （在对耳轮下脚前端与耳轮内缘交界处，即对耳轮 6 区前端）	Autonomic neurologic diseases and gastrointestinal, heart, bile, ureter diseases （自主神经功能疾病及胃肠、心、胆、输尿管等疾病）

Acupoint name （穴名）	Location （定位）	Indications （主治）
Gluteus（AH$_7$） （臀（AH$_7$））	On the posterior 1/3 of the inferior antihelix crus （在对耳轮下脚的后 1/3 处，即对耳轮 7 区）	Sciatica and hip pain （坐骨神经痛，臀部疼痛）
Abdomen（AH$_8$） （腹（AH$_8$））	On the upper 2/5 of the anterior part of the body of the antihelix （在对耳轮体前部上 2/5 处，即对耳轮 8 区）	Digestive system and pelvic diseases （消化系统、盆腔疾病）
Lumbosacral Vertebrae（AH$_9$） （腰骶椎（AH$_9$））	On the body of the anterior part of the antihelix posterior to Abdomen（AH$_8$） （在腹区后方，即对耳轮 9 区）	The corresponding site diseases （相应部位疾病）
Chest（AH$_{10}$） （胸（AH$_{10}$））	On the middle 2/5 of the anterior part of the body of the antihelix （在对耳轮体前部中 2/5 处，即对耳轮 10 区）	The corresponding chest and hypochondrium area diseases （相应胸胁部位疾病）
Thoracic Vertebrae（AH$_{11}$） （胸椎（AH$_{11}$））	On the body of the antihelix posterior to Chest（AH$_{10}$） （在胸区后方，即对耳轮 11 区）	The corresponding site diseases （相应部位疾病）
Neck（AH$_{12}$） （颈（AH$_{12}$））	On the lower 1/5 of the anterior part of the body of the antihelix （在对耳轮体前部下 1/5 处，即对耳轮 12 区）	Neck stiffness and other diseases at the corresponding areas （落枕等颈项部疾病）
Cervical Vertebrae（AH$_{13}$） （颈椎（AH$_{13}$））	On the body of the antihelix posterior to Neck（AH$_{12}$） （在颈区后方，即对耳轮 13 区）	Cervical vertebral disease and other related site diseases （颈椎病等相应部位疾病）

6. Partition and auricular points of triangular fossa（Fig. A-8, Tab. A-4）

There are 5 points in 5 areas in triangular fossa.

The triangular fossa is divided into three equal parts from the edge of helix to the bifurcation of the antihelix. The middle third is TF$_3$（area 3 of the triangular fossa）. The anterior third is further divided into three subparts: the upper third is TF$_1$, and the middle and lower two-thirds are TF$_2$. The posterior third near the bifurcation is divided into two subparts: the upper half is TF$_4$ and the lower half is TF$_5$.

六、三角窝部分区与耳穴（图 A-8，表 A-4）

三角窝部分为 5 区，共有 5 穴。

将三角窝由耳轮内缘至对耳轮上、下脚分叉处分为前、中、后三等份，中 1/3 为三角窝 3 区；再将前 1/3 分为上、中、下三等份，上 1/3 为三角窝 1 区，中、下 2/3 为三角窝 2 区；再将后 1/3 分为上、下两等份，上 1/2 为三角窝 4 区，下 1/2 为三角窝 5 区。

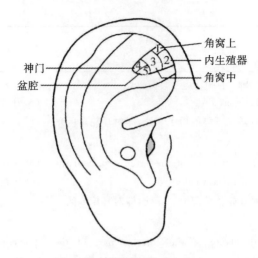

图 A-8　三角窝部分区与耳穴

Tab. A-4　Acupoints on the triangular fossa(表 A-4　三角窝穴位)

Acupoint name (穴名)	Location (定位)	Indications (主治)
Superior Triangular Fossa(TF$_1$) (角窝上(TF$_1$))	In the upper part of the superior 1/3 of the triangular fossa (在三角窝前 1/3 的上部,即三角窝 1 区)	Hypertension (高血压)
Internal Genitals(TF$_2$) (内生殖器(TF$_2$))	In the lower part of the superior 1/3 of the triangular fossa (在三角窝前 1/3 的下部,即三角窝 2 区)	Gynaecological diseases and male diseases (妇科病、男性病)
Middle Triangular Fossa(TF$_3$) (角窝中(TF$_3$))	In the middle 1/3 of the triangular fossa (在三角窝中 1/3 处,即三角窝 3 区)	Asthma,cough,liver disease,etc. (哮喘,咳嗽,肝病等)
Shenmen(TF$_4$) (神门(TF$_4$))	In the upper part of the posterior 1/3 of the triangular fossa (在三角窝后 1/3 的上部,即三角窝 4 区)	Insomnia, dreaminess, various pain, cough, asthma, dizziness, hypertension, allergic disease,withdrawal syndrome (失眠,多梦,各种痛证,咳嗽,哮喘,眩晕,高血压,过敏性疾病,戒断综合征)
Pelvis(TF$_5$) (盆腔(TF$_5$))	In the lower part of the posterior 1/3 of the triangular fossa (在三角窝前 1/3 的下部,即三角窝 5 区)	Pelvic inflammation,attachment inflammation and other in-pelvic diseases (盆腔炎、附件炎等盆腔内病证)

7. Partition and auricular points of tragus (Fig. A-9,Tab. A-5)

There are 9 points in 4 areas in tragus.

The external surface of the tragus is divided into two parts;the upper part is TG$_1$(area 1 of the tragus) and the lower part is TG$_2$. The internal surface of the tragus is divided into two parts, the upper part is TG$_3$,and the lower part is TG$_4$.

七、耳屏部分区与耳穴 (图 A-9,表 A-5)

耳屏部分为 4 区,共有 9 穴。

耳屏外侧面分为上、下两等份,上部为耳屏 1 区,下部为耳屏 2 区。将耳屏内侧面分上、下两等份,上部为耳屏 3 区,下部为耳屏 4 区。

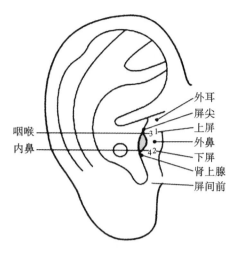

图 A-9　耳屏部分区与耳穴

Tab. A-5　Acupoints on the tragus（表 A-5　耳屏穴位）

Acupoint name （穴名）	Location （定位）	Indications （主治）
Upper Tragus（TG_1） （上屏（TG_1））	On the upper 1/2 of the external surface of the tragus （在耳屏外侧面上 1/2 处，即耳屏 1 区）	Pharyngitis and simple obesity （咽炎，单纯性肥胖）
Lower Tragus（TG_2） （下屏（TG_2））	On the lower 1/2 of the external surface of the tragus （在耳屏外侧面下 1/2 处，即耳屏 2 区）	Rhinitis and simple obesity （鼻炎，单纯性肥胖）
External Ear（TG_{1u}） （外耳（TG_{1u}））	It is inferior to the crus of helix and anterior to the supratragic notch on the upper edge of Upper Tragus（TG_1） （在屏上切迹前方近耳轮部，即耳屏 1 区上缘处）	All kinds of ear diseases, such as tinnitus and dizziness （各类耳病，如耳鸣、眩晕）
Apex of Tragus（TG_{1p}） （屏尖（TG_{1p}））	On the projection of the upper tragus at the posterior edge of Upper Tragus（TG_1） （在耳屏游离缘上部尖端，即耳屏 1 区后缘处）	Facial inflammation and pain syndrome （五官炎症，痛证）
External Nose（$TG_{1,2i}$） （外鼻（$TG_{1,2i}$））	At the midpoint of the external surface of the tragus at the juncture of the TG_1 and TG_2 （在耳屏外侧面中部，即耳屏 1、2 区之间）	All kinds of nasal diseases, such as sinusitis （各类鼻病，如鼻渊等）
Adrenal Gland（TG_{2p}） （肾上腺（TG_{2p}））	On the end of the inferior edge of the tragus at the posterior edge of TG_2 （在耳屏游离缘下部尖端，即耳屏 2 区后缘处）	Hypotension, fainting, shock, inflammation, asthma, allergic diseases, pulseless diseases, etc. （低血压，晕厥，休克，炎症，哮喘，过敏性疾病，无脉症等）
Pharynx-Larynx（TG_3） （咽喉（TG_3））	On the upper 1/2 of the internal surface of the tragus （在耳屏内侧面上 1/2 处，即耳屏 3 区）	Sore throat, hoarse voice, pharyngitis, etc. （咽喉肿痛，声音嘶哑，咽炎等）

续表

Acupoint name （穴名）	Location （定位）	Indications （主治）
Internal Nose(TG$_4$) （内鼻(TG$_4$)）	On the lower 1/2 of the internal surface of the tragus （在耳屏内侧面下 1/2 处,即耳屏 4 区）	All kinds of nasal diseases, such as sinusitis, nasal congestion, and runny nose （各类鼻病,如鼻渊、鼻塞流涕等）
Anterior Intertragic Notch(TG$_{21}$) （屏间前(TG$_{21}$)）	On the lowest part of the front surface of the intertragic notch on the inferior edge of TG$_2$ （在屏间切迹前方耳屏最下部,即耳屏 2 区下缘处）	Eye diseases （眼病）

8. Partition and auricular points of antitragus (Fig. A-10,Tab. A-6)

There are 8 points in 4 areas in antitragus.

Draw two lines, one extending vertically from the apex of the antitragus to the superior line of the ear lobe, the other vertically from the midpoint of the antitragus to the helix notch. The external surface of the antitragus is thus divided into three areas. The anterior area is AT$_1$ (area 1 of the antitragus), the intermediate is AT$_2$, and the posterior is AT$_3$.

八、对耳屏部分区与耳穴（图 A-10,表 A-6）

对耳屏部分为 4 区,共有 8 穴。

由对屏尖及对屏尖至轮屏切迹连线之中点,分别向耳垂上线作两条垂线,将对耳屏外侧面及其后部分成前、中、后 3 区,前为对耳屏 1 区,中为对耳屏 2 区,后为对耳屏 3 区,对耳屏内侧面为对耳屏 4 区。

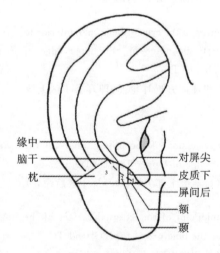

缘中　脑干　枕　对屏尖　皮质下　屏间后　额　颞

图 A-10　对耳屏部分区与耳穴

Tab. A-6　Acupoints on the antitragus（表 A-6　对耳屏穴位）

Acupoint name （穴名）	Location （定位）	Indications （主治）
Forehead(AT$_1$) （额(AT$_1$)）	In the anterior area of the lateral side of the antitragus （在对耳屏外侧面的前部,即对耳屏 1 区）	Sinusitis, headache, dizziness, insomnia, and dreaminess （额窦炎,头痛,头晕,失眠,多梦）

续表

Acupoint name （穴名）	Location （定位）	Indications （主治）
Posterior Intertragicus(AT_{11}) （屏间后（AT_{11}））	At the anteroinferior part of the antitragus, posterior to intertragicus and the lower edge of AT_1 （在屏间切迹后方对耳屏前下部，即对耳屏 1 区下缘处）	Eye diseases （眼病）
Temple(AT_2) （颞（AT_2））	At the midpoint part of the lateral side of the antitragus （在对耳屏外侧面的中部，即对耳屏 2 区）	Migraine （偏头痛）
Occiput(AT_3) （枕（AT_3））	At the posterior part of the lateral side of the antitragus （在对耳屏外侧面的后部，即对耳屏 3 区）	Headache, dizziness, asthma, epilepsy, and neurasthenia （头痛，眩晕，哮喘，癫痫，神经衰弱）
Subcortex(AT_4) （皮质下（AT_4））	On the medial side of the antitragus （在对耳屏内侧面，即对耳屏 4 区）	Pain, tertian malaria, neurasthenia, pseudo myopia, stomach ulcers, diarrhea, hypertension, coronary heart disease, arrhythmia, and insomnia （痛证，间日疟，神经衰弱，假性近视，胃溃疡，腹泻，高血压，冠心病，心律失常，失眠）
Apex of Antitragus($AT_{1,2,4i}$) （对屏尖（$AT_{1,2,4i}$））	At the free end of the apex of the antitragus at the juncture of AT_1, AT_2 and AT_4 （在对耳屏游离缘的尖端，即对耳屏 1、2、4 区交点处）	Asthma, mumps, itching of the skin, orchitis, and epididymitis （哮喘，腮腺炎，皮肤瘙痒，睾丸炎，附睾炎）
Central Rim($AT_{2,3,4i}$) （缘中（$AT_{2,3,4i}$））	On the free rim at the midpoint of the apex of the antitragus and antihelix-antitragus notch at the juncture of AT_2, AT_3 and AT_4 （在对耳屏游离缘上，对屏尖与轮屏切迹之中点处，即对耳屏 2、3、4 区交点处）	Enuresis, inner ear vertigo, and functional uterine bleeding （遗尿，内耳眩晕症，功能性子宫出血）
Brain Stem($AT_{3,4i}$) （脑干（$AT_{3,4i}$））	At the antihelix-antitragus notch at the juncture of AT_3 and AT_4 （在轮屏切迹处，即对耳屏 3、4 区之间）	Headache, dizziness, and pseudomyopia （头痛，眩晕，假性近视）

9. Partition and auricular points of concha (Fig. A-11, Fig. A-12, Tab. A-7)

There are 21 points in 18 areas in concha.

The part formed by the inferior edge of the helix crus and the

九、耳甲部分区与耳穴（图 A-11、图 A-12，表 A-7）

耳甲部分为 18 区，共有 21 穴。

将BC 线前段与耳轮脚下缘间

anterior part of line BC is divided into three equal areas, CO_1 (area 1 of the concha), CO_2 and CO_3, from front to back. In front of the ABC line, the fan-shaped area at the end of the helix crus is CO_4. The part formed by the superior edge of the helix crus and the anterior part of line AB is divided into three equal areas. From the posterior to the anterior are CO_5, CO_6 and CO_7, respectively.

CO_8 is anterior to a line drawn form point C to the junction of the anterior third and the posterior two-thirds of the lower edge of the inferior antihelix crus. The part posterior to CO_8 and superior to CO_6 and CO_7 is divided into two equal areas, the anterior is CO_9 and the posterior is CO_{10}. The part posterior to CO_{10} and superior to line BD is divided into two equal areas; the superior is CO_{11} and the inferior is CO_{12}. The area marked off by a line drawn from the antihelix-antitragus notch to line BD is CO_{13}. Taking the midpoint of the cavum concha as the center of a circle with a radius of half the distance from the center to line BC gives us CO_{15}. The area between two parallel lines drawn respectively from the highest and lowest points of the orifice of the external auditory meatus to the highest and lowest points of CO_{15} is CO_{16}. The area external to CO_{15} and CO_{16} is CO_{14}. The area inferior to a line drawn from the lowest point of the orifice of the external auditory meatus to the midpoint of the concha edge of the antihelix is divided into two equal areas; the upper is CO_{17} and the lower is CO_{18}.

分成三等份,前 1/3 为耳甲 1 区,中 1/3 为耳甲 2 区,后 1/3 为耳甲 3 区。ABC 线前方,耳轮脚消失处为耳甲 4 区。将 AB 线前段与耳轮脚上缘及部分耳轮内缘间分成三等份,后 1/3 为耳甲 5 区,中 1/3 为耳甲 6 区,前 1/3 为耳甲 7 区。

将对耳轮下脚下缘前、中 1/3 交界处与 A 点连线,该线前方的耳甲艇部为耳甲 8 区。将 AB 线前段与对耳轮下脚下缘间耳甲 8 区以后的部分分为前、后两等份,前 1/2 为耳甲 9 区,后 1/2 为耳甲 10 区。在 AB 线后段上方的耳甲艇部,将耳甲 10 区后缘与 BD 线之间分成上、下两等份,上 1/2 为耳甲 11 区,下 1/2 为耳甲 12 区。由轮屏切迹至 B 点作连线,该线后方、BD 线下方的耳甲腔部为耳甲 13 区。以耳甲腔中央为圆心,圆心与 BC 线间距离的 1/2 为半径作圆,该圆形区域为耳甲 15 区。过 15 区最高点及最低点分别向外耳门后壁作两条切线,切线间为耳甲 16 区。耳甲 15、16 区周围为耳甲 14 区。将外耳门的最低点与对耳屏耳甲缘中点相连,再将该线下的耳甲腔部分为上、下两等份,上 1/2 为耳甲 17 区,下 1/2 为耳甲 18 区。

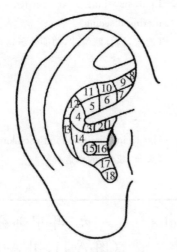

图 A-11　耳甲部分区与耳穴 1

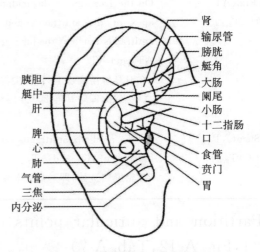

图 A-12　耳甲部分区与耳穴 2

Tab. A-7 Acupoints of concha(表 A-7 耳甲穴位)

Acupoint name （穴名）	Location （定位）	Indications （主治）
Mouth(CO_1) （口（CO_1））	In the concha inferior to the anterior 1/3 of the helix crus （在耳轮脚下方前 1/3 处，即耳甲 1 区）	Facial paralysis, stomatitis, choleystitis, cholelithiasis, withdrawal syndrome, periodontitis, and glossitis （面瘫，口腔炎，胆囊炎，胆石症，戒断综合征，牙周炎，舌炎）
Esophagus(CO_2) （食管（CO_2））	In the concha inferior to the intermediate 1/3 of the helix crus （在耳轮脚下方中 1/3 处，即耳甲 2 区）	Esophagitis and esophageal spasms （食管炎，食管痉挛）
Cardia(CO_3) （贲门（CO_3））	In the concha inferior to the posterior 1/3 of the helix crus （在耳轮脚下方后 1/3 处，即耳甲 3 区）	Stoic spasms and neurotic vomiting （贲门痉挛，神经性呕吐）
Stomach(CO_4) （胃（CO_4））	At the end of the helix crus （在耳轮脚消失处，即耳甲 4 区）	Gastritis, stomach ulcers, insomnia, toothache, indigestion, nausea and vomiting （胃炎，胃溃疡，失眠，牙痛，消化不良，恶心呕吐）
Duodenum(CO_5) （十二指肠（CO_5））	In the posterior 1/3 of the region between the helix crus and line AB （在耳轮脚及部分耳轮与 AB 线之间的后 1/3 处，即耳甲 5 区）	Duodenal bulb ulcer, choleystitis, cholelithiasis, pylorospasm, abdominal distension, diarrhea, and abdominal pain （十二指肠球部溃疡，胆囊炎，胆石症，幽门痉挛，腹胀，腹泻，腹痛）
Small Intestine(CO_6) （小肠（CO_6））	At the intermediate 1/3 of the region between the helix crus and line AB （在耳轮脚及部分耳轮与 AB 线之间的中 1/3 处，即耳甲 6 区）	Indigestion, abdominal pain, tachycardia, and cardiac arrhythmia （消化不良，腹痛，心动过速，心律不齐）
Large Intestine(CO_7) （大肠（CO_7））	At the anterior 1/3 of the region between the helix crus and line AB （在耳轮脚及部分耳轮与 AB 线之间的前 1/3 处，即耳甲 7 区）	Diarrhea, constipation, dysentery, cough, and acne （腹泻，便秘，痢疾，咳嗽，痤疮）
Appendix($CO_{6,7i}$) （阑尾（$CO_{6,7i}$））	At the juncture of CO_6 and CO_7 （在小肠区与大肠区之间，即耳甲 6、7 区交界处）	Simple appendicitis, diarrhea, and abdominal pain （单纯性阑尾炎，腹泻，腹痛）
Angle of Superior Concha(CO_8) （艇角（CO_8））	In the cymba concha below the anterior region of the inferior antihelix crus （在对耳轮下脚下方前部，即耳甲 8 区）	prostatitis and urethritis （前列腺炎，尿道炎）
Bladder(CO_9) （膀胱（CO_9））	In the cymba concha below the intermediate region of the inferior antihelix crus （在对耳轮下脚下方中部，即耳甲 9 区）	Cystitis, enuresis, urinary retention, low back pain, sciatica, and posterior headache （膀胱炎，遗尿，尿潴留，腰痛，坐骨神经痛，后头痛）

续表

Acupoint name (穴名)	Location (定位)	Indications (主治)
Kidney(CO_{10}) (肾(CO_{10}))	In the cymba concha below the posterior region of the inferior antihelix crus (在对耳轮下脚下方后部,即耳甲 10 区)	Low back pain, tinnitus, neurasthenia, edema, asthma, enuresis, irregular menstruation, seminal emission, impotence, premature ejaculation, eye diseases, and predawn diarrhea (腰痛,耳鸣,神经衰弱,水肿,哮喘,遗尿,月经不调,遗精,阳痿,早泄,眼病,五更泻)
Ureter($CO_{9,10i}$) (输尿管($CO_{9,10i}$))	At the juncture of CO_9 and CO_{10} (在肾区与膀胱区之间,即耳甲 9、10 区交界处)	Ureteral calculus and colic (输尿管结石绞痛)
Pancreas and Gallbladder(CO_{11}) (胰胆(CO_{11}))	In the posterosuperior part of the cymba concha (在耳甲艇的后上部,即耳甲 11 区)	Cholecystitis, cholelithiasis, biliary ascariasis, migraine, herpes zoster, otitis media, tinnitus, hearing loss, pancreatitis, bitter taste in mouth pain, and hypochondriac pain (胆囊炎,胆石症,胆道蛔虫症,偏头痛,带状疱疹,中耳炎,耳鸣,听力减退,胰腺炎,口苦,胁痛)
Liver(CO_{12}) (肝(CO_{12}))	In the postero-inferior part of the cymba concha (在耳甲艇的后下部,即耳甲 12 区)	Hypochondriac pain, vertigo, premenstrual tension, irregular menstruation, climacteric syndrome, hypertension, pseudomyopia, simple glaucoma, swelling and pain in the eyes (胁痛,眩晕,经前期紧张症,月经不调,更年期综合征,高血压,假性近视,单纯性青光眼,目赤肿痛)
Center of Superior Concha($CO_{6,10i}$) (艇中($CO_{6,10i}$))	At the juncture of CO_6 and CO_{10} (在小肠区与肾区之间,即耳甲 6、10 区交界处)	Abdominal pain, abdominal distention, and mumps (腹痛,腹胀,腮腺炎)
Spleen(CO_{13}) (脾(CO_{13}))	In the region inferior to line BD, posterosuperior to the cavum concha (在 BD 线下方,耳甲腔的后上部,即耳甲 13 区)	Abdominal distention, diarrhea, constipation, loss of appetite, functional uterine bleeding, excessive leucorrhea, vertigo, edema, and splanchno ptosis (腹胀,腹泻,便秘,食欲不振,功能性子宫出血,白带过多,内耳眩晕症,水肿,内脏下垂)
Heart(CO_{15}) (心(CO_{15}))	In the center of the depression of the cavum concha (在耳甲腔正中凹陷处,即耳甲 15 区)	Tachycardia, arrhythmia, angina pectoris, pulse less syndrome, spontaneous sweating, night sweats, hysteria, mouth sores, palpitation, insomnia, forgetfulness (心动过速,心律不齐,心绞痛,无脉症,自汗盗汗,癔病,口舌生疮,心悸怔忡,失眠,健忘)

续表

Acupoint name （穴名）	Location （定位）	Indications （主治）
Trachea(CO_{16}) （气管（CO_{16}））	Between the CO_{15} and the orifice of the external auditory meatus （在心区与外耳门之间，即耳甲 16 区）	Cough, asthma, acute and chronic pharyng-itis （咳嗽，气喘，急慢性咽炎）
Lung(CO_{14}) （肺（CO_{14}））	In the cavum concha in the region surrounding CO_{15} and CO_{16} （在心、气管区周围处，即耳甲 14 区）	Cough, asthma, chest tightness, hoarseness, acne, pruritus, urticaria, flat wart, constipation, withdrawal syndrome, spontaneous sweating, night sweats, and rhinitis （咳喘，气喘，胸闷，声音嘶哑，痤疮，皮肤瘙痒，荨麻疹，扁平疣，便秘，戒断综合征，自汗盗汗，鼻炎）
Triple Energizer(CO_{17}) （三焦（CO_{17}））	Between CO_{14} and CO_{18} in the region posteroinferior to the orifice of the external auditory meatus （在外耳门后下，肺区与内分泌区之间，即耳甲 17 区）	Constipation, abdominal distention, edema, tinnitus, deafness, diabetes （便秘，腹胀，水肿，耳鸣，耳聋，糖尿病）
Endocrine(CO_{18}) （内分泌（CO_{18}））	Inside of the inter tragus notch in the anteroinferior region of the cavum concha （在屏间切迹内，耳甲腔的底部，即耳甲 18 区）	Dysmenorrhea, irregular menstruation, menopausal syndrome, acne, tertian malaria, and diabetes （痛经，月经不调，更年期综合征，痤疮，间日疟，糖尿病）

10. Partition and auricular points of ear lobule (Fig. A-13, Tab. A-8)

There are 8 points in 9 areas in ear lobe.

The ear lobe is divided by two equidistant vertical lines extending from superior to inferior border. Two equidistant horizontal lines, parallel to the superior border, cross the verticals to divide the lobe into nine areas. From the anterior to the posterior the upper three areas are LO_1 (area 1 of the lobe), LO_2 and LO_3. The middle three areas are LO_4, LO_5 and LO_6. The lower three areas are LO_7, LO_8 and LO_9.

十、耳垂部分区与耳穴（图 A-13，表 A-8）

耳垂部分为 9 区，共有 8 穴。

在耳垂上线至耳垂下缘最低点之间划两条等距离平行线，于该平行线上引两条垂直等分线，将耳垂分为 9 个区，上部由前到后依次为耳垂 1 区、2 区、3 区；中部由前到后依次为耳垂 4 区、5 区、6 区；下部由前到后依次为耳垂 7 区、8 区、9 区。

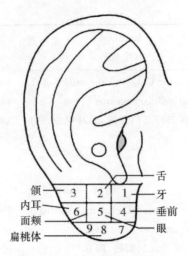

图 A-13　耳垂部分区与耳穴

Tab. A-8　Acupoints of the ear lobe(表 A-8　耳垂穴位)

Acupoint name （穴名）	Location （定位）	Indications （主治）
Tooth(LO_1) （牙(LO_1)）	In the anterosuperior area of the anterolateral surface of the ear lobe （在耳垂正面前上部,即耳垂 1 区）	Toothache,periodontitis,hypotension （牙痛,牙周炎,低血压）
Tongue(LO_2) （舌(LO_2)）	In the superior intermediate area of the anterolateral surface of the ear lobe （在耳垂正面中上部,即耳垂 2 区）	Glossitis and stomatitis （舌炎,口腔炎）
Jaw(LO_3) （颌(LO_3)）	In the posterosuperior area of the anterolateral surface of the ear lobe （在耳垂正面后上部,即耳垂 3 区）	Toothache and temporomandibular joint functional disorder （牙痛,颞颌关节紊乱症）
Anterior Ear Lobe(LO_4) （垂前(LO_4)）	In the anterior intermediate area of the anterolateral surface of the ear lobe （在耳垂正面前中部,即耳垂 4 区）	Neurasthenia and toothache （神经衰弱,牙痛）
Eye(LO_5) （眼(LO_5)）	In the central of the anterolateral surface of the ear lobe （在耳垂正面中央部,即耳垂 5 区）	Pseudomyopia, swelling and pain in the eyes, and tears when facing wind （假性近视,目赤肿痛,迎风流泪）
Internal Ear(LO_6) （内耳(LO_6)）	In the intermediate posterior area of the anterolateral surface of the ear lobe （在耳垂正面后中部,即耳垂 6 区）	Vertigo,tinnitus,and hearing loss （内耳眩晕症,耳鸣,听力减退）
Cheek($LO_{5,6i}$) （面颊($LO_{5,6i}$)）	In the intermediate posterior part of the anterolateral surface of the ear lobe at the juncture of LO_5 and LO_6 （在耳垂正面,眼区与内耳区之间,即耳垂 5、6 区交界处）	Peripheral facial paralysis, trigeminal neuralgia, acne,and verruca plana （周围性面瘫,三叉神经痛,痤疮,扁平疣）
Tonsil($LO_{7,8,9}$) （扁桃体($LO_{7,8,9}$)）	Three divisions of the inferior anterolateral surface of the ear lobe （在耳垂正面下部,即耳垂 7、8、9 区）	Tonsillitis and pharyngitis （扁桃体炎,咽炎）

11. Partition and auricular points of posterior surface of auricle and ear root（Fig. A-14，Tab. A-9）

There are 9 points in 5 areas in posterior surface of auricle and ear root.

Two horizontal lines passing through the back corresponding to the bifurcation of the antihelix crus and the antihelix-antitragus notch were drawn to divide the posterior surface into three parts，the upper being P_1 (area 1 of the posterior surface of the auricle)and the lower being P_5. The middle part is divided into three equal areas：the medial area is P_2，the middle is P_3，and the lateral is P_4.

十一、耳背及耳根部分区与耳穴（图 A-14，表 A-9）

耳背及耳根部分为 5 区，共有 9 穴。

分别过对耳轮上、下脚分叉处耳背对应点和轮屏切迹耳背对应点作两条水平线，将耳背分为上、中、下 3 部，上部为耳背 1 区，下部为耳背 5 区，再将中部分为内、中、外三等份，内 1/3 为耳背 2 区，中 1/3 为耳背 3 区、外 1/3 为耳背 4 区。

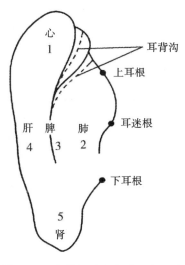

图 A-14　耳背及耳根部分区与耳穴

Tab. A-9　Acupoints of the posterior surface of auricle and the ear root（表 A-9　耳背及耳根穴位）

Acupoint name （穴名）	Location （定位）	Indications （主治）
Heart，Posteromedial Surface of the Ear(P_1) （耳背心（P_1））	P_1 is located on the superior area of the posteromedial surface of the ear （在耳背上部，即耳背 1 区）	Palpitations，insomnia，and dreaminess （心悸，失眠，多梦）
Lung，Posteromedial Surface of the Ear(P_2) （耳背肺（P_2））	P_2 is located on the intermediate medial area of the posteromedial surface of the ear （在耳背中内部，即耳背 2 区）	Cough and asthma，and cutaneous pruritus （咳喘，皮肤瘙痒）
Spleen，Posteromedial Surface of the Ear(P_3) （耳背脾（P_3））	P_3 is located at the center of the posteromedial surface of the ear （在耳背中央部，即耳背 3 区）	Stomachache，indigestion，loss of appetite，abdominal distension，and diarrhea （胃痛，消化不良，食欲不振，腹胀，腹泻）
Liver，Posteromedial Surface of the Ear(P_4) （耳背肝（P_4））	P_4 is on the intermediate lateral area of the posteromedial surface of the ear （在耳背中外部，即耳背 4 区）	Cholecystitis，cholelithiasis，and flank pain （胆囊炎，胆石症，胁痛）

续表

Acupoint name （穴名）	Location （定位）	Indications （主治）
Kidney, Posteromedial Surface of the Ear(P_5) （耳背肾（P_5））	P_5 is located in the inferior area of the posteromedial surface of the ear lobe （在耳背下部，即耳背 5 区）	Headache, dizziness, and neurasthenia （头痛，眩晕，神经衰弱）
Groove, Posteromedial Surface of the Ear(P_s) （耳背沟（P_s））	P_s is the groove on the posteromedial surface of the ear formed by superior and inferior antihelix crura （在对耳轮沟和对耳轮上、下脚沟处）	Hypertension and cutaneous pruritus （高血压，皮肤瘙痒）
Upper Ear Root(R_1) （上耳根（R_1））	R_1 is the highest point at which the ear attaches to the head （在耳郭与头部相连的最上处）	Epistaxis and asthma （鼻衄，哮喘）
Root of Ear Vagus(R_2) （耳迷根（R_2））	R_2 is located on the ear root at the posteromedial groove formed by the helix crus （在耳轮脚沟的耳根处）	Cholecystitis, cholelithiasis, biliary ascariasis, rhinitis, tachycardia, abdominal pain, and diarrhea （胆囊炎，胆石症，胆道蛔虫症，鼻炎，心动过速，腹痛，腹泻）
Lower Ear Root(R_3) （下耳根（R_3））	R_3 is the lowest point on the ear root （在耳郭与头部相连的最下处）	Hypotension and paralysis of the lower extremities （低血压，下肢瘫痪）

Note: From the annex table A-1 to A-9, capital letters indicate the abbreviation of the anatomic division where the acupoint is located; subscript numbers indicate the number of the division where the acupoint is located; subscript letters represent the following meanings: "i" is stand for the junction of the two acupoint areas; "a" is stand for the front end of the acupoint area; "p" is stand for the rear edge of the acupoint area; "l" is stand for the lower edge of the acupoint area, "u" is stand for the upper edge of the acupoint area. (注：大写字母标示该穴位所在解剖分区英文缩写；下标数字为该穴位所在分区编号；下标字母代表含义：i——两穴区交界，a——该穴区前端，p——该穴区后缘，l——该穴区下缘，u——该穴区上缘。)

Appendix B Common Terms of Acupuncture (Chinese and English comparison)

附录B 常用针法技法术语（中英文对照）

1. Classics of acupuncture & moxibustion	针灸古典文献
Moxibustion Canon of Eleven Channels on the Foot and Arm	《足臂十一脉灸经》
Moxibustion Canon of Eleven Channels of Yin-Yang System	《阴阳十一脉灸经》
Huangdi Neijing	《黄帝内经》
Plain Questions	《素问》
Miraculous Pivot	《灵枢》
Classic of Questioning	《难经》
Grand Simplicity of Inner Canon of Huangdi	《黄帝内经太素》
Treatise on Cold Pathogenic and Miscellaneous Diseases	《伤寒杂病论》
Treatise on Cold Pathogenic Diseases	《伤寒论》
Synopsis of the Golden Chamber	《金匮要略》
A-B Classic of Acupuncture and Moxibustion	《针灸甲乙经》
Illustrated Manual of Acupuncture Points of the Bronze Figure	《铜人腧穴针灸图经》
Precious Writings of Bianque	《扁鹊心书》
Classic of Nourishing Life with Acupuncture and Moxibustion	《针灸资生经》
Guide to the Acupuncture Classics	《针经指南》
Elucidation of Fourteen Meridians/Channels	《十四经发挥》
Collection of Gems of Acupuncture and Moxibustion	《针灸聚英》
Compendium of Acupuncture and Moxibustion	《针灸大成》
Questions & Answers About Acupuncture and Moxibustion	《针灸问对》
Introduction to Medicine	《医学入门》
Rhythm of Golden Needle	《金针赋》
Song to Elucidate Mysteries	《标幽赋》
2. Ancient needles & needling	古代针具针法
nine classical needles	九针
shear needle	镵针
round-pointed needle	圆针
spoon needle；blunt needle	鍉针
lance needle	锋针
round-sharp needle	员利针
stiletto needle	铍针
long needle	长针
big needle	大针
great needle	巨针
filiform needle	毫针
stone needle	砭石
flint needle	砭针
needling	针法
acupuncture technique	刺法
techniques of acupuncture and moxibustion	刺灸法

stone needle therapy	砭刺疗法
five needling methods	五刺
nine needling methods	九刺
twelve needling methods	十二刺
half needling	半刺
leopard-spot needling	豹文刺
joint needling	关刺
join valley needling	合谷刺
transport point needling	输刺
meridian needling	经刺
distant needling	远道刺
collateral needling	络刺
intermuscular needling	分刺
great drainage needling	大泻刺
skin needling	毛刺
red-hot needling	焠刺
contralateral meridian needling	巨刺
contralateral collateral needling	缪刺
paired needling	偶刺
successive trigger needling	报刺
relaxing needling	恢刺
triple needling	齐刺
centro-square needling	扬刺
perpendicular needling	直针刺
short thrust needling	短刺
superficial needling	浮刺
yin needling	阴刺
proximatal needling	傍针刺
repeated shallow needling	赞刺
3. Filiform needle therapy	**毫针法**
silver needle	银针
stainless steel needle	不锈钢针
disposable needle	一次性针
the needle tip	针尖/针芒
the needle body	针身/针体
the needle root	针根
the needle handle	针柄
the needle tail	针尾
filiform needle therapy	毫针疗法
needle insertion	进针
needling hand;needle-holding hand	刺手
pressing hand	押手
hand-pressing method	押手法
needle insertion method	进针法

single-handed needle insertion;needle-inserting with a single hand	单手进针法
double-handed needle insertion;needle-inserting with both hands	双手进针法
fingernail-pressing needle insertion;fingernail-pressure needle inserting	指切进针法
hand-holding needle insertion	夹持进针法
pinching needle insertion;skin-pinching up needle inserting	提捏进针法
skin spreading needle insertion;skin stretching needle inserting	舒张进针法
insertion of needle with tube;insert the needle within a guide tube	管针进针法
posture	体位
supine body position	仰卧体位
lateral recumbent	侧卧体位
prone body position	俯卧体位
angle of insertion	针刺角度
depth of insertion	针刺深度
perpendicular insertion of needle;inserting straightly	直刺
transverse/horizontal insertion of needle;inserting horizontally	横/平刺;沿皮刺
oblique insertion of needle;needling obliquely	斜刺
qi arrival	气至
qi extending affected parts	气至病所
arrival of qi	得气
waiting for qi arrival	候气
promoting arrival of qi	催气
needle sensation/needling response/acu-esthesia	针感
painful sensation	酸感
numb sensation	麻感
distending sensation	胀感
meridian phenomenon	经络现象
running course of the meridian	经脉循行
transmission of sensation along meridian	循经感传
needle manipulation;manipulating needle	行针
twirling of needle	捻转
twirling method	捻转法
lifting and thrusting of needle	提插
lifting-thrusting method	提插法
handle-scraping method	刮柄法
handle-twisting method	搓柄法
handle-waggling method	摇柄法
handle-flicking method	弹柄法
trembling method	震颤法
mild pressing meridian course	循法
supplementation and draining	补泻
reinforcing and reducing manipulations of acupuncture therapy	针刺补泻
even reinforcing-reducing method;uniform reinforcing-reducing method	平补平泻
reinforcing and reducing by twirling and rotating the needle	捻转补泻
reinforcing and reducing by lifting and thrusting the needle	提插补泻

directional supplementation and draining method	迎随补泻
rapid-slow reinforcing and reducing method	徐疾补泻
respiratory supplementation and draining method	呼吸补泻
the open-closed supplementation and draining method	开阖补泻
neutral supplementation and draining	平补平泻
meridional reinforcing and reducing	子午补泻
comprehensive reinforcing and reducing method	复式补泻手法
heat-producing needling	烧山火（法）
cool-producing needling	透天凉（法）
Feijing Zouqi acupuncture；the four traditional methods of flying meridians and moving qi	飞经走气
Qinglong Baiwei acupuncture	青龙摆尾
Baihu Yaotou acupuncture	白虎摇头
Canggui Tanxue acupuncture	苍龟探穴
Chifeng Yingyuan acupuncture	赤凤迎源
Zi-wu Daojiu needling	子午捣臼
yang occluding in yin	阴中隐阳
yin occluding in yang	阳中隐阴
induction qi method	导气法
dragon-tiger fighting needling method；dragon and tiger warring	龙虎交战法
Chou tian method	抽添法
mother-supplementing child-draining method	补母泻子法
midnight-noon ebb-flow acupoint selection	子午流注法
deep multiple abscess	流注
heavenly stem-prescription of point selection	纳甲法
earthly branch-prescription of point selection	纳子法
eightfold methods of intelligent turtle	灵龟八法
pathway of qi	气街
four seas	四海
needle retention/retention of needle	留针
kinetic acupuncture	运动针刺法
needle withdrawal	出针
needle withdrawal method	出针法
acupuncture indications	针灸适应证
non-indication of acupuncture	针灸不适应证
acupuncture contraindications	针灸禁忌证
acupuncture syncope reaction；fainting during acupuncture treatment	晕针
bending of the needle；bent needle	弯针
needle breakage；broken needle	折针/断针
stucking needle	滞针
hematoma	血肿
4．Moxibustion	艾灸法
moxibustion	灸法
moxa	艾
argy wormwood leaf	艾叶

moxa floss/moxa wool	艾绒
moxa cone	艾炷
incense thread	线香
common rush	灯心草
moxa-cone moxibustion	艾炷灸
direct moxibustion	直接灸
moxibustion with seed-sized moxa cone	麦粒灸
one moxa-cone；Zhuang	壮
number of moxa cones	壮数
indirect moxibustion；sandwiched moxibustion	间接灸/隔物灸
moxibustion on ginger；ginger-partitioned moxibustion	隔姜灸
moxibustion on salt；salt partition moxibustion	隔盐灸
moxibustion on garlic；garlic partition moxibustion	隔蒜灸
moxibustion on monkshood cake；monkshood cake-separated moxibustion；monkshood cake partition moxibustion	隔附子饼灸
moxa stick	艾条
moxa stick moxibustion	艾条灸
moxa roll	艾卷
moxa roll moxibustion	艾卷灸
gentle moxibustion；mild-warm moxibustion	温和灸
circling moxibustion；revolving moxibustion	回旋灸
sparrow-pecking moxibustion	雀啄灸
suspended moxibustion；over skin moxibustion；suspension moxibustion	悬起灸
pressing moxibustion	实按灸
Governor vessel moxibustion；spreading moxibustion；long snake moxibustion	督灸/铺灸/长蛇灸
moxibustion scar	灸痕
purulent moxibustion/scarring moxibustion	化脓灸/瘢痕灸
non-purulent moxibustion/non-scarring moxibustion	非化脓灸/无瘢痕灸
natural moxibustion	天灸
medicinal moxibustion	药物灸
Taiyi miraculous moxa roll	太乙神针
thunder-fire miraculous moxa roll	雷火神针
warm needling；warming needle moxibustion；needle warming through moxibustion	温针/温针灸
moxa burner；moxibustioner	温灸器
rush-fire cauterization；burning rush moxibustion	灯火灸

5. Cupping　　拔罐

cupping	拔罐
cupping method	拔罐法
bamboo cup/jar	竹罐
glass cup	玻璃罐
suction cup	抽气罐
retained cupping；retaining the cup；cup retaining	留罐
medicated cupping	药罐
fire cupping	火罐法

fire-insertion cupping	投火法
flash-fire cupping	闪火法
cotton fire cupping	贴棉法
slide cupping；moving cupping；cup moving	走罐
quick cupping；successive flash cupping	闪罐
needle cupping	针罐法
pricking-cupping bloodletting method	刺血拔罐法
cupping with boiling water method	煮罐法
suction cupping method	抽气罐法
lining-up cupping	排罐法
cup lifting	起罐
cupping skin marks	罐斑

6. Scrapping　　　　刮痧法

scrapping therapy	刮痧法
scraping plate	刮痧板
buffalo horn	水牛角
jade made scraping plate	玉质刮痧板
surface-scrapping method	面刮法
angle-scraping method	角刮法
point-pressing method	点按法
flap method	拍打法
rubbing method	揉按法
pinching scrapping method	撮痧法
picking scrapping method	挑痧法
letting blooding scrapping method	放痧法
Sha disease	痧症

7. Specific Region Acupuncture　　　　特定部位刺法

microsystem acupuncture	微针系统
ear acupuncture manipulation	耳针刺激方法
auricular point	耳穴
ear acupuncture stimulation method	耳针刺激方法
scalp acupuncture therapy	头针/头皮针
eye acupuncture	眼针
facial acupuncture	面针
nose acupuncture	鼻针
hand needle therapy	手针
hand-finger acupuncture technique	手指针术
wrist-ankle needle；winkle and ankle needle therapy	腕踝针
foot needle therapy	足针
abdominal acupuncture	腹针
navel needling therapy；navel acupuncture therapy	脐针
tender point	压痛点
tender point needling	压痛点针刺
trigger point	激痛点

trigger point needling	激痛点针刺
intramuscular stimulation needling	筋肉针刺
paraneural needling	傍神经针刺

8．Special Needle Acupuncture　特种针具刺法

dermal needle	皮肤针
dermal needle therapy	皮肤针疗法
plum-blossom needle;percussopunctator;pyonex(5 needles)	梅花针
plum-blossom needle therapy	梅花针疗法
seven-star needle(7 needles)	七星针
eighteen arhat needles(18 needles)	十八罗汉针
roller needle	滚刺筒
three-edged needle	三棱针
three-edged needle therapy	三棱针疗法
swift pricking blood	点刺
pricking therapy;swift pricking blood therapy	点刺疗法
pricking bloodletting method	刺络法
collateral vessel pricking therapy	刺络疗法
bloodletting therapy	刺血法/放血法
pricking blood therapy	挑刺法
pricking method	挑治法
cutting method	割治法
scattered needling method;surrounding pricking	散刺法
intradermal needle	皮内针
intradermal needle therapy	皮内针疗法
subcutaneous needle retention method	皮下留针法
needle-embedding method	埋针法
thumbtack needle	揿针
thumbtack type intradermal needle	揿钉型皮内针
grain-like type intradermal needle;grain-shaped type intradermal needle	麦粒型/颗粒型皮内针
heated needling	火针(烧针、燔针、焠针)
fine heated needle	细火针
thick heated needle	粗火针
three-headed heated needle	三头火针
concentrated needling method	密刺法
surround needling method	围刺法
elongated needle	芒针
spoon needle;blunt needle	鍉针
superficial needle therapy;Fu's subcutaneous needling(FSN)	浮针法

9．Unique Therapeutical Methods of Acupoints　腧穴特种疗法

electro-acupuncture;electric acupuncture	电针
electrotherapy	电针法
electrothermic needle	电热针
electro-acupuncture therapeutic apparatus	电针仪
laser needles for acupuncture	激光针

magnetic therapy needle	磁疗针
herbal acupuncture	药针
acupoint application therapy	穴位贴敷
acupoint thread-embedding therapy	穴位埋线
auricular points plaster therapy	耳穴贴压法
ear acupoint pressure bean method	耳穴压豆法
acupuncture point injection;point injection	穴位注射
acupuncture point injection therapy	穴位注射疗法
acupoint magnet plastering therapy	穴位磁疗法
acupoint laser therapy	穴位激光照射疗法